ORGANIZATION THEORY: TENSION AND CHANGE

D0166509

FIRST EDITION

ORGANIZATION THEORY: TENSION AND CHANGE

David Jaffee
University of North Florida

Boston   Burr Ridge, IL   Dubuque, IA   Madison, WI
New York   San Francisco   St. Louis
Bangkok   Bogotá   Caracas   Lisbon   London   Madrid   Mexico City
Milan   New Delhi   Seoul   Singapore   Sydney   Taipei   Toronto

McGraw-Hill Higher Education

*A Division of The **McGraw-Hill** Companies*

ORGANIZATION THEORY: TENSION AND CHANGE
Published by McGraw-Hill, an imprint of The McGraw-Hill Companies, Inc. 1221 Avenue of the Americas, New York, NY, 10020. Copyright © 2001, by The McGraw-Hill Companies, Inc. All rights reserved. No part of this publication may be reproduced or distributed in any form or by any means, or stored in a database or retrieval system, without the prior written consent of The McGraw-Hill Companies, Inc., including, but not limited to, in any network or other electronic storage or transmission, or broadcast for distance learning.

Some ancillaries, including electronic and print components, may not be available to customers outside the United States.

This book is printed on acid-free paper.

3 4 5 6 7 8 9 0 DOC/DOC 0 9 8 7 6 5 4

ISBN 0072341661

Editorial director: *Phillip A. Butcher*
Sponsoring editor: *Sally Constable*
Developmental editor: *Katherine Blake*
Marketing manager II: *Leslie A. Kraham*
Project manager: *Susanne Riedell*
Production associate: *Gina Hangos*
Freelance design coordinator: *Craig E. Jordan*
New media: *Kimberly Stark*
Cover designer: *Crispin Prebys*
Compositor: *Carlisle Communications, Ltd.*
Typeface: *10.5/13 Times Roman*
Printer: *R. R. Donnelley & Sons Company*

Library of Congress Cataloging-in-Publication Data

Jaffee, David.
   Organization theory: tension and change/David Jaffee.
   p. cm.
   ISBN 0-07-234166-1 (softcover: alk. paper)
   1. Organization. 2. Management. I. Title

HD31 .J243 2001
658.4'02--dc21

00-031852

www.mhhe.com

ABOUT THE AUTHOR

David Jaffee received his B.A. in Political Science from the University of Florida and his M.A. in Political Science from Washington University in St. Louis. He received his Ph.D. in Sociology from the University of Massachusetts at Amherst. Professor Jaffee has published articles on a variety of topics, including international development, gender inequality, industrial location, organization theory, and instructional technology. He is the author of *Levels of Socio-Economic Development Theory* (Praeger, 1998). He is currently an associate professor of sociology at the University of North Florida.

For my parents

CONTENTS

Chapter   3   The Rise of the Factory System   42

Chapter   4   The Human Organization   64

PREFACE

As a sociologist, I was first attracted to the study of organizations because they seemed to hold the key to understanding so many other aspects of social life.

Organizations affect us as individuals, as well as at the group, community, national, and international levels. For example, definitions of self and human identity are shaped by the kinds of work people do and the roles they assume within organizations. To understand inequality among members of society, one must look at the ways in which organizations reward people in terms of income, prestige, and authority. To understand the dynamics of power, it is impossible to ignore organizations. Power stems from positions held within organizations and/or from the ownership and control of organizations. People who seek political power use organizations and mobilize organizational resources. International development is heavily influenced by the actions of transnational corporations and international agencies. In short, it seems that everywhere we look, organizations play some role in shaping social structures and influencing social change.

Another unique aspect of organizations is the fact that people spend most of their lives working in, moving between, and being influenced by organizations. The entire life course—from birth, to family life, to schooling, to work, to death—takes place within organizational settings.

When they come to class, students are operating within the organizational setting of higher education. Most students are—or have been—employed by some type of a work organization. In this context, many of the seemingly abstract ideas, concepts, and theories come to life because students are able to connect them to their own concrete experiences. Not only do students benefit, but this makes teaching a course on organizations very rewarding and exciting!

Because one of the central objectives of a liberal education is to develop the capacity to interpret and analyze our personal lives using theoretical ideas and perspectives, studying and writing about organizations contributes to this vital educational mission as well.

Another appealing aspect about the study of organizations is that the subject matter is inherently **interdisciplinary.** When we talk about organizations and try to understand why and how they work, we can benefit by borrowing insights from psychology, sociology, political science, economics, geography, management, history, and even biology. For example, it is difficult to make sense of what goes on within organizations without considering the *psychological* component people bring to them and the way organizations might shape personality. Similarly, from a *sociological* perspective, we see that organizations influence behavior through the roles and norms associated with the different positions people occupy within an organization.

Organizations are *political* arenas, because people and groups develop different goals and interests, engage in conflict, and compete for resources. As places where goods and services are produced, organizations are *economic* entities. They are located in *geographic* locations and thus draw on and influence resources in different regions, communities, and societies. As goal-directed entities, organizations must be managed and coordinated, and a great deal of the literature on organizations is closely connected to the topics of *business* and *management.* There is also a *historical* dimension. History provides insights into the development of organization theories as they have evolved as tools for analyzing organizations from the rise of the factory to the emergence of post-modern forms. Finally, *biological* models have been used to describe and understand the workings of organizations as organisms.

It is difficult to imagine another subject area in sociology with so many connections to so many different fields of intellectual inquiry and analysis. To write and teach about organizations is to advance the cause of interdisciplinary thinking.

In short, I view organizations as an exciting and stimulating topic. I, therefore, enjoy writing about organizational issues and sharing these ideas with others. Much of my motivation for writing this book stems from my commitment to the subject matter and to my desire to provide a fresh and contemporary view of organizational theories and developments. It is exciting to discover the ways in which organizations connect not only with our daily experiences but also with larger events that indirectly influence our human existence. In an academic context, it is vital to integrate the work of different disciplines in developing an understanding of organizations. I have written this book in the hope that students will develop an interest in organizations as well as a capacity for sound and rigorous organizational analysis.

What Makes This Text Different?

There are already many fine books about organization theory, so one might ask, why do we need another one? Or, to put it in more positive terms, if one is going to write another text, what special features should it offer that will differentiate it in some meaningful way from the existing crop? Let me highlight what I believe are some distinctive aspects of this book.

The Approach

I have always believed that one of the best ways to engage student interest in a topic is to link the subject matter to a set of questions, issues, problems, or controversies. Because ideas, concepts, and theories are generated as tools with which to address these intellectual and practical challenges, one must try to determine what these central problems or questions are and also explain how the theoretical literature grapples with them. As I have taught and studied organization theory over the past fifteen years, I have identified two fundamental tensions that have stimulated much of the work in this field. These tensions serve as a theoretical framework throughout the book.

First, there is the tension posed by the human factor. How to control and manage human beings poses a perpetual organizational problem. As conscious, reflective, and reactive creatures, humans are able—and often willing—to resist organizational pressures. Consequently, a large portion of organization and management theory is devoted to explaining how humans are effectively controlled or managed in organizational settings. If humans were passive *objects,* rather than active *subjects,* they would readily conform to organizational dictates. Because humans are neither passive nor objects, an endless series of organization theories and management strategies have been developed to explain and mobilize the human factor. The history and evolution of organization theory is heavily shaped by this tension.

A second tension is generated by the organizational decision to *differentiate* activities in terms of jobs, occupations, departments, and units. This differentiation is an attempt to rationally structure organizational processes and thus gain the benefits of specialization. At the same time, however, organizations must also make sure that people, jobs, and production units fit well together. They must be coordinated, and they must be connected to the larger mission of the organization. This constitutes the problem of *integration.* The tension between differentiation and integration has also provided fertile ground for significant theorizing, organizational analysis, and management strategy.

As noted above, these tensions posed by the human factor and the differentiation-integration tradeoff will serve as a thematic framework for the material presented in this book. As we consider the ways in which organization theories develop and evolve, and how they are transformed, we will see how these tensions are a constant source of theoretical and practical concern. This theme will also emphasize the fact that organizations are characterized by conflict, contradiction, and paradox—the harbingers of organizational change.

Illustrations and Examples

A second feature of this book which distinguishes it from other texts, particularly sociological, is its use of illustrations and examples derived from the real world of organization and business. It is important for students to appreciate the integral relationship between theory and reality (or practice). This point has special relevance for organizations, because many theories directly inform organizational and management practices and, in turn, organizational experiences and management problems stimulate new theoretical approaches.

In Chapter 2 the tensions and contradictions inherent in organizations are illustrated with case material focusing on an auto parts manufacturer, a quality improvement program, and higher education. In Chapter 4 we consider the way human relations and resource theories are translated into actual management practices. Chapter 5 explores the diffusion of bureaucracy in the context of the fast-food model known as McDonaldization. In Chapter 6 emerging organizational forms revolve around the contrasting practices of Ford Motor Company and Toyota Motors. In Chapter 7 postbureaucracy is illustrated with examples from a chemical company, a hearing aid manufacturer, and an office furniture firm. Interspersed throughout the text, there is also a wide assortment of illustrations derived from the business press.

Content

The core content of organization theory revolves around scientific management, bureaucracy, human relations, technology, the environment, and culture. In addition to these standard themes, this text will introduce topics that are often neglected but which are increasingly vital for organization theory and analysis. These include the literature on:

- emerging organizational forms (e.g., post-Fordism, Toyotaism, the keiretsu, and flexible and lean manufacturing);
- emerging organizational paradigms (e.g., postbureaucracy, strong corporate cultures, the learning/knowledge organization, and postmodernism);
- emerging inter-organizational arrangements (e.g., networks, partnerships, alliances, and joint ventures);

- the role of information technologies and the rise of the "virtual organization";
- the highly interdisciplinary work analyzing the political-economic environment, the role of geographic space, and the emergence of globalized production systems.

Book Website

An important pedagogical feature of this book is the corresponding website that will help instructors and students get the most out of the material in this book. The website will be easily accessible through the McGraw-Hill website [www.mhhe.com/jaffee]. It will contain exercises, discussion questions, additional content, and links to websites that have a direct connection to the topics covered in each chapter. The website will be a learning environment that will emphasize the application of theory, the synthesis of ideas, and active learning processes. Instructors can direct their students to particular items, or students may use the site as a way to further their own learning and understanding of the organizational issues.

Softcover Format/Manageable Length

This book is intentionally designed to be shorter in length than the standard hardcover text, which can often run 500 pages or more. For many instructors who like to assign additional readings, such as an anthology or a research monograph, this text would be an ideal companion to these other learning resources. The shorter length and softcover format will also ease the strain on the student's budget.

Acknowledgments

I would like to express my appreciation to the panel of reviewers who took the time to read the manuscript and provide constructive suggestions that have produced a better final product. They are: Paul S. Ciccantell, Kansas State University; Lisa A. Keister, University of North Carolina-Chapel Hill; Geoffrey Grant, South Dakota State University; David Olday, Moorhead State University; Teresa Scheid, University of North Carolina-Charlotte; and William E. Snizek, Virginia Polytechnic Institute and State University.

I would also like to thank my student at SUNY-New Paltz, Kathy Warner, who devoted an entire independent study to reading and recommending ways to make this book more student-friendly.

Thanks are also due, once again, to Marilyn Glass, who typed the entire manuscript and tolerated my endless revisions, changes, reorganizations, and wholesale substitutions.

Finally, there is my loving family—my wife, Marianne, and my daughters, Katy and Anna—who always wonder why I spend my time writing these things but support my efforts nonetheless.

David Jaffee
University of North Florida

1 INTRODUCTION: DEFINITIONS AND CONCEPTIONS

Many books on organization theory begin with a definition of organization. This definition may even be what most people expect. However, in this first chapter we will avoid the one-sentence definition of organization in favor of a different approach. Instead, we will review some of the existing contributions to the study of organization theory. These come in the form of conceptualization, frameworks, and even some definitions. Thus, we will follow the advice of two well-known organization theorists who claimed, "It is easier, and probably more useful, to give examples of formal organizations than to define the term . . . We are dealing with empirical phenomena, and the world has an uncomfortable way of not permitting itself to be fitted into clean classifications" (Simon and March 1958).

Even if we wanted to arrive at a single definition of organization, it would be extremely difficult to include all the components or satisfy all the different perspectives. Organizational theory has become a multiperspective or multiparadigmatic field of study (Burrell and Morgan 1979; Schultz and Hatch 1996). This means that there are a wide variety of ways to approach, or get a grip on, the central elements of an organization. These different approaches and points of entry generate a great deal of debate and argument over the essential and defining features of organizational life. Should we focus on the techniques that enhance organizational efficiency? the differences in power and influence between organizational members? the decision-making processes used to initiate organizational behavior? the language and culture of the organization? the dehumanizing aspects of bureaucratic organization? the interdependent relationships between organizations? or the human interaction and communications that occur in the organization? I am just getting started, but I hope you get the point. There are different levels and places to look when we study organizations. No single or concise definition can hope to encapsulate all of these different analytical angles.

Another good reason not to formulate a definition is that too many already exist. You will find hundreds, maybe thousands, of these definitions in books on organization and management theory. A lot of hard work has gone into defining and conceptualizing organizations. It seems nonsensical to simply ignore all these previous efforts or to develop definitions as if they never existed. Therefore, I will provide some examples of the way various theorists have attempted to introduce and define the concept of organization. One can learn a lot from their efforts. In the next chapter I will offer some of my own ideas on how to approach organization theory.

Organization: Elements, a Definition and Images

As an indication of the lack of consensus over the meaning of organization, we can consider several of the leading texts on organization theory. It is notable that each approaches the conceptualization issue in a very different way and, in so doing, reveals important insights on organization.

Scott's Elements of Organization

Rather than presenting a single definition of organization, W. Richard Scott (1987) outlines the central elements. These include social structure, participants, goals, technology, and the environment.

In sociology we use the term *social structure* to refer to those activities, relationships, and interactions that take on a regular pattern. Most organizations have standard techniques, practices, and methods that are repeated day in and day out. There are also patterned and recurring forms of human interaction among organizational members. Many of these aspects of the social structure are explicitly defined in job descriptions and organizational charts. They are often formally specified because they are designed to accomplish a particular organizational task. This is the *formal social structure.* The *informal social structure* contains those patterned activities and relationships that emerge naturally and which are created by organizational members. They do not exist in written documents, organizational charts, or job descriptions. The social structure is the fundamental building block of organization. It is what distinguishes a spontaneous and temporary collection of people from an actual organizational entity that comes together on a regular basis for a specific purpose.

The second element in Scott's scheme is *participants*. These are the humans who "people" the organization. While there has been a great deal of discussion and a few minor examples of "peopleless" organization—inhabited by machines and robots—most organizations rely heavily on the human factor of production. We will have much more to say about the unique nature of this factor and the challenges it creates for organization theory and management practice. Because organizations depend on human labor power (physical and mental) and because humans ("participants") do not automatically exert their labor when they enter an organization, organizations and their owners face the endless challenge of trying to figure out how to extract this human energy. This is a persistent organizational problem.

The *goals* of the organization are the "conceptions of desired ends" (Scott 1987:18); that is, what is the organization trying to achieve? This could be the production of a reliable product, high-quality customer service, or the efficient distribution of social services. We often speak of these as "the goals of the organization." This phrase is so widely used by organizational and management theorists, and anyone who talks about organizations, that it is rarely scrutinized. However, organizations do not have goals, purpose, or intent. Rather, "organizational goals" are human goals. The goals of the organization are usually the goals of those who own or control the organization. Once we acknowledge this fact, we begin to see the more problematic aspects of this concept. Since goals are formulated by humans, organizational participants may not share the same goals. The goals of owners may not be the goals of managers, production workers, or support staff. The fact that humans will have different goals, and that goal conflict will take place, is further evidence of the challenge posed by organizational participants.

Technology is the means used by the organization to transform the raw materials of the organization—physical, informational, or human—into some final product. All organizations use particular techniques—methods, machines, hardware, software, computers—to process resources and materials. Technology is significant because it shapes many other aspects of the organization such as the labor process, social structures, and participants.

The *environment* refers to all things outside the boundaries of the organization that are either shaped by or influence a particular organization. This book devotes an entire chapter to this element of organization. Environmental factors can include, for example, other organizations with which the organization interacts (suppliers, distributors) and competes, or political and legal regulations that are imposed on organizations.

Scott's elements can be used to conduct a basic analysis of any organization. In Table 1–1 we present a hypothetical firm called ModParts, Inc., which produces modular auto parts, like dashboard control panels, for car manufacturers. Examples of each organizational element are identified.

It is also important to note that each element of organization points to a critical feature that has attracted theoretical interest. Some theories of organization would place the greatest emphasis on the relationships between

TABLE 1–1   **Elements of Organization: ModParts, Inc.**

Elements	Examples
Social structure	Decision-making process, authority structure, relationships between workers on assembly line
Participants	Line supervisors, middle managers, production workers
Goals	Low-cost assembly of high-quality modular auto parts
Technology	Team-based assembly line
Environment	Suppliers of components for modular parts; large automakers who purchase the finished product

participants (social structure), other theories would examine the impact of assembly-line production techniques (technology), and still other approaches would consider the relationship between ModParts and the larger auto manufacturers (environment).

Scott also took on the difficult task of devising a scheme for categorizing the vast number of organization theories. The scheme is based on three major perspectives used to analyze organizations: the rational system, natural system, and open systems perspectives.

The *rational system perspective* has been the most widely employed approach to organizational analysis, especially in management. In this perspective, "organizations are collectivities oriented to the pursuit of relatively specified goals and exhibiting relatively formalized social structures" (Scott 1987:22). Goals and formal social structures are the key organizational elements emphasized in this perspective.

The *natural system perspective* views "organizations as collectivities whose participants share a common interest in the survival of the system and who engage in collective activities, informally structured, to secure this end" (Scott 1987:23). This perspective is more sociological with its emphasis on the informal activities of participants, the way behavior in organizations deviates from formal rules and structures, and the role human participants play in creating organizational values and cultures.

In the *open systems perspective,* "organizations are coalitions of shifting interest groups that develop goals by negotiations; the structure of the coalition, its activities, and its outcomes are strongly influenced by environmental factors" (Scott 1987:23). As the open-systems terminology suggests, organizations in this perspective are not hermetically sealed entities but collectivities that depend on and are influenced by environmental agents and resources. The emphasis on the environmental element denotes an organization that must negotiate with both human participants and other organizations.

These three perspectives represent a metatheoretical framework for classifying organization theories. The term *metatheoretical* implies a grand theory of how people theorize about organizations. Such a framework seeks to identify the major fundamental criteria that can distinguish one theory from another. In Scott's scheme, theories can be distinguished on the degree to which they emphasize the rational, natural, or environmental elements of organization.

Hall's Definition of Organization

While we have thus far avoided a one-sentence definition of organization, we can now consider one such attempt. This particularly comprehensive definition is provided by Richard H. Hall (1999:30):

> An organization is a collectivity with a relatively identifiable boundary, a normative order (rules), ranks of authority (hierarchy), communications system, and membership coordinating systems (procedures); this collectivity exists, on a relatively continuous basis in an environment, and engages in activities that are usually related to a set of goals; the activities have outcomes for organizational members, the organization itself, and for society.

Don't memorize this! As Hall himself admits, "This is a cumbersome and perhaps unwieldy definition, but then so too is the subject matter" (1999:32). Therefore, it might prove useful to dissect this definition and highlight the key themes.

When sociologists use the term *collectivity,* they are suggesting a group of humans who have something in common. In the case of organizations, it may be no more than a common objective. However, there will always be some tension between the particular interests of individual members and the larger organizational objective or goal. The additional characteristics of organization that are listed by Hall—boundaries, norms, authority, communication, and coordination—are the mechanisms designed to reconcile the potential conflict between collective and individual interests.

Boundaries distinguish who is inside and who is outside the organization. This establishes common membership. The normative order, which is the cultural dimension, implies shared beliefs and values about the appropriate way to behave and accomplish organizational activities. This suggests that the collectivity is not simply an assortment of individuals who happen to occupy the same organizational space but a cohesive social group with a common set of ideas. Authority, communication, and coordination systems are additional means to convert individuals into a cohesive collectivity.

Because the "collectivity exists on a regular continuous basis," it is a social structure. The "activities that are usually related to a set of goals" provide direction for the organization and its members. Reference to the "continuous basis" suggests the repeated achievement of goals such as producing a particular product or providing a service. It is not a one-shot deal but an ongoing enterprise.

The final component of the definition—the outcome of organizational activities for members, the organization, and society—highlights the way organizational processes can shape organizational members, transform the organization itself, and influence the environment or larger society.

This definition also represents Hall's attempt to identify three distinct but interrelated aspects of organizational reality: *structures, processes,* and *outcomes.* The first part of the definition emphasizes the social structural elements (boundaries, norms, hierarchy, communications, and coordination mechanisms); the second part highlights active processes that are goal directed; the third part considers the consequences of organizational structure and process on members, the organization, and society at large.

Morgan's Images of Organization

A third popular approach to studying organization theory uses metaphors, images, or mental models. Gareth Morgan (1997) has argued that how we define, understand, and conceptualize organizations depends on our mental images of the essential shape and feature of organizations. Morgan believes that most definitions and theories of organization can be associated with a particular organizational metaphor. The most common metaphors view organizations as machines, organisms, brains, cultures, political systems, psychic prisons, or instruments of domination. We can take each of these metaphors and show how they are reflected in different definitions of organization.

The *machine metaphor* views organizations as technical instruments used to produce some outcome. The elements of the organization, including humans, are parts of a structure that work together with mechanical-like efficiency to achieve a particular goal. The following definitions embody this metaphor:

> An organization is a tool used by people to coordinate their actions to obtain something they desire or value (G. Jones 1993:4).

> There does appear to be some agreement about the fact that organizations generally develop as instruments for attaining specific goals (A. Bedeian 1984:2).

Each definition is consistent with a machine metaphor, as well as a rational system perspective, in viewing organizations as "tools" or "instruments." Both also come from mainstream textbooks used in management courses. Thus, they present a standard and widely accepted definition of organization. The organization does not emerge accidentally or informally but is constructed a priori to achieve an objective. This is the defining feature of a formal organization.

A second metaphor identified by Morgan is the organization as an *organism.* This implies that organizations are akin to living things that need resources to stay alive and flourish. An example:

> Most books about organizations describe how they operate, and the existence of the organizations is taken for granted. This book discusses how organizations

manage to survive. Their existence is constantly in question, and their survival is viewed as problematic.

The key to organizational survival is the ability to acquire and maintain resources (Pfeffer and Salancik 1978:2).

As in biology, the survival of the organizational organism is heavily dependent upon the level of competition and resources in the ecosystem. Those who employ the organism metaphor, therefore, place a great deal of emphasis on the ability of organizations to manage and cope with environmental conditions. Organizations can only obtain the necessary nourishment for survival if they have the appropriately complex structure that is able to access and process resources. The organism metaphor combines features of both the natural system and open-systems perspectives.

Organizations are also conceptualized as *brains*. They are defined as information-processing, decision-making, or learning entities. The primary focus in this metaphor is on the ability to access, use, and process information for the purpose of learning, decision making, and assessment.

> Organizations make decisions. They make decisions in the same sense in which individuals make decisions. The organization as a whole behaves as though there existed a central coordination and control system capable of directing the members of the organization sufficiently to allow the meaningful imputation of purpose to the total system (Cyert and March 1992).

In this metaphor, organizational success requires the right kind of decision-making structures, data gathering apparatus, analytical tools, and collective mind-set able to translate information into improved organizational processes.

Organizations are also *cultural systems*. As collectivities of human beings who act and interact, some shared set of values and beliefs emerges. Using the culture metaphor, organizations are:

> a network of intersubjectively shared meanings that are sustained through the development and the use of a common language and everyday social interaction (Walsh and Ungson 1991:60).

> a set of people who share many beliefs, values, and assumptions that encourage them to make mutually reinforcing interpretations of their own acts and the acts of others (Smircich and Stubbart 1985:727).

In these definitions, organizations are not objective structures designed to achieve a measurable goal but collections of humans who construct reality with shared meanings and assumptions. This metaphor shares many assumptions with Scott's natural system perspective. In order for organizations to operate, members must define a problem to be solved. They must also come to some mutually agreeable understanding about the best and most appropriate way to solve the problem. In short, for people to act and organizations to function, there must be a definition or construction of reality.

Others use the metaphor of *political systems* to describe organizations.

The organization is characterized as a complex network of competing and cooperating individuals and coalitions in which conflict is the natural occurrence. The central variable of the political model is power, and understanding of its nature and consequences is essential if the mysteries of the organization are to be unraveled (Lee and Lawrence 1991:42–43).

In all organizations, individuals and groups compete for resources, for attention, for influence; there are differences of opinion as to the priorities and objectives to be attained; clashes of values and belief occur with common frequency. All of these factors lead to the formation of pressure groups, vested interests, cabals, personal rivalries, personality clashes, hidden deals and bonds of alliance (Kakabadse 1983:3).

In viewing organizations as political systems, these definitions place the greatest emphasis on conflict and competition for resources between groups that have different values, interests, and priorities.

Organizations can also be conceptualized as *psychic prisons* because, in demanding physical and emotional energy, their rules and methods may shape our psyche and control our mental processes. The analogy to a prison suggests that the organizations we create and in which we participate, limit our freedom of thought and constrain not just our body, but our soul. This metaphor can be used to launch a radical critique of all organizational systems or it can be used to identify the way we develop patterns of thought that hamper effective organizational learning and performance. Pay close attention to the language used in the following examples.

Organizations are human-made environments. They are produced and reproduced by groups of people as particular ways of relating to each in order to get work done. Institutionally supported authoritarian and totalitarian acts are organizational, psychosocial, and political phenomenon. But psychologically these forms of systemic oppression would not exist without group consensus (or collusion) about a set of unconscious feelings that support specific values, norms, ideas, actions. . . where an organization prizes unilateral decision making, this value can elicit and reinforce needs for obsessional control and compulsive dominance (Diamond 1993:57).

To begin with, since complex organizations play such a large part in our lives, the way in which we construct reality is obviously guided by our experiences and our training in organizations. . .

The result of this socialization process is the widespread assumption of a particular viewpoint, a sort of organizational ethic. . . we will come to value discipline, regulation and obedience in contrast to independence, expressiveness and creativity. . .

What is especially important is that this new ethic of organization does not just instruct our activities in organizations; rather, its power is so great that it recommends those same patterns of thought and behavior for our lives generally (Denhardt 1981:3–5).

In these two passages, organizational experience can spawn obsessive-compulsive behavioral tendencies and a general orientation toward discipline and obedience.

Finally, organizations can be seen as *instruments of domination*. This combines the machine metaphor of the organization-as-a-tool with the political metaphor's image of competition and power. The organization becomes the instrument that advances the interests of one group at the expense of another. Those who are able to own, control, and manage organizations are able to exercise domination and power over others. In this view, organizations do not advance the collective will or the general interest; they advance particular interests. Organizations control, exploit, dominate, and dehumanize. Like the psychic prison perspective, this metaphor is employed by radical critics of large bureaucracies and global corporations.

> In so far as bureaucracy is a "necessity" of capitalist industry, it is largely due to the continuing need to deny workers' control over their productive lives and by the monopolistic tendencies of the capitalist system which result in gigantic, relatively centralized corporations operating on a worldwide scale (Goldman and Van Houten 1988:62).

> [T]his analysis does not see bureaucracy as something which capitalists want in and of itself. . . If workers did not resist, if they were fully and truly socialized to be happy and obedient, capitalists would not need the enormous and complex apparatus that is bureaucracy, nor would they need to distort the entire labor process to ensure exploitation. . . if workers tried always to do what their masters wanted, then bureaucracy would be unnecessary (Clawson 1980:24).

Morgan's images and metaphors provide an additional framework for sorting organizational theories, and we will see how these metaphors are embedded in various theories of organization. It is important to recognize that metaphors both illuminate and obscure. They focus our attention on particular realities of organizational life while at the same time blinding us to other equally important components. The assortment of metaphors is also compelling testimony to the way we socially create mental models of abstract entities. The infinite complexity of organizations yields a wide range of metaphorical images.

If, as Morgan argues, the study and analysis of organizations is driven by metaphors, it is only fair to ask whether any particular metaphor will inform the analysis in this text. There is an eighth metaphor that I have thus far omitted— *organization as flux and transformation*. This metaphor comes closest to capturing the framework I will use in this text. The primary assumption driving this metaphor is that organizations are in a constant state of flux or change. There are many reasons why this might be the case. I will argue that flux and transformation is generated by several fundamental organizational tensions or contradictions. These tensions affect not only organizations but the theories and strategies designed to explain and guide organizations.

Classical Social Theory and Organizational Analysis

Our understanding of organizational structure and process can also be enhanced by considering the contribution of classical sociological theory. This usually refers to the work of Karl Marx, Émile Durkheim, and Max Weber. The significance of their writings is reflected in their continuing relevance for organizational analysis. The three theorists were living through the historically monumental transition from feudalism to capitalism, or from an agricultural to an industrial society. This had a profound impact on their social theory and each tended to focus on a particular aspect of this transition. We shall briefly consider each of the theorists' sociological insights and their relationship to issues in organization theory.

Marx

The work of Karl Marx (1818–83) has had an enormous influence on organization theory (Marx 1963; 1964). This can largely be explained by the role he assigned to the organization of production. He believed that an understanding of the human relationships guiding economic production was the key to social analysis. This leads directly to a focus on organizations and work.

In terms of the transition from feudalism to capitalism, Marx emphasized the shifting foundation of social power from the ownership of land to the ownership of capital. The means of production in the industrial capitalist society are the machines, factories, and organizations that produce goods for sale in the market. Ownership of the means of production defines the dominant social class, in this case the *capitalist class* (capital). Those who do not own this productive property must sell their labor power for a wage by entering into an employment relationship with the capitalist owners. This defines the *working class* (labor). The relationship between capital and labor, defined by their respective role in the production process, is played out in the "hidden abode" of the organization. Because labor depends on capital for its survival, it is an asymmetric and dependent relationship that allows for the subordination and exploitation of the working class. The ability of the capitalist class to exploit workers and extract "surplus value" is the basis for profitable production, further investment, and capital accumulation.

An analysis of this relationship between capital and labor (or owners and workers, or management and labor) generates many of the central concepts in organization theory. One of the most widely employed concepts is *control* (Marglin 1974; Braverman 1974; Clawson 1980; Edwards 1979). It is assumed that profitable production requires the control of workers by capitalists. Therefore, organizational structures and strategies are designed primarily to control the mental and physical labor of workers. In this view, organizational structures that are assumed to evolve naturally, or to be the most efficient, are actually intended to socially control and dominate labor. Organization theories influenced by Marx typically employ the organization-as-instrument-of-domination metaphor.

The emphasis on class domination and control has tended to obscure another equally important element in the Marxist equation—*struggle and resistance.* While capitalists and their organizations are interested in the maximization of profit and the social control of labor, it is equally true that labor is capable of individually and collectively resisting the efforts of owners and managers. According to Marx, the development of increasingly effective organizational means of exploitation had the paradoxical effect of galvanizing the collective opposition of the working class. This dynamic embodies a fundamental organizational tension between the effort to increase efficiency and profitability, on the one hand, and the human labor reaction to these efforts, on the other. The struggle to manage and control these human reactions is an important dynamic in understanding the evolution of organizational theory and management strategy. It will be a consistent theme as we review various theories of organization.

Marx's analysis also rests on a particular set of assumptions about the unique nature of the human species. Workers under capitalism suffer from *alienation*—a sense of separation and detachment—because they are unable to exercise their distinctive abilities. These involve the capacity of humans to abstractly conceptualize a finished product, gather the necessary materials to build the product, and engage in a sequential production process. Under capitalism these capacities are not fully realized because production is subjected to a division of labor, and workers have no control over the process. This means that workers engage only in a small piece of a larger production process. Further, most of the mental labor will be placed in the hands of engineers and managers. The worker, left with a single manual task, is thus alienated from the larger labor process that defines the distinctive capacity of the human species. Alienation is another factor contributing to working-class organization and resistance.

Durkheim

For Émile Durkheim (1858–1917), the most general concern was the bases of order and solidarity in society (Durkheim 1933). The question, What holds society together? was then and remains today a fundamental concern of social theory. Durkheim believed that social solidarity in traditional agricultural society was based on the similarity in life experiences derived from common activities in a rural community. People doing the same kinds of work develop a common set of beliefs and sentiments that serve to encourage consensus and integration while minimizing individual differences and social conflict. He referred to this as *mechanical solidarity.*

In the transition from an agricultural to industrial society, a more complex division of labor develops. The similarity and common experience derived from rural, agricultural activities are replaced by growing differences as individuals take on a variety of different economic roles. As individuals pursue different jobs and occupations, distribute themselves in rural and urban areas, and occupy different social class positions, similarity is replaced by differentiation. This undermines the basis of mechanical solidarity and, therefore, threatens social order and social integration. The different outlooks and perspectives can produce opposing interests and generate social conflict. In this environment, Durkheim believed that a new form of solidarity would emerge based on interdependence. This interdependent division of labor—where some people grow food, others produce clothing and tools, others sell goods and services—means that the members of society depend upon each other for the fulfillment of their needs. The network of interdependence results in the rise of *organic solidarity*. More generally, Durkheim concluded that all forms of social organization required social integration and social solidarity. This would be based on a *collective conscience* of shared beliefs and sentiments among organizational members that would serve as a normative form of social control.

Durkheim's analysis of, and problem associated with, the transition from an agricultural to an industrial society has a direct application to one of the most persistent organizational problems: the difficulty in balancing the dual but often conflicting objectives of differentiation and integration. Almost all organizations are structured around a division of activities. There is differentiation and specialization which are often viewed as fundamental prerequisites for organizational efficiency. However, these divisions can prove problematic when they undermine a common mission by promoting particularistic identification with an occupation, a department, or a social class. People in a single organization can begin to pursue very different interests and objectives that defeat collective organizational goals. Thus, in all organizations there is a constant balancing act between divisions of labor and differentiation, on the one hand, and building community and integration, on the other. This tension will be a driving theme throughout this text.

Weber

Max Weber's (1864–1920) impact on organizational theory derives heavily from his work on bureaucratic organization. We will examine this topic in greater detail in Chapter 5.

For the moment, we can devote our attention to Weber's broader concern with the rise of rationality in the transition from traditional agricultural to modern industrial society.

Weber's (1946; 1947) historical analysis of different societies focused upon the forms of social organization and their corresponding forms of *authority*. In most organizations some people command and some people obey. Weber was especially interested in the way these authority differences were granted legitimacy; that is, how some people are able to exercise the right to command while others are willing to accept their duty to obey.

The foundations for legitimate authority varied historically. Previous societies established authority on the basis of charisma (based on the personality characteristics of leaders) or tradition (based on custom or inherited status, as in a monarchy or family succession). What distinguished modern industrial society, according to Weber, was the rise of rationalization as the dominant operating principle. Under this system, authority was *rational-legal*—based on the application of rational principles linking means and ends. Authority relations were accepted because they were regarded as the necessary means to accomplish specific goals. Authoritative commands were not arbitrary and capricious. Rather, they were part of the organizational rules and procedures designed to maximize efficiency. Those occupying positions of authority did so on the basis of their knowledge and ability to rationally direct social action. This form of authority was regarded by Weber as the most historically advanced and efficient and was a central element in his theory of bureaucracy. In this sense, bureaucracy is the organizational embodiment of rationality in modern society.

However, while bureaucracy advanced efficiency and was based on a rational-legal foundation, Weber also believed it was a dominating force that stifled individual freedom and creativity. This points to the important fact that objective structures designed for efficiency may conflict with the subjective desires of humans for freedom and autonomy. The human consequences of bureaucracy was a major theme in Weber's work. This also represents a fundamental organizational tension generated by human actors who struggle to resist the "iron cage" of bureaucratic control. This is another organizational tension that will inform the analysis of organizations in subsequent chapters.

Taken together, the three classical theorists identify important organizational contradictions. Durkheim noted that the process of economic development and progress, through a more complex division of labor, threatened social order and solidarity. The paradox for Weber stems from the organizational superiority of bureaucracy that allows for high efficiency while at the same time creating the iron cage that imprisons human participants. Marx revealed how the process of exploitation contributed to the accumulation of capitalist wealth while at the same time fueling the resistance and opposition of the working class. Paradox, contradiction, and tension are built into their analyses of social structure and change. These are valuable analytical devices that will assist in our review of organization theories and management strategies.

Contemporary Social Theory and Organizational Analysis

Three major theoretical perspectives in sociology have been applied to a wide variety of social phenomena including organizations. These are structural functionalism, conflict theory, and symbolic interactionism.

Structural Functionalism

Functionalism is most closely associated with the work of Talcott Parsons (1902–79), who also had a great deal to say about organizations. Parsons (1960) employed a model of social system functions that was designed to demonstrate how all societies and social organizations carry out a necessary set of functions to ensure survival. The now classic acronym AGIL delineates the four functions: adaptation, goal attainment, integration, and latency. Adaptation refers to the way systems gain access to the resources they need. Goal attainment refers to the establishment and achievement of objectives. Integration refers to the problem of ensuring the cohesiveness and coordination of society's members and activities. Latency refers to the way the system sustains and reproduces itself over time through the transmission of culture and values.

This simple list of basic functions has generated a wide variety of ideas and theories of organization. For example, each of these functions can be carried out by the elements of a single organization. Adaptation points to the way an organization will interact with its environment to access resources required for production. Goal attainment is a central objective of rational bureaucratic organizations that construct formal structures to achieve specified goals. Integration, already discussed in the context of Durkheim's classical sociological theory, is necessary if organizations are to retain social solidarity and articulate their various activities. Latency would involve the socialization and cultural processes designed to ensure organizational longevity. Organizations, in this scheme, implement structures and processes to fulfill these essential functions. An assessment of organizational performance might then be linked to the degree to which these functions have been successfully carried out.

Alternatively, Parsons conceived of organizations as institutions within the larger society that were responsible for carrying out a particular function. Firms engaged in economic production carry out the adaptation function by providing resources for consumption. Government organizations fulfill the goal attainment function through public policies. Criminal justice organizations perform the integration function through the enforcement of laws. Educational organizations socialize members of society, thereby contributing to long-term cultural stability. Together, these organizations contribute to the maintenance of social order.

This kind of functionalist analysis of organizations highlights the positive functions and apparent objectives of different social organizations. These are what Robert Merton referred to as the *manifest functions*—the obvious and officially stated purpose of an organization or institution. But there are also, according to Merton, *latent functions*. These are the unintended, unexpected, and unannounced functions of an organization (Merton 1957).

We can take the example of educational institutions. The manifest function is to train and educate the population to be productive members of society. However, there are also some other consequences of educational institutions that may be equally important for the society, yet are rarely stated or discussed. For example, educational institutions keep a large portion of the population out of the labor force, thus reducing the unemployment rate and, with that, the likelihood of social unrest; educational institutions prepare people for life in bureaucratic and hierarchical organizations; educational institutions sort people at an early age on the basis of academic ability which is later used as a socially legitimate means to allocate people into high-paying and low-paying jobs. While none of these functions are mentioned in the organizational mission statement, they may be as socially significant as those functions that are publicly pronounced. A sound functionalist analysis of organizations will examine both the manifest and latent functions.

A second problem with the functionalist model, as presented by Parsons, is its failure to consider the tensions and contradictions produced by organizations that ultimately contribute to social disorder and instability. We simply need to refer back to the insights of Marx, Durkheim, and Weber to illustrate this point. Marx showed how economic production in a class society entails exploitation and alienation which in turn generate class conflict. Durkheim believed a division of labor that enhanced productive efficiency also threatened social solidarity. Weber argued that bureaucratic organizational techniques, while technically rational, were also dehumanizing. In each of these cases, the methods used to satisfy one function produced negative or dysfunctional consequences. Such contradiction and paradox are a fundamental dynamic of all organizations.

Conflict Theory

In sociology, conflict theory is a very broad perspective used to understand social structures and social change. Unlike structural functionalism, which tends to emphasize stability and order, conflict theory is based on the assumption that all societies are characterized by ongoing conflict between groups and persistent social change. This is due to the fact that (1) individuals develop different political interests based on racial, ethnic, class, religious, gender, occupational, or regional affiliation; (2) socially valued resources tend to be relatively scarce, which generates conflict and competition over access to and the distribution of these resources; (3) social institutions are organized to serve the interests of those who own and control the scarce resources; (4) the struggle between those who possess and those who do not possess the resources creates instability and change.

If this perspective is applied to organizations, it is likely to yield a political system metaphor that emphasizes conflict, competition, and the exercise of power. It is also likely to conjure up the instrument-of-domination metaphor because those who are successful at securing "ownership" of the scarce resource use organizations as a way to dominate and exercise control over those who lack these resources. Further, emphasis on instability and change is consistent with the metaphorical notions of flux and transformation.

Like the larger society, organizations are made up of members who occupy different positions—they carry out different roles, work in different departments and units, and possess different levels of authority and decision-making power, and receive different levels of reward such as income. For all these reasons, organizational members will develop a variety of conflicting political interests and may engage in various forms of competition. Organizational analysis must acknowledge that in almost all organizations such divisions and conflicts are inevitable. A large bulk of organization and management theory is designed to explain how these conflicts are controlled and managed.

As noted above, Marxist analyses of organizations emphasize the role of valued resource ownership—particularly ownership of the means of production—as the foundation for the domination and control of one social class (the capitalist class) by another social class (the working class). The two classes develop divergent political interests and struggle over control of the workplace and the distribution of profits. This conflict in turn stimulates changes in labor-management relations, wages, working conditions, and the larger organization of production.

Symbolic Interactionism

In contrast to structural functionalism and conflict theory, which are *macrolevel* theories focusing on society-level institutions and change, symbolic interactionism is a *microlevel* approach aimed at analyzing individual-level social interaction. As a general social theory, symbolic interactionism assumes that social order is based on the interpretations we assign and the meanings we transmit in the process of social interaction. Without a shared understanding of verbal and body language, nonverbal cues, gestures, expressions, and demeanor, there would be no social life as we know it. All of these forms of communication entail symbolic messages that have to be understood in the same way by the person transmitting as well as the person receiving the symbolic action.

The symbolic language and behavior that a person employs will depend upon the role or identity that he or she wants to assume or the context in which that person is operating. In the college classroom, for example, a student who wants to be identified as a serious intellectual might sit in the front row, attend all classes, ask many questions, carry a large number of books, and speak with the instructor after class. All of these forms of behavior send a message to the instructor and other students. We associate these actions with a particular student identity.

More generally, all the students who enter the classroom are operating in a *context* that demands symbolic forms of behavior associated with the generic student role. Students walk into class, find a seat, open a notebook, direct their attention toward the front of the room, assume a passive rather than proactive presence, and engage in "civil attention." The instructor, likewise, enters the room communicating an important purpose, assumes a position at the front of the room, commands the attention of the class, and takes responsibility for initiating and directing the learning process. The ultimate success of the classroom interaction hinges on conformity with these symbolic role behaviors. Such behaviors are employed in all organizational settings.

A second organizational application of symbolic meaning is captured in Karl Weick's (1995) notions of "enactment" and "sensemaking." Human organizations place events and stimuli in a framework that is commonly understood and widely shared (intersubjective) in order to motivate and generate human action. A language, a sense of mission, objectives, and particular ways to achieve these objectives, are constructed and defined (or "enacted") so that organizational members can make sense of what it is they do and explain what it is they have done. In higher education, for example, instructors will define or make sense of their activities in the context of educating and teaching students. Instructors engage in a wide variety of organizational activities that may seem to have little relation to this objective. However, if instructors are pressed to explain why they did this or that, they are likely to place their actions in the context of, and use language emphasizing, teaching and the instruction of students. In this way, organizations provide a setting, context, language, and set of routines that fuel the cognitive energy of organizational members.

Just as individuals and activities are situated in a symbolic context, so is the larger organization. As a final way to apply symbolic interactionism to the study of organizations, we should note that how an organization "looks," the way it is structured, and its methods and techniques for achieving some goal, are subjected to symbolic interpretation. A university that has no campus, no academic departments, no student union building, or delivers courses online instead of in lecture halls and classrooms, violates the symbolic expectations of higher education consumers. For this reason, many organizations work very hard to establish and communicate symbols that consumers and clients associate with a legitimate operation.

The contemporary sociological perspectives that emphasize social functions, conflict, and symbols have shaped the study of organizations. They provide a further set of frameworks, like Scott's elements and Morgan's metaphors, that shape our understanding of and direct our attention to particular aspects of organizational life. But much of what we call contemporary social theory is not so contemporary anymore. More recent theoretical developments, particularly postmodernist theory, question whether organizations have functions, or groups have interests, or people have clear-cut roles and identities. These challenges to the basic assumptions underlying models of social and organizational life will be discussed in greater length in the concluding chapter. It is important to emphasize, however, that most of the existing organization theory has been influenced by "modernist" assumptions that assume identifiable functions, roles, identities, goals, and outcomes of social organization. As our review of organization theory moves from the rise of the factory system to the virtual organization, we will be better equipped to also see how the old assumptions associated with "modernism" give way to "postmodern" conceptions.

Summary

This chapter introduced the various ways organizations have been conceptualized and defined. The main points are as follows:

1. A single widely accepted definition of organization is difficult to establish because of the complex nature of the object of study and the multiple perspectives that inform organizational analysis.

2. The "elements of organization" can be regarded as focal points on which to construct a theory of organization. Images of organization are mental constraints that direct our attention to particular aspects of organizational life. As we study and analyze organizations, we should reflect on and be cognizant of our mental images and focal points and how these shape our understanding of organization.

3. The classical sociological theories of the "big three"—Durkheim, Weber, and Marx—have shaped contemporary organization theory and also provided useful conceptual tools to analyze contemporary organization. Each also offers a lesson about the tensions and contradictions of organizational systems.

4. Each of the three major contemporary theoretical perspectives in sociology—functionalism, conflict theory, and symbolic interactionism—have influenced the conceptualization of organization. Functionalism highlights the functions played by parts of a single organization in advancing organizational survival as well as the functions played by different social institutions in ensuring social order. Conflict theory denotes the competition and conflict among groups in organizations who struggle over valued resources. Symbolic interactionism directs our attention to the symbolic messages that are transmitted among organizational members and between organizations and environmental constituents.

2

CONCEPTUAL FRAMEWORK FOR THE ANALYSIS OF ORGANIZATION THEORY

Throughout this book we will be considering a wide variety of organizational theories and their application to different settings. As noted in Chapter 1, there is a range of definitions and conceptualizations of organization. In this chapter I will again eschew a single definition or approach in favor of a more flexible analytical framework. This framework has two dimensions. The first addresses the level of analysis of an organizational theory. Does the theory focus on the internal characteristics of an organization or the way organizations interact with the environment? The second dimension identifies the two fundamental organizational transactions that generate tension and change within organizations and in relation to the environment and other organizations.

Levels of Organizational Analysis and Transactions

We can make a distinction between two levels of organizational analysis. The *intraorganizational level* refers to the internal interactions and characteristics of an organization. These include labor-management relations, formal and informal interactions among employees, internal organizational design, methods of organizational control, and organizational culture. At this level the organization is viewed as a largely closed system.

20

The *interorganizational level* refers to the external interactions among organizations and between organizations and their environment. These include relationships with suppliers and distributors, markets and clients, government regulatory agencies, labor organizations, financial institutions, and competitors. At this level the organization is viewed as a largely open system.

A large portion of the organizational and managerial literature can be placed into one of these two levels of analysis. Many theories of organization, particularly those pertaining to organizational behavior and formal structure, focus upon intraorganizational dynamics. Other theories are more concerned with the way organizations manage their relations with other organizations and agencies, and how they secure needed resources from other organizational units. While these levels can be distinguished conceptually and many theories of organization can be squarely placed in one level or another, a complete organizational analysis must integrate the two levels and specify their mutual influence.

Interorganizational relations can have a direct influence on an organization's internal structure. For example, a highly competitive interorganizational environment can prompt a restructuring of internal organizational relationships. Likewise, internal organizational dynamics can shape interorganizational relations. For example, internal conflicts between parties, such as labor and management, might prompt the establishment of an outsourcing strategy with external firms or subcontractors. We shall consider many of these possibilities and also point out the means to integrate the interorganizational and intraorganizational levels of analysis.

Since we have now established the fundamental interorganizational and intraorganizational distinction, we can move to a consideration of the central organizational dilemmas, tensions, or problematics that have shaped the evolution of organization theory.

If there is a single process that is central to the operation of organizations, it is the transaction. A *transaction* is the exchange relationship between the provider and the recipient of a labor, service, or product (Tilly and Tilly 1998:71). Taking the two levels of analysis outlined above, we can think of two basic types of transactions. At the intraorganizational level are the transactions among owners, managers, and workers. At the interorganizational level are the transactions between organizations or interdependent production units (see Table 2-1).

We might say that the conceptualization and management of these transactions lies at the core of organization theory and management strategy. However, the management of these transactions is forever problematic given two enduring tensions facing all organizations. The first involves the *unique nature of the human factor,* the second involves balancing the dual demands for *differentiation* and *integration*.

TABLE 2–1 Levels of Organizational Analysis

	Levels of Analysis	
	Intraorganizational	*Interorganizational*
Definition	Within the organization	Between organizations
Structures	Bureaucracy	Network of Firms Interorganizational Relations
Relationships	Workers–managers–co-workers	Suppliers-manufacturers-distributors-regulators
Transactions	Employment contract	Market exchange/subcontracting

Tension #1: Controlling the Human Factor

The most fundamental intraorganizational transaction involves the *employment relationship.* We can think of this as the relationship between an organizational owner (or the owner's representative) and a worker—an employer hires a worker for a wage or salary. What makes this basic transaction so special is that the owner is not purchasing a tangible commodity that can be detached from the worker. Instead, the commodity or service is labor power—mental and physical energy. It cannot be purchased and owned by the employer like a piece of technology or a raw material. Because the service (labor energy) and the provider (the worker) are indivisible, the owner will usually hire the worker as a regular member of the organization in order to get the labor service. While the worker may be physically and mentally able, there is no guarantee that he or she will be willing. Thus, workers have considerable control over how much physical and mental energy they will exert. This seemingly rudimentary fact about the employment relation has enormous consequences for organization when coupled with the unique interpretative capacities of the human resource.

When we refer to the *unique nature of the human resource,* we are noting its status as a conscious, reflective, and reactive entity compared with other things found inside organizations. When humans employ their unique abilities to observe, evaluate, reflect, and react to organizational conditions, they often invalidate organization theories and frustrate management strategies. For this reason, the human factor has posed the greatest challenge for organization theory and management practice.

The centrality of the human factor as a conceptual focus and problematic point for organization theory is reflected in the attention disparate theoretical perspectives give to it. As a preliminary illustration we can consider conventional managerial and Marxist views on the human factor.

Organizational Behavior and the Human Factor

The managerial literature on organizational behavior, directed toward managers who seek to organize, coordinate, and control the elements of organization, notes that the human factor presents some especially difficult problems. One difficulty stems from what is referred to as "the law of individual differences" (Davis 1981). This law states that "all people are different." As the organizational consequences of this simple "law" are explained, the unique human properties are revealed.

First, people are different because of their distinct backgrounds, experiences, perceptions, and expectations. There are also variations along the lines of race, ethnicity, and gender. This means that humans within an organization, even if they share the same job title, represent a very heterogeneous factor of production. Further, all people will not respond in the same way to the same stimuli or managerial techniques. Humans are not standardized but rather highly distinct entities. The lesson for managers is that methods for controlling organizational behavior cannot be applied universally but must be modified, altered, revised, or discarded, depending on the situation, person, or group of workers in question. This diversity makes the regulation and control of human behavior much more complicated. The effectiveness of a particular human resource strategy may depend upon the particular individuals or type of labor force employed.

A second point raised by organizational behavior specialists is that the organization "employs the whole person" (Davis 1981). While workers package themselves and their credentials in the standard categories demanded by personnel administrators—based on particular skills, formal credentials, experience, and technical capacities—these represent only a small slice of the whole person. While this might be the most relevant slice from the perspective of the personnel department, it may not necessarily be the most significant for organizational behavior. Given the indivisibility of the human resource, a worker will always transport into the organization some "excess baggage," such as personality quirks, personal problems, and external social obligations and commitments. Organizational behavior specialists are quick to note that these may detract from a worker's performance and be so significant as to negate the potentially positive organizational contributions indicated by an employee's résumé and experience. It is also possible that these "hidden factors" can enhance one's organizational effectiveness. In either case, this kind of uncertainty and unpredictability make the human resource a very unique organizational element.

Marxist Theory and the Unique Nature of Labor

Marxist theories of organization also emphasize the unique nature of the human factor. They begin by rejecting the neoclassical economic argument that labor is like other factors of production, such as land and capital. Rather than seeing labor as just another commodity that is "bought" and "sold" in a market, Marxists view labor as a "pseudo-commodity" that can be distinguished from "true commodities" in four critical ways (Storper and Walker 1983).

First, unlike true commodities, human labor can collectively and/or individually *react* to their environment. After they have been hired, workers can decide that they should be paid more money, that working conditions are unsafe, and that fringe benefits are required. Through strikes, work stoppages, and union organization, people are able to "up the ante" after an employment relationship has been established, and demand changes that increase the cost to the employer. In contrast, machines do not demand better working conditions nor have they ever been known to stage a walkout.

Second, because people possess variable levels of creativity and cognitive skill that are difficult to measure, market-based wages and salaries can never be an objective indicator of one's productive worth to the organization. Humans can also decide to be more or less creative, or develop increasing skill capacities over time. In contrast, machine and raw material commodities have a fixed price and are not able to self-transform their basic characteristics.

Third, with the "pseudo-commodity" of labor, there is no guarantee that the employer will get what it paid for. Workers have the ability to consciously reduce or increase their work effort. Workers can intentionally withhold and refuse to exercise their energies, skills, and know-how. A great deal of organization theory and management strategy is devoted to an analysis and determination of the methods to control and maximize work effort.

Last, workers leave the enterprise at the end of the day to engage in leisure and sustenance, to reflect on their life, to develop new ideas, to involve themselves in their communities and cultures, and to consume material goods with the monetary rewards of their labor. All of these processes further influence the work orientation and performance of human labor.

Together, these four points reveal the unique nature of the human factor compared to other organizational inputs and indicate some of the special problems this poses for organizations.

Philosophical Status of the Human Factor

To reiterate, the central and defining characteristic of labor that distinguishes it from other organizational fixtures is its status as a *conscious and reflective* factor of production. Humans are aware of their environment, the way that they are treated, and the conditions under which they live and work. Human behavior is affected by these factors and often is directed toward changing or alleviating unpleasant conditions. Land and machines, on the other hand, are not conscious and reflective; therefore, they cannot respond and react to their experiences, cannot make demands, intentionally avoid work, or develop ideas away from the organization.

Walter Weisskopf's concept of "existential alienation" strikes at a key feature of these distinctly human qualities:

> Man is finite and mortal; he is conditioned by heredity and environment and by his physique, his life history, the accidents of time and place of birth and by social and historical factors. But man can transcend the given situation because he is aware of this situation and can look at it from the outside. Man "is" and at the same time knows that he is. Through the various forms of consciousness—thought, language, memory, imagination and vision of the future—he can emancipate himself from what is. . . He can transcend his position in time by remembering what was and by imagining the possibilities of the future. He can transcend the immediate sensory experience by his conceptual thought. This transcendence of the immediately given experience is the source and the cause of existential alienation. (Weisskopf 1971:19)

Organizations may seek to control and constrain the human resource, but physical presence at work does not preclude psychic emancipation. Humans may feel trapped by organizational structures, but they have the capacity to imagine alternative arrangements. For Weisskopf (1971:22), human existence is a "continuous conflict between the wide realm of envisioned possibilities and the limited realm of actuality."

The Human Factor and the Reformulation of Organization Theory and Management Practice

For all of the reasons outlined above, the human factor creates challenges and problems for those who try to understand and theorize about organizations (theorists) and for those who try to run and manage organizations (managers and administrators). This means that theories have to be revised and reformulated and that methods of administration have to be altered and modified. Those who are in the business of actually managing an organization are usually the first to face this challenge. Because there is a strong link between theory and practice in the organizational and management literature, organization theory both shapes and is shaped by the strategies and experiences of managers and administrators.

One of the most famous examples of this theory-practice linkage comes from the industrial relations experiments carried out at the Hawthorne Western Electric plant in the late 1920s (this case will be presented in detail in Chapter 4). The experiments were originally designed to gauge the impact of physical working conditions at the factory on worker performance and productivity. This involved manipulating the working conditions and measuring the changes in output. In the course of conducting the experiments, the researchers observed, communicated, and socialized with the workers and the different work groups. As it turned out, the factor that had the greatest influence on increasing output and productivity was not changes in the physical working conditions but the attention paid to, and the interaction with, the workers. As a conscious and reflective factor of production, the workers responded to human interaction, adjusted behavior accordingly, and built bonds of productive solidarity with their fellow workers. This practical "discovery" laid the groundwork for a whole new theoretical approach to organizations, known as human relations theory, that prescribed principles of management that emphasized interaction and communication between workers and managers.

A similar dynamic operates in bureaucratic organizational structures. Methods involving differentiation, specialization, chains of command, and evaluation/accounting systems place limits on the freedom and autonomy of employees. Administrators realize that the subjective and behavioral reaction of employees to these organizational systems (low morale, distrust, alienation, absenteeism, minimal effort) can counteract the potential advances in efficiency and productivity (see Hodson 1999). Thus, managers and administrators must develop additional formal and informal mechanisms that facilitate subjective attachment to the organization such as symbolic rewards, ideological appeals, organizational cultures, human relations strategies, or participatory programs.

Today we see organizational developments that often seem inconsistent. Elaborate technological systems of workplace accounting and surveillance exist alongside efforts to involve workers in decisions about quality and the organization of work. Each of these tendencies are the product of different but coupled forces. The imperative to plan and control production encourages the drive to rationalize; the human subjective response to rationalization, which often defeats the purpose of rationalization, prompts the implementation of alternative management strategies. The evolution of organizational theory and strategy is driven by this basic contradiction or paradox.

In highlighting the role of the human factor in shaping organization theory and management practice, we are treading on a central debate in social theory. This sometimes goes under the heading of *structure and agency*. As it applies to organizational analysis, the question is whether organizational structures determine and control human behavior, or whether humans can determine and shape the organizational structure. Those who emphasize "structure" argue that formal organizational structures are imposed on, shape, and control human behavior. Those who emphasize "agency" argue that the organizational structures are shaped by human action.

Much of our discussion about the role of the human factor suggests the importance of agency. More precisely, while those who own and control

organizations do create structures of control over subordinates, human reactions and resistance to these structures may force organizational owners
and managers to revise these structures.

This relationship between superordinates and subordinates has been described by Anthony Giddins as a "dialectic of control"; that is, organizational structures, designed by organizational owners and administrators to
advance their goals and shape organizational behavior, depend upon the actions of employees for their success. The fact of this dependence "offers
some resources whereby those who are subordinate can influence the activities of their superiors," or what Giddens called "the *dialectic of control* in
social systems" (Giddens 1984:16).

In the relationship between owners (superordinates) and workers (subordinates), the latter are able to influence the former because the former depend on
the latter. Or, as Ira Cohen argued, "no superordinate agent who attempts to
achieve outcomes through the doings of subordinates is so autonomous that she
can achieve their outcomes without depending upon subordinates to respond one
way or another" (Cohen 1989:152). The human factor in this scenario may decide to toe the line, ignore procedures, develop its own procedures, actively resist the formal procedures, withhold mental and physical labor, or stay home.
The form of response will obviously influence superordinate staff and the administrative structure. This influence may manifest itself in the development and
emergence of different management strategies and theories of organization.

To summarize, a central organizational tension stems from the ability of the
human factor to respond—subjectively and behaviorally—to organizational
arrangements. These reactions and responses prompt changes in both managerial
strategies and organization theory (see Figure 2–1). As real organizations, and

FIGURE 2–1

Role of human factor in shaping organization theory and management strategy

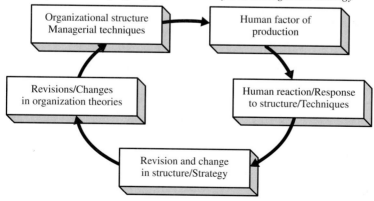

working managers and administrators, grapple with the task of developing rational, efficient, and predictable systems of control, they are constantly faced with constraints imposed by the human factor. This results in revised strategies and the development of alternative systems of management. This in turn influences and reshapes organization theory and management strategy. The newly developed theories are then communicated to managers who attempt to implement the theories in practice.

Tension #2: Differentiation and Integration

A second tension in organizations exists between the strategies for achieving a rational division of economic activities and, at the same time, ensuring that these activities are coordinated and integrated. Differentiation, divisions of labor, and specialization are fundamental organizational principles. When individuals or organizations are unable to assume responsibility for all productive activities, they must depend upon and enter into transactions with other parties.

This raises the issue of integration. How do different workers, jobs, departments, units, and organizations coordinate and integrate their interdependent activities? Does a highly differentiated and specialized division of labor undermine the ability to work together or share a common vision? Does the division of labor create problems of coordination? These questions have posed a major challenge for both organization theory and management practice in terms of conceptualizing and implementing organizational changes and strategies.

This organizational problem can be closely tied to the insights of the classical sociological theorist, Émile Durkheim, who counterposed divisions of labor and differentiation against social integration and regulation. Durkheim argued that the foundations of social solidarity in preindustrial agriculture societies would be threatened by industrialization and the increasingly complex division of labor. As you read in Chapter 1, solidarity in rural agricultural settings was fostered by common economic activities and beliefs. As societies became more industrialized, people would migrate to urban areas, specialize in different economic activities, and develop different interests and ideologies. While the division of labor and increasing differentiation was a necessary condition for industrial modernization, it tended to weaken the factors that fostered social solidarity. This created a need for mechanisms that would facilitate the social integration of the industrial society.

We can think of two divisions of labor (see Table 2–2). The first operates at the intraorganizational level involving the division of activities within the firm, enterprise, or organization. This is the *technical division of labor.* This includes not only the *horizontal dimension,* where humans carry out different kinds of

TABLE 2–2   Tension between Differentiation and Integration

Organizational Level	Tension between:	
	Differentiation	*Integration*
Intraorganizational/ within the firm	**Technical Division of Labor** Different tasks, jobs, occupations, departments	**Social Integration**—integrating humans through communication, interaction, culture
Interorganizational/ among firms	**Social Division of Labor** Different firms, producers, suppliers, distributors	**Functional Integration**— integrating organizational units involved in the stages of the production and distribution process

tasks at the same level of the organization, but also the *vertical dimension* involving differences in power, authority, rewards and decision making.

A second division of economic activities takes place at the interorganizational level between separate production units. This is the *social division of labor.* It involves the exchange of inputs and outputs, the buying and selling, and the supplying and distributing relationships *between firms.* The general challenge for both divisions of labor stems from the interdependent nature of economic activity within and among firms and the need to coordinate and integrate production activities.

The Technical Division of Labor: Intraorganizational Dynamics

The tension between differentiation and integration within the firm can be introduced with a familiar organizational problem. Most organizations employ a division of labor and job specialization as a means to enhance efficiency. This represents one form of differentiation. People engage in different and specialized tasks. However, this technical division of labor can undermine social integration because specialized work disconnects people from the larger objectives of the organization or leads people to identify less with the organization and more with their particular occupation or department. For this reason, most organizations also employ methods to enhance attachment and commitment to the larger organizational mission. The tension is reflected in management literature that tends to alternate between emphasizing structural arrangements that rationally differentiate and normative approaches that foster solidarity and integration (Barley and Kunda 1992).The centrality of the tension between differentiation versus integration can be further illustrated with some examples from managerial and sociological literature.

In a widely used organizational theory text designed for management students, Gareth Jones argued that one of the "basic challenges of organizational design" is to balance differentiation and integration (Jones 1997:Chapter 2). Differentiation is defined as the "process by which an organization allocates people and resources to organizational tasks and establishes the task and authority relationships that allow the organization to achieve its goals" (Jones 1997:47).

While differentiation is an organizational imperative that "enables people to specialize and thus become more productive" it also "limits communication between subunits and prevents them from learning from one another" (Jones 1997:47). This requires implementing strategies that promote integration, which Jones (1997:56) defined as "the process of coordinating various tasks, functions, and divisions so that they work together and not at cross-purposes." The fundamental challenge facing managers therefore is to "match the level of integration with the level of differentiation." The task of managers is to create the right balance between the two levels.

Paul Lawrence and Jay Lorsch's (1967) classic study of organizations and environments begins: "It is on the states of differentiation and integration in organizational systems that this study places major emphasis" (p. 8). They defined differentiation as "the difference in cognitive and emotional orientation among managers in different functional departments." Integration is "the quality of the state of collaboration" existing between departments which are forced by the demands of the environment to unify their efforts (1967:11). In describing the tension between the two, they wrote: "As the early organization theorists did not recognize the consequences of the division of labor on the attitudes and behaviors of organizational members, they failed to see that these different orientations and organizational practices would be crucially related to problems of achieving integration (1967:11).

In his organizational model, Talcott Parsons (1956) pointed out that the development of internal mechanisms for the mobilization of resources is one of the major problems facing organizations. The mechanisms include three decision-making processes: (1) *policy* decisions over the general goal-attainment process, (2) *allocative* decisions about the distribution of responsibilities and the allocation of physical and human capital, and (3) *integration/coordination* decisions facilitating cooperation and motivation. Parsons saw a clear conflict between the allocative and integration/coordination decisions. He refers to an "inherent centrifugal tendency" among the subunits of the organization, based on the different personalities of the participants, and the special demands of particular job situations. In this scenario, management must "implement measures that counteract the centrifugal pull and integrate the subunits and individuals within the organization. Managing this integrative "problem" requires ultimately a distinctly social solution. In Parsons' scheme, this means "institutionalized *norms* which can effectively bind the actions of individuals in their commitments to organizations" (p. 74).

One does not have to leave the university to find an example of this organizational tension. The division of academic labor into disciplines and departments produces loyalty and attachment to a part rather than the whole. Academic departments compete with each other for monetary resources, faculty positions, and students. Administrative divisions between the university's student advising and registration units produces conflict over the desire to serve the unique scheduling needs of each student and the equally strong interest in making sure students are registered in a timely and efficient fashion. In attempting to integrate various and regularly conflicting interests and commitments, universities search for a common integrative cement such as the "student-centered" orientation.

For many theorists, such as Andrew Sayer and Richard Walker (1992), the division and integration of labor is *the* organizational problem. They noted that "The organizational problem in the industrial economy begins with production . . . the puzzle of piecing together the complex divisions of labor inherent in all modern production. The mirror image of the division of labor is, therefore, the *integration of labor*" (1992:111).

It should be noted that the problem of social integration within the firm can arise from two very different structural situations. One problem of integration can stem from a highly bureaucratic structure that divides, fragments, and departmentalizes the labor process. The example of the university falls into this category. Human relations and organizational mission strategies, designed to improve organizational morale, cohesiveness, and job satisfaction, have been the most widely adopted solution to problems stemming from this form of differentiation.

A second type of integration problem can stem from organizational structures that allow high levels of worker discretion and autonomy, with minimal forms of bureaucratic coordination. These kinds of organizations must often rely on the more encompassing "corporate culture" strategies that extend beyond bureaucratic mechanisms. In this case, as organizations weaken formal bureaucratic controls, there is a growing emphasis on developing intensive normative-based mechanisms that ensure conformity, cooperation, and compliance.

The two situations suggest the hypothetical relationship presented in Figure 2–2. When the level of differentiation is high, there is the risk of fragmentation and the potential loss of unity of purpose. When the level of differentiation is low, structural mechanisms of control are absent and individual self-interest might prevail over an attachment to the common mission. Each will be elaborated in subsequent chapters.

FIGURE 2–2

Relationship between organizational differentiation and social integration

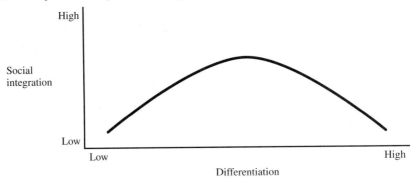

The Social Division of Labor: Interorganizational Dynamics

Just as organizational and management literature has struggled with the tensions between the optimal forms of internal organization of the labor process and the social integration of human labor, there are parallel tensions related to the functional integration among production units. A consideration of the social division of labor involves transactions among interdependent but distinct phases of a production process and the functional integration of these interdependent production units.

The social division of labor is often based on the principle of specialization and expertise, such as, for example, a parts producer supplying customized components to a manufacturing enterprise. This kind of interdependence always poses an integration problem. Will the inputs from the supplier be delivered on time? Will the supplier produce a high-quality component that meets the manufacturer's specifications? Can the manufacturer be guaranteed a constant supply of the component at a stable price?

A division of labor that is mediated through a market exchange and contractual arrangements between organizations can pose uncertainties that threaten the ability to carry out a well-coordinated production process. This creates pressures for a more tightly integrated chain of production.

A manufacturing firm may decide to vertically integrate the production process through the buying up of suppliers. In this way it will gain greater control over delivery, price, and quality. Or the manufacturer may attempt to forge a more tightly connected network of firms that can join together and collectively develop product and process standards. Tension may arise whether the organization should specialize in what it does best and rely on the social division of labor to access needed resources, or integrate the entire process under a single organizational umbrella, or develop an alliance of independent but affiliated firms.

Each of these strategies represents different points on the differentiation-integration trade-off. As we shall see, there are advantages and disadvantages to each of these arrangements and these are what contribute to the tension between differentiation and integration. A significant portion of organization theory and management strategy centers on this tension at the interorganizational level.

A Note on Organizational Tensions and Ascribed Characteristics

In thinking about the characteristics of the human factor and the division of labor, the issues of race, ethnicity, and gender may be significant. While the framework for organizational analysis used in this text does not assume that organizational theories are inherently race- or gender-biased (for alternative views, see Martin and Knopoff 1997; Calas and Smircich 1996), these factors can play a significant role in organizational dynamics.

We have already noted that one feature of the human factor is its heterogeneous character; that is, humans cannot be standardized prior to their entry into an organization. Race and gender are significant factors shaping prior experiences, biography, and orientation toward work. Recognition of this demographic fact and the associated organizational challenge is reflected in the growing organizational and management literature on diversity and multiculturalism (Prasad, Mills, Elmes, and Prasad 1997; Tayeb 1997; Ritvo, Litwin, and Butler 1995).

Furthermore, where racial, ethnic, and gender characteristics are associated with positions in the division of labor, differentiation is enforced at the expense of integration. Such segregated patterns of human resource deployment—shaped by a combination of worker choices and employer discrimination (England and Farkas 1986)—will tend to increase the salience of the group (racial, ethnic, gender) as opposed to other forms of identity (Wharton 1992). What impact this will have on larger organizational objectives depends on whether one is interested in pursuing a divide-and-rule approach to administration or attempting to create a cohesive workforce. If identities with sub-groups override the common organizational identity, teamwork among members of different groups will be difficult to achieve (Nkomo and Cox 1996:342).

In their application of the work of Clayton Alderfer and K. K. Smith (1982), Nkomo and Cox distinguished between identity groups and organization groups. Race, gender, and ethnicity are widely recognized as identity groups. To be a member of the group has social significance and consequences and, therefore, shapes an individual's definition of his or her self-identity. Organizational groups are those associated with intraorganizational differentiation that share a common occupational, task, or work experience. Given forms of inequality and discrimination based on race, gender, and ethnicity, these identities tend to be salient prior to organizational participation. Because "individuals don't leave their racial, gender, and ethnic identities at the door when they enter an organization" (Nkomo and Cox 1996: 342), identity group membership will influence perceptions of and behavior within the organizational landscape. If the identity group overlaps with the organizational group, mutually reinforced pressures toward ever-greater identity group identification will be generated. On the other hand, if there is no relationship between identity group membership and organizational group location, the salience of race, ethnicity, and gender will tend to diminish in relation to other organizational divisions or dynamics.

Paradox: The Underlying Source of Organizational Tension

As noted in Chapter 1, the metaphor that drives the analysis of organization theories in this text is flux and transformation. The tensions outlined above conform with this approach. A variety of terms have been used to capture this dynamic model—contradiction, dilemma, dialectic, tension, and paradox (see Aram 1976; Hampden-Turner 1990; McWhinney 1992; Tenner 1996; Mitroff and Emshoff 1979). We shall discuss paradox here since it has become one of the central concepts in current organization and management studies. The contemporary literature on both public and private organization theories and management strategies places a great deal of emphasis on the growing number of paradoxes challenging organizations (Handy 1994; Quinn and Cameron 1988; Nutt and Backoff 1992).

Models of Organizational Paradox

There are many ways to think about and conceptualize paradox. One simple model is presented in Figure 2–3a. The model shows that paradox stems from the multiple consequences of a single action which seem to contradict or work at cross-purposes with one another. In the organizational context, there are the *intended consequences* (Merton 1957) of the action which are directed toward improving performance and profit. On the other hand, there are the *unintended consequences* of the same action which may actually undermine performance, productivity, and profit and thus cancel out the intended "positive" consequences. Paradox is captured by both the positive and negative effects on the organizational objective that are produced by the same action. In this paradoxical scenario, we can incorporate both forms of tension outlined above.

The human factor tension is illustrated in the paradox model in Figure 2–3b. Managers implement an organizational strategy which has two consequences. The first, labeled the objective structural consequence, restructures

FIGURE 2–3

Organizational paradox and tension

***a.* Paradox model**

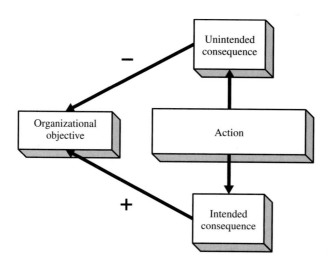

***b.* Paradox: The human factor tension**

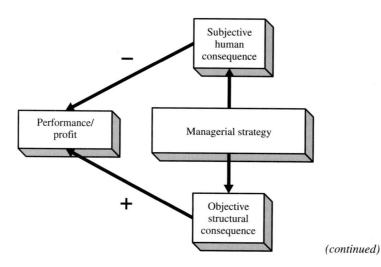

(continued)

organizational tasks and relationships to enhance efficiency and productivity. The second, the subjective human consequence, weakens or counteracts the intended efficiency and productivity of the structural arrangement. The managerial action, therefore, has paradoxical effects on the ultimate organizational objective of enhanced performance and productivity.

FIGURE 2–3

Organizational paradox and tension (continued)

c. **Paradox: The differentiation-integration tension**

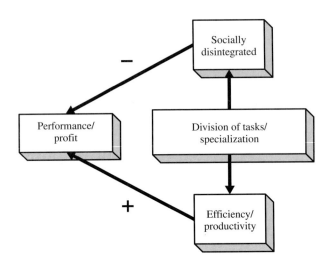

The differentiation-integration tension is illustrated in the paradox model in Figure 2–3c. The initial action implements a strategy of differentiation involving a rigid division of labor and highly specialized tasks. The intended consequence is to rationalize and make the actions of organizational members more efficient and productive, which should enhance organizational performance. The unintended consequence is the creation of a socially disintegrated organizational climate that produces departmentalism, parochialism, attachment to a particular position within the organization, and low levels of common purpose or cross-communication. This can ultimately weaken the positive contribution of the rational division of tasks.

It should be emphasized that the unintended consequence need not always be negative. In our example of the Hawthorne experiments, discussed earlier in the chapter, the unintended consequence of conducting the experiments and interacting with workers was enhanced output and productivity. This was an unexpected but positive consequence. When we use the term paradox, however, this usually implies that an action has contradictory consequences.

Figure 2–4a presents a second way to conceptualize paradox. Paradox can be conceptualized as a kind of *"inverted symbiosis"* (Etzioni 1996) in which two mutually desirable and enhancing states develop a negative, or inverse, relationship with one another. This means the advancement of one desired state (point 1 to point 2 on the horizontal axis) can result in the diminution of, or detraction from, the other desired state (point 2 to point 1 on the vertical axis).

FIGURE 2–4

Organizational paradox and tension

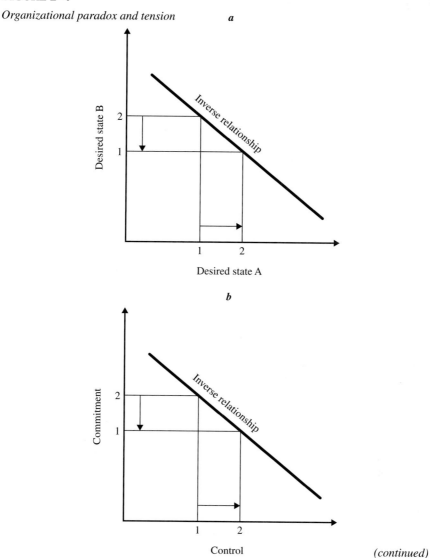

(continued)

In *The Age of Paradox*, Charles Handy (1994) captured this "paradox of organization" in outlining the dilemma of trying to "reconcile what used to be opposites. . . Firms must be planned yet flexible, differentiated yet integrated, mass marketers and niche marketers."

Figure 2–4b applies the inverted symbiosis logic to the human factor tension. This example shows two desired states or conditions: control and commitment. The first is an objective structural system of managerial control over labor. This might be accomplished through bureaucratic systems of control

FIGURE 2–4

Organizational paradox and tension (continued)

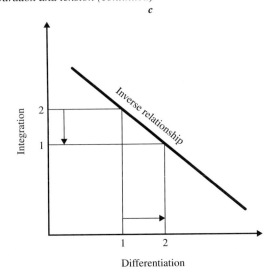

and supervision. The second desired state is a positive subjective commitment to the organization. While both conditions must exist to some degree in all organizations, the implementation of the control strategy might result in a weakened commitment to the organization because it could undermine a climate of trust. Control and commitment exist in a symbiotically inverted relationship.

Figure 2–4c applies the inverted symbiosis model to the differentiation-integration tension. The desired state of differentiation for the purpose of efficiency and specialization works to undermine the equally desired state of integration. In both cases, one mutually desirable condition is advanced, the other is diminished.

Three Cases of Organizational Paradox

Quality Improvement Programs.   The abstractions presented in Figures 2–3 and 2–4 can be further illuminated with some concrete cases and examples. Studies of quality improvement programs in a variety of firms report an interesting "improvement paradox" (Sterman et al. 1996; Sterman, Repenning, and Kofman 1994). Lucent Technology, Ford Motor Company, Harley-Davidson, and National Semiconductor have instituted quality improvement programs aimed at reducing product defect rates and manufacturing cycle time, and responding to customer needs through systematic and continuous product development. This is the intended action designed to improve quality. Such quality efforts are common throughout manufacturing firms. However, many of these quality initiatives have been unsuccessful or have produced mixed results. The failure is due not to poor implementation or leadership, but to the "unanticipated consequences of successful improvement arising from feedback between quality programs and other functions and organizational routines in the firm" (Sterman et al. 1996). More specifically, quality improvement programs that have yielded rapid productivity gains have also created a problem of excess capacity caused by the inability of a firm's marketing department to expand its customer base at a proportional rate. This unintended consequence of the quality improvement program can potentially nullify the positive consequences. When capacity is expanded faster than demand, management is confronted with a paradox or dilemma. In the short run, costs can be reduced by laying off excess labor. However, this will have the negative effect of disrupting quality work groups, eroding morale, and creating the perception that workers can "improve themselves out of a job." Retaining labor, on the other hand, will preserve the organizational climate on which the quality programs depend, despite negative short-term financial results.

A Piecework Wage System.   In the early 1980s, A.O. Smith Corporation, a manufacturer of car and truck frames, had implemented a wage system based on piecework designed to increase work effort and productivity. This was the intended consequence. The more frames that were produced, the more money the workers received. Output increased under this system but at a heavy cost. Up to 20 percent of the frames had to be repaired before they could be shipped to Ford Motor Company. An assembler summed up the prevailing worker orientation—"get 'em out the door, junk or not." The piecework system, which also included a rigid division of labor based on an assembly line, had created enormous unanticipated negative consequences.

The quality problems became so severe that A. O. Smith decided in the late 1980s to redesign the entire workplace. Self-managing, job-rotating, production teams were formed, which doubled the productivity rate and reduced defects to 3 percent. Many first-line foremen, made redundant as production teams assumed management duties, were retired or fired. This had another unintended effect: undermining the morale of the remaining supervisors. This "second-order" unintended consequence required the development of a training program for supervisors on the value of participative-style management practices.

Teaching vs. Research in Higher Education.   Higher education has been struggling for many years with a trade-off between teaching and research. Historically, the large comprehensive university has defined quality on the basis of the faculty's research activity and scholarly productivity. To encourage these efforts, the primary academic rewards—such as tenure, promotion, reappointment, and merit pay—were based on the publication of research articles and books. The intended consequence of this reward structure was greater scholarly productivity and enhanced prestige for the university. However, it is now widely recognized that the means and rewards employed to achieve this goal have had the unintended consequence of neglect for teaching. If one's professional status is based on contributions to scholarly journals, the publication of research monographs, and the acquisition of grants, there is little reason to expect a concerted commitment to classroom teaching. These "organized contradictions of academe" (Rau and Baker 1989) not only generate unintended consequences but also undermine one of the central missions of higher education: excellence in undergraduate education.

In each of these three examples, the methods used to realize intended consequences produced paradoxical unintended consequences. The paradoxical outcomes have their source in (1) the often unpredictable human reaction to organizational initiatives (the A.O. Smith example); and (2) the interdependent nature of organizational activities that means changes in one area will have consequences for other areas (the quality improvement program and higher education reward systems).

From a managerial or administrative vantage point, this paradox perspective poses a "dilemma of trade-offs." The pursuit of any strategy will produce unintended consequences or will result in a likely reduction of some other desired state or objective. Thus, every decision involves a trade-off between mutually desired states and objectives. As Handy (1994) suggested, managers must reconcile the paradoxical relationships and establish some middle-ground strategies that maximizes each. Those who study organizational paradoxes such as these do not believe they can ever be resolved, only managed. But managing requires the establishment of some kind of balance or a conciliatory position between two potentially contradictory points. As we review the various theories of organization, we shall see that most theories tend to simplify organizational relationships by stressing only the intended and expected consequence of a particular action or strategy.

Summary

1. Two levels of organizational analysis can be used to classify theories of organization. *Intraorganizational* level theories tend to focus on the internal structures and processes within the organization. *Interorganizational* theories focus on the external relationships among organizations and between the organization and its environment.

2. Transactions are fundamental organizational processes that pose challenges for and generate tensions in organizations. There are

human transactions embodied in the employment relationship between an owner and an employee. There are interdependent transactions between functional units of an organization and between organizations exchanging goods and services.

3. Managing these transactions reveals two major tensions inherent in all organizations. The first is the tension generated by attempts to control and extract work effort from the human factor of production. The second is the tension generated by the conflict between differentiation and integration of independent organizational activities.

4. The management of these tensions has a direct impact on the development and evolution of management strategies and organization theories. Changes in organizational techniques and theories stem from practical organizational problems and dilemmas. Unlike many other areas of social science, there is a close relationship between the practice of administration and the development of organization theory.

5. Most generally, effective organizational analyses require the acknowledgement of unanticipated consequences and paradoxical outcomes. The intended purposes of organizational structures and administrative processes often go unrealized because they create unexpected and counterproductive consequences. These stimulate further changes, adjustments, and revisions in managerial practices and organizational theorizing.

THE RISE OF
THE FACTORY
SYSTEM

*It is, therefore, excessively the interest of every mill-owner to organize his
moral machinery on equally sound principles with his mechanical, for
otherwise he will never command the steady hands, watchful eyes, and
prompt cooperation, production requires.*

(Andrew Ure. *The Philosophy of Manufactures.* 1861, p. 417.)

In this chapter we will take an historical approach to the rise of industrial organization. This will allow us to appreciate some of the immediate problems
that emerged, along with the various theories and methods that were developed to deal with the fundamental organizational challenges. The greatest emphasis will be placed on the organizational tension generated by the effort to
subordinate the human factor of production.

Introduction

The beginnings of industrial organization can be linked to the *formal subordination of labor.* In this process, those who own or have access to productive
property that provides an independent means of subsistence—peasants, farm-
ers, craftsmen, and artisans—gradually lose control or access to the property.
This can occur as independent producers sell off their assets, are bought out,
or outcompeted by larger producers, or as peasants are evicted from the land.
This process, also referred to as *proletarianization,* forces increasing numbers
of people into a labor market to sell their labor power to a capitalist for a wage.
It therefore involves the creation of the proletariat or working class. The for-

mal subordination of labor is an essential stage in the evolution of industrial capitalism, though it is hardly a once-and-for-all process. It is simply the beginning of a long and hard struggle between organizational owners and the human factor of production.

Separating people from productive property does not mean they will automatically accept their working-class status and enter the factory. As E. P. Thompson (1963:241) wrote in his historical account of the English working class, "there were many halfway stages before the workhouse door was reached." Human roles and identities had to be redefined. A traditional way of life was disrupted. This provoked intense resistance and conflict over the emerging organization of production.

The eventual establishment of the factory and wage labor system did not signal the end of the battle with labor—only a shift in terrain. Once labor was gathered in the factory, owners and managers instituted the *real subordination of labor.* These were the various managerial strategies designed to control and extract work from labor. Since there was no final solution or one best way to achieve this objective, the struggle and process is ongoing. A large part of the evolution of organization theory and management strategy can be chronicled as a history of trial and error in developing methods and techniques for the real subordination of labor.

This chapter will chart these early efforts to manage the often insubordinate human resource and the special problems this posed for the emerging class of owners and industrialists. The discussion will revolve around some familiar themes that have shaped the development of organization theory: the rise of the factory system, the collective resistance among segments of labor, the early problems of labor discipline and control, and the various strategies employed, including scientific management.

The Formal Subordination of Labor: Creating a Human Factor of Production

There are many descriptions of the transition to industrial capitalism. A familiar image in sociological accounts compares precapitalist craftsmen—possessing rare skills and exercising total control over the labor process—with the industrial factory worker—who has been de-skilled and reduced to a mere machine tender. While perhaps heuristically useful, this dichotomous image of work life under precapitalist and capitalist societies suffers from a comparative historical bias: the glorification of the past and the degradation of the present. As most sociologists are well aware, not all workers prior to capitalism were craftspeople nor does everyone under modern capitalism work on an assembly line. Nonetheless, the rise of capitalism certainly *did* threaten and destroy an established way of work life. What is interesting about this process is not that the good old system was replaced by the bad new system but the way threatened segments of the population reacted in opposition to the new arrangement. This made the transition to a factory system difficult and conflict-ridden.

There are at least two ways to tell the story—from the perspective of labor or from the perspective of the emerging capitalist class. In this chapter we will consider both. To understand the unprecedented collective response and struggle against the onslaught of industrialization, we must consider the culture and interests of labor. Likewise, organizational and managerial strategies are best viewed from the perspective of the owners' objectives. The overall struggle is shaped by the tactics of the two parties and the resources at their disposal. Labor historians, such as David Montgomery (1979:113), have attempted to incorporate both sides of the action.

> From one side, the craftsmen themselves develop increasingly collective and formal practices for the regulation of their trades, both openly through union work rules and covertly through group enforced codes of ethical behavior on the job.
>
> From the other side, the owners and managers of large enterprises developed more direct and systematic controls over the production side of their firms.

It is important to emphasize that the human resource required by the emerging factory system could not simply be purchased, collected, and controlled like other factors of production. Humans develop traditions, identities, bonds of solidarity, and routines that cannot be easily abandoned and replaced. These traditions provided the basis for collective political struggle and forced industrial owners to devise strategies for labor recruitment and social control.

There are two broad struggles worth noting when we evaluate the response of labor to the rise of capitalism. The first struggle was the reaction against the formal subordination of labor, primarily by artisans and craftsmen who did not want to be reduced to "wage slaves." The second struggle was the reaction against the real subordination of labor by those who ultimately entered the factory and did not want to conform to the rhythms of factory discipline.

The historical account of the Industrial Revolution in England provided by E. P. Thompson in *The Making of the English Working Class* (1963) offers important insights into the human response to the rise of the factory system. Thompson's analysis is essentially the history of struggle against the formal subordination of labor that focuses on the cultural traditions disrupted and the political tactics employed during the late-18th and early-19th centuries.

> The general rebellion was based on the following set of grievances related to changes in the character of class exploitation: . . . the rise of a master-class without traditional authority or obligations: the growing distance between master and man: the transparency of the exploitation at the source of their new wealth and power: the

loss of status and above all independence for the worker, his reduction to total dependence on the master's instruments of production: the partiality of the law: the disruption of the traditional family economy: the discipline, monotony, hours and conditions of work: loss of leisure and amenities: the reduction of the man to the status of an "instrument" (Thompson 1963:202–3).

In Thompson's documentation of the emergence of industrial capitalism and the reaction of various groups to the new system, he developed a theory of class formation, class consciousness, and class action. In many ways the central argument of his book revolves around a certain definition of social class that emphasizes common subjective experience, identity, and interests. Class, in this view, is not a category but a "happening." The Industrial Revolution, according to Thompson, initiated a set of conditions that unified the "laboring classes" and transformed them into a "working class" (for a compelling critique and alternative analysis see Calhoun 1982).

Thompson's analysis of class and class formation points to the subjective nature of labor. It is not an *object* that can be shaped, despite such intentions by industrial owners but a *subject* with emotion and sentiment. Accordingly, what Thompson emphasized is the capacity of labor to assess the loss of tradition and culture, to communicate shared interests, and to act as an organizational force with an alternative conception of social arrangements. As Thompson noted, labor is not a "raw material" nor a mere commodity that can be collected, controlled, and shaped into a proletariat.

The collective opposition to the new organizational forms was based on the strength of the traditional communities of artisans and craftsmen. This gave power and cohesiveness to their collective actions and reflects the broader human capacity to develop bonds of solidarity based on traditional routines, common patterns of interaction, and mutual social relationships. These became the resources that were mobilized in the struggles and movements that Thompson identified. Calhoun (1982:220) argued that the issue was not one of an aggregate of individuals but of a social organization. "With a social organization, collective action, not merely similar actions, becomes possible." It is social organization that distinguishes labor from the other factors of production.

The Real Subordination of Labor: Disciplining the Human Factor

The political struggles and movements, stimulated by the rise of capitalism and the formal subordination of labor, eventually subsided and were replaced by conflicts between workers and owners over the real subordination of labor. The monumental challenge of coordinating and controlling large numbers of workers within a single factory had never been confronted on such a scale. "In many respects the rational and methodological management of labor was the *central management problem* in the Industrial Revolution, requiring the fiercest wrench from the past" (Pollard 1965:160, emphasis added).

Traditional Habits and Cultures

There was no easy *technical* remedy to this managerial problem because cultural traditions and habits are *social* obstacles that require not mechanical but social solutions. "The concept of industrial discipline was new, and called for as much innovation as the technical innovations of the age" (Pollard 1965:185). Others believed that the taming of the human factor was a more formidable challenge than any of the technical obstacles that might be confronted. In comparing the cotton loom with labor, one observer wrote:

> The main difficulty did not, to my apprehension, lie so much in the invention of a proper self-acting mechanism for drawing out and twisting cotton into a continuous thread, as in the distribution of the different members of the apparatus into one cooperative body, in impelling each organ with its appropriate delicacy and speed, and above all, in training human beings to renounce their desultory habits of work, and to identify themselves with the unvarying regularity of the complex automaton (Ure 1861:15-16; cited in Bendix 1956:59).

The social habits and ways of life of the past could not be easily erased from the minds of this new mass of labor. The emerging factory system stood in stark contrast to the earlier modes of economic activity that permitted greater freedom and autonomy for many workers. For those who grew up before the introduction of the factory system, adaptation to the new discipline did not come easily. This is one reason that child labor offered a partial solution for owners. Young workers were easier to coerce and control; they had not yet developed a tradition of work so they did not sense the affront to their way of life as did older workers. Thus, the second generation of workers, uncontaminated by preindustrial habits of work and leisure, posed a different set of problems for management. Managers and owners were beginning to realize that cultural normative systems die hard. In lamenting the perpetual managerial problem of worker commitment, Wilbert Moore (1963: 174) noted that it "involves both the performance of appropriate actions and the acceptance of the normative system that provides the rules and rationale. Whether such a commitment can be achieved in a single generation is debatable. . ." First-generation capitalists, unfortunately, had to contend with the existing generation of workers who were the most able and most skilled, though hardly the most willing. This was clearly expressed by the industrialists of the day.

> Even at the present day, when the system is perfectly organized, and its labor lightened to the utmost, it is found nearly impossible to convert persons past the age of puberty, whether drawn from rural or from handicraft operations, into useful factory hands (Ure 1861: 15–16; cited in Bendix 1956:59).

The general problem, as Reinhard Bendix (1956) described it, was "traditionalism"—the ideological way of life among labor prescribing pre-capitalist customs, norms, routines, and work habits. This stood as the major obstacle to the enforcement of the "new discipline" within the factory. American labor historians, such as David Montgomery (1979) and Herbert Gutman (1975), also found the source of industrial conflict and struggle in the persistence of traditional culture. In the United States, the heterogeneity of the labor factor, fueled by the constant flow of immigrants, resulted in a variety of cultural norms that did not fit smoothly into the emerging industrial machine. This posed a double challenge for management: the need to transform both the traditional work habits as well as the "foreign" cultural obstacles to managerial control.

The organizational dynamics involved a complex interaction between conflicting forces—traditional work habits, the emerging factory system, managerial strategies to break traditions and impose discipline, and the reaction and resistance of labor. The special difficulties posed by the human factor are continually emphasized in the historical accounts of this period. A major problem was the human tendency to carry the cultural baggage:

> Men and women who sell their labor power to an employer bring more to a new . . . changing work situation than their physical presence (Gutman 1975:18).
>
> [I]mmigrant laborers were not passive clay to be molded by the requirements of American industry, but brought with them preindustrial work habits that shaped their responses to the environment they found here (Montgomery 1979:40).

In addition to the cultural norms transported from the rural community or other shores, there were those that developed within the factory. Even when workers were willing to enter the factory, submit to rules and regulations, and perform for a set number of hours, there was still the individual and collective capacity to restrict output and set informal quotas. This emerging normative order was acknowledged by the industrial engineers of the time, such as Harvey Gantt, who surmised that "there is in every workroom a fashion, a habit of work, and the new worker follows that fashion, for it isn't respectable not to" (cited in Montgomery 1979:13). It was this problem that prompted the eventual development of scientific management systems of control.

Early Strategies and Assumptions

In the early stages, however, the primary strategy was to develop techniques congruent with traditional culture. Montgomery has used the term *corporate welfare* to describe strategies that rested on a paternalistic orientation toward labor. This involved a personalized system of labor employment, recruitment, and control within a familial-like environment. It was hoped that this would ease the transition to the factory system and circumvent the opposition to impersonal and contractual forms of servitude.

In many emerging shops and factories, the system of paternalism gave way to a "subcontracting system" (see Littler 1982; Clawson 1980). This strategy was utilized not only because it retained the familial relationships between workers and, in this case, the subcontractor or middleman (Bendix 1956), but also because owners lacked sufficient knowledge about production techniques and the labor process (Clawson 1980). Thus, the subcontractor, who often hired friends and relatives, assumed the managerial tasks of organization and motivation. The subcontracting system can be seen as a transitional stage toward a more bureaucratic system of labor control. The viability of the system hinged on the desire of master craftsmen to retain control of production, and the willingness of owners to permit a quasi-traditional system of work relations. More generally, this arrangement stemmed from the dependence of owners on the knowledge possessed by the craftsmen.

Among other, less paternalistic, methods designed to overcome problems of factory discipline were the beating of children, the firing of workers or the threat of dismissal, and monetary fines for lateness, absenteeism and insubordination (Pollard 1965).

Payment by results and piecework were also used as a means to entice labor to maximize work effort. The motivational logic driving the piecework system rested on a particular view of human behavior that was of relatively recent vintage. Pollard (1965) and Bendix (1956) have emphasized the importance of shifting assumptions about human motivation and its impact on evolving systems of management. The conventional wisdom assumed the best way to motivate effort was through the maintenance of subsistence wage levels. Under this arrangement, workers would submit to the rigors of the factory system to secure the financial means of survival. If levels of remuneration exceeded subsistence, owners feared that workers would lose their motivation to work.

In contrast, the payment-for-results system hinged on a different view: that human acquisitiveness and insatiability, rather than satisfaction with subsistence, would generate continuous effort in exchange for continuous reward. Even when a certain level of subsistence was reached, people would still want to make more money in order to consume more goods. Therefore, work effort could be elicited beyond the payment of a subsistence wage.

If this new set of assumptions about human motivation matched reality, a fundamental economic dilemma of capitalism would also be addressed: the balancing of supply and demand. On the supply side, monetary incentives would stimulate the *production of goods*. On the demand side, the expanded cash rewards would stimulate the *consumption of goods*. In this way, many of the changing assumptions about humans can be related to the shifting ideologies and requirements of the developing capitalist system. As Weisskopf (1971:60) suggested, "The moral problem of early capitalism consisted of convincing people that their self-interest lay in the pursuit of economic gain, and not in noneconomic goals as was believed in previous periods."

Another set of ideological assumptions can be linked to the emerging authority relations in the factory. There is no better account of the ideological strategies of management than that presented by Bendix in *Work and Authority in Industry* (1956). Bendix identified not only the pervasive "traditionalism" of labor noted above, but the tactics used by management to rid labor of its disposition toward irregular work habits. Further, in the process of eliminating the old traditional culture, the new system had to be legitimated. Here Bendix's (1956:13) notion of "managerial ideology" remains a powerful analytic tool defining not only early managerial efforts but those that have followed to the present day. Managerial ideologies are:

> such ideologies that interpret the facts of authority and obedience so as to neutralize or eliminate the conflict between the few and many in the interest of a more effective exercise of authority. To do this, the exercise of authority is either denied altogether on the grounds that the few merely order what the many want; or it is justified with the assertion that the few have qualities of excellence which enable them to realize the interests of the many.

For the nonhuman objects of organization, ideology is a nonissue. For the subjects—human labor—it is a central element of the social organization of the production process. Workers had to be convinced and motivated, to some extent, if production was to proceed. Bendix argued that the differentiation in authority between worker and manager had to be reconciled through a set of assumptions about the inherent nature of managers and workers—their needs, skills, and desires. The emerging formal bureaucratic authority structure had to be accompanied by an ideological massage.

> Managers have typically resorted to ideological appeals, not as a substitute for material incentives and organizational improvements, but as a means by which to increase, if possible, the cooperation of employees, given the organizational environment in which they had to work (Bendix 1956:248).

Broadly speaking, Bendix diagnosed the phases of industrial organizational development in a Weberian framework that centered on the relationship between organizational arrangements and legitimate authority. The immediate point that needs to be emphasized is that predictable control could not be assured by the formal structure and authority system. The human capacity for subjective and behavioral resistance remained. As Bendix (1956:251) put it, "Beyond what commands can effect and supervision control, beyond what incentives can induce and penalties prevent, there exists an exercise of discretion important even in relatively menial jobs, which managers of economic enterprises seek to enlist for the achievement of managerial ends." The ability to "exercise discretion" means that labor always retains some control over its exertion of mental and physical energy. This has posed a continuing dilemma for organizational theory and management strategy. For employers and managers at the end of the 19th century, the desire was for a "human" input that could be shaped and molded without negative consequences. The failure of the human factor to conform to such a system produced the following opinion in *The Review,* an employer trade association publication:

> Now when we purchase a machine tool and find it slightly unfitted for requirements, we can usually make a change in construction, which will convert the difficulty in it. Why? Because the machine tool is never supersensitive, it is never obstinate, perverse, discouraged.
>
> If the human machine could be controlled by the set of rules that govern machine tool operation, the world would be a much different place . . . (cited in Bendix 1956:271).

Such were the utopian musings of the early managerial class. As it turned out, Frederick W. Taylor and his colleagues were on their way to formulating such a human machine that would draw on both the principles of engineering and the scientific method.

Scientific Management in Theory

Motivation for the Theory

Scientific management can be viewed as one of the first, and surely the best known, attempts to deal systematically with the "labor problem." Under the emerging factory system, the unique and problematic nature of labor is manifested in (1) its possession and control of knowledge about the methods of production, and (2) its capacity to exercise discretion in its exertion of work effort. These twin and associated problems, from the perspective of owners, were directly confronted by Frederick Winslow Taylor (1856–1915) and his theory of scientific management.

Taylor was trained as an industrial engineer. He began his career working for the Midvale Steel Company. When he became foreman of the plant, he developed an intense interest in industrial productivity and efficiency. Taylor believed that worker control over production knowledge and know-how placed owners at a serious disadvantage. Skilled workers and foremen, rather than the owners, determined the organization and pace of production. The owners had to depend on these employees to organize production in what they hoped was the most efficient manner. However, there were no independent and reliable means for determining whether output was reaching an optimal level. In this context, as others have noted (see Goldman and Van Houten

1988), the knowledge of workers was a potent source of power. Though workers depended on owners for employment, owners depended on the craft knowledge of workers for production to proceed. To shift the balance of power decisively in favor of owners required the elimination of this residual dependence on worker knowledge. Taylor viewed this as one of the fundamental objectives of scientific management.

> The mass of rule-of-thumb or traditional knowledge may be said to be the principal asset or possession of every tradesman . . . a large part of which is not in the possession of management . . . their own knowledge and skill falls far short of the combined knowledge and dexterity of all the workmen under them . . . The management must take over and perform much of the work that is now left to the men (Taylor 1911:26, 33).

The ability to use knowledge as a source of power represented the first unique capacity of labor that scientific management targeted for attack. Once management had wrestled productive knowledge from workers, a second labor problem could be confronted.

> The problem before the management, then, may be briefly said to be that of obtaining the best *initiative* of every workman . . . the workers believe it to be directly against their interests to give their employers their best initiative, and that instead of working hard to do the largest possible amount of work and best quality of work for their employers, they deliberately work as slowly as they dare while they at the same time try to make those over them believe that they are working fast (Taylor 1911:33).

Here Taylor is referring to what he called "soldiering" by workers—that is, pretending to work while in reality loafing.

Taylor's challenge, then, was to reduce labor to an *object* in the production process. Rather than having labor determine the organization of production or the pace of work, managers would determine them based on the principles of scientific management. This could be achieved by dissolving the bases of independent action or, more specifically, the leverage obtained by virtue of possessing technical knowledge. Curtailing this source of power would transform labor into an object that would be more similar to other, more controllable, factors of production. As labor takes on the character of an object, it is more prone to manipulation and malleability.

For Taylor, only the application of science could realize this purpose. Science would additionally remove the variability and uncertainty characterizing the methods of production and replace them with a "one best way" to complete any given task. Much of this variability was the direct result of hiring workers who brought their particular habits, backgrounds, and training to the factory. Instead of a standard method, there were a variety of techniques and assorted rule-of-thumb routines that workers developed during apprenticeship or by trial and error. This craft knowledge mirrored the unstandardized and variegated nature of the humans who carried it. This presented a problem for those, like Taylor, who preferred machinelike uniformity and predictability.

> The workmen in all our trades have been taught the details of their work by observation of those immediately around them, there are many ways in common use for doing the same thing . . . Now, among the various methods and implements used in each element of each trade there is always one method and one implement which is quicker and better than any of the rest. And this one best method and best implement can only be discovered or developed through a scientific study and analysis of all the methods and implements in use, together with accurate, minute, motion and time study. This involves the gradual substitution of science for rule-of-thumb throughout the mechanic arts (Taylor 1911:15).

The one best way represented an effort to reorganize work so that the labor input could be inserted into the production process like a part into a machine. Just as parts do not determine the design of the machine, so labor does not determine the operation of production. Labor conforms to the existing scientifically determined tasks already in place.

The principles of scientific management are, in essence, principles of engineering applied to the social organization of production. Taylor was simply applying *his* special craft knowledge—machine design—to a factory system that included some rather cumbersome and devious parts—humans. Humans possess properties that engineers find the least attractive—temperament, resistance, friction, and nonuniformity. Taylor's science of management was aimed at minimizing the problems posed by this variable and unpredictable factor of production.

The Principles and Stages

The central elements of Taylor's system involved four basic steps.

1. Analysis of each element in the labor process including rules of motion for each worker and standardization of working conditions.
2. Scientific selection, training, and development of workers.
3. Cooperation of managers and workers.
4. Equal division of work and responsibility between management and workers.

The first step was the development of a science for each element of the labor process that encompassed rigid rules of motion for every man and the standardization and perfection of working conditions. The infamous "time and motion" studies were an integral component of this first stage. Taylor believed that each and every physical act of labor could be subjected to scientific analysis, and that the single best way to carry out each act could eventually be discovered. This applied to the most mundane forms of physical labor. Taylor insisted that:

> [E]very single act of every workman can be reduced to a science . . . the writer has never met a single shovel contractor to whom it had ever occurred that there was such a thing as the science of shoveling. This science is so elementary as to be almost self-evident (Taylor 1911:64–65).

Once each task had been sufficiently analyzed and perfected, the second duty of management involved the scientific selection, training and development of the workers. Taylor did not believe that a worker could do any task; he recognized that labor was variable in its capacities and talents and that management must be able to detect these differences and assign workers to the tasks most appropriate to them. In this sense Taylor was a firm believer in the axiom, "there is a proper tool for every job." Humans were viewed as tools, instruments, or parts to be fit into the production process. The challenge was to determine the dimensions of the labor parts and the most appropriate location in the machine. Again, science was called upon, this time to measure human specifications with regard to reaction time, physical prowess, and mental alertness.

For example, Taylor spoke of physiological experiments and the measurement of the "personal coefficient" that gauged the "quick powers of perceptions accompanied by quick responsive action" (Taylor 1911:89). On the basis of these types of experiments, managers could select the best worker for a particular job. For those tasks that required little mental or perceptual skill, Taylor described the need for something less than human:

> Now one of the first requirements for a man who is fit to handle pig iron as a regular operation is that he should be so stupid and so phlegmatic that he more nearly resembles in his mental make-up the ox than any other type (Taylor 1911:59).

While Taylor made reference to training and development, it is clear that his primary concern was to create relatively simple tasks on the basis of time and motion analysis and to select workers appropriate for the performance of these simple tasks. These might range from handling pig iron to shoveling coal—and for those gifted with the best "personal coefficients"—to inspecting bicycle ball bearings. The scientific analysis of the labor process had reduced all jobs to a series of simple and repetitive physical motions. Placement into these undemanding manual tasks was, for all practical purposes, terminal. If a worker exhibited exceptional efficiency at a particular task, it simply vindicated and justified the procedure of scientific selection. There would certainly be no incentive for management to remove a worker from a task that was being performed well, or to promote that worker to a higher level; after all, "if the part fits, keep it."

The third major principle of Taylor's system invoked the notion of cooperation. Managers should cooperate with workers to see that all jobs are carried out according to scientifically determined guidelines or, as Taylor described it, "bringing the science and the workers together."

The fourth and final stage of scientific management was the maintenance of an equal division of work and responsibility between management and workers. In contrast to earlier systems of management where the whole problem was left largely to the workman, management now took up fully one-half of the problem under principles of scientific management. While the 50-50 split can be viewed as an "equal division," quantitatively, there is a clear qualitative division between mental and manual labor. Managers conceive and workers execute.

Assessment and Consequences

The net effect of this analysis and reorganization of production was to reduce an extended labor process down to a series of discrete activities (or motions) that laborers could repeat. The division of labor with the assignment of workers to specialized tasks was the hallmark of scientific management and is a component of all bureaucratic models of organization. The division of labor is both horizontal—dividing workers across an interdependent series of tasks—and vertical—dividing the mental labor of management from the manual labor of workers.

Scientific management also represents one of the sharpest examples of the machine metaphor of organization (Morgan 1997). As we have already noted, the engineering model employed by Taylor is a mechanical model that conceptualizes human tasks as analogous to the actions of different parts of a machine. A wristwatch, for example, is a very simple machine that involves a detailed division of labor among the pieces that make up the larger device. The pieces of the watch "specialize" in repeated actions. Together, the repetitive movement of specialized parts produces the synchronized motion of the hands of the timepiece. This is a highly efficient and simple metaphor that serves as a model for the human labor process.

Taylor's prescribed system of management is clearly aimed at controlling the inevitable uncertainties that arise when humans enter the production process. His so-called science is designed to reduce these uncertainties. This is accomplished by limiting the discretion and variability in human action through the application of engineering principles.

In Taylor's various comments on the fundamental challenges of management, he addressed a variety of sociological and psychological issues directly related to the unique status of human labor. In his discussion of soldiering, for example, he described the emergent nature of collective behavior. He made a distinction between "natural" and "systematic" soldiering (Taylor 1911:30–34). Natural soldiering refers to the tendency or "natural instinct" of workers to take it easy. He assumed that humans are basically lazy and that they usually have to be motivated, coerced, or persuaded to exercise initiative. This is essentially an argument about human nature. The notion of systematic soldiering, in contrast, refers to soldiering that results "from more intricate second thought and reasoning caused by their relations with other men" when workers carry out group tasks. Taylor viewed this form of soldiering as the most pernicious.

> As another illustration . . . the loss of ambition and initiative . . . takes place in workmen when they are herded into gangs instead of being treated as separate individuals . . . as far as possible each laborer should be given a separate individual task (Taylor 1911:72–73).

The implied *natural* laziness of humans is contradicted by Taylor's focus on the systematic form of soldiering. More important, however, is that systematic soldiering stems from the fact that human labor is simultaneously a supplier and controller of labor power. Unlike other organizational inputs, workers are copresent when they supply their labor. This allows for the communication of norms and expectations, including limits on output and sanctions against "ratebusting." As Taylor suggested in the above quote, individuals in isolation are driven by a different set of motives that management can more easily manage. The key is to prevent individual workers from developing group norms and standards. In Taylor's account, emergent norms and properties serve to hinder the effectiveness and efficiency of the organization. Thus, management should divide the workforce and bargain with workers on an individual basis rather than relying on collective forces.

> Personal ambition always has been and will remain a more powerful incentive to exertion than a desire for the general welfare. The few misplaced drones, who do the loafing and share equally in the profits with the rest, under cooperation are sure to drag the better men down to their level (Taylor 1911:95).

Again, the reference to personal ambition contradicts the inherent laziness argument embodied in the "natural soldiering" concept.

It should also be noted that Taylor's position in isolating the worker differs sharply from those that follow, such as Chester Barnard's notion of "common moral purpose," Fritz Roethlisberger and William Dickson's informal groups, or the contemporary concept of "synergy" (Barnard 1938; Roethlisberger and Dickson 1939). While all agree that the whole is *different* from the sum of the parts, there is dispute over whether the whole promotes *greater or less* organizational efficiency.

In spite of the contradictory arguments on the issue of human motivation, Taylor ultimately relied heavily on a reinforcement model that was consistent with his individualist orientation toward management-labor relations. He argued at various points that the most valuable law of motivation is the "task idea."

> . . . It is absolutely necessary, then, when the workmen are daily given their task which calls for a high rate of speed on their part, that they should also be ensured the necessary high rate of pay whenever they are successful . . . These two elements, the task and the bonus constitute two of the most important elements of the mechanism of scientific management (Taylor 1911:121–22).

Taylor totally disregarded any potential intrinsic rewards that might stem from the work itself and, as noted, he was suspicious of motives deriving from the cooperative effort among workers. The "bonus" is the only carrot in Taylor's model. The powerful incentive of personal ambition is thus reduced to the exertion of physical effort in return for a material bonus. The material bonus in turn ensures that a worker's physical exertion will be repeated.

Taylor depicted and encouraged in these principles a very *asociological* labor process. Workers are viewed as individual parts. Tasks are fragmented and segregated. Unity and cohesiveness is discouraged. Communication is confined to interaction between the manager and the individual worker. Energy is exerted in return for a material bonus.

The system also ignores social norms of solidarity, loyalty, or commitment. The organization is devoid of any developmental opportunities—there is virtually no allowance for the growth of intellectual capacity, expanded skills, or a transformed consciousness. In spite of the socially barren organizational landscape embodied in Taylor's prescriptive principles, his summary (1911:140) of the basic message of scientific management suggested a different reality.

> Science, not rule of thumb.
>
> Harmony, not discord.
>
> Cooperation, not individualism.
>
> Maximum output, in place of restricted output.
>
> The development of each man to his greatest efficiency and prosperity.

As we have already seen, cooperation and development are hardly integral elements of the scientific management scheme. Nonetheless, as the next section highlights, scientific managers attempted to present their system in a manner that would promote its acceptance and encourage its adoption. The public relations rhetoric, however, was not supported by the system in practice.

Scientific Management in Practice: The Hoxie Study

A remarkable study of scientific management was published in 1915 by Robert Hoxie, who was appointed special investigator for the U.S. Commission on

Industrial Relations. Hoxie's research was connected to a larger U.S. House of Representatives investigation and set of hearings, conducted in 1911, on Taylor's system of factory management. Hoxie interviewed managers who were employing scientific management procedures and visited machine shops to observe scientific management in practice. The purpose of his report was to assess the claims made by management advocates and their labor opponents regarding the effects of the scientific management system.

The advocates of scientific management claimed the system served the interests of workers, owners, managers, and society through the reduction of waste, the improvement of methods of production, and the development of a scientific basis for distributing the fruits of production (Hoxie 1966:7–13). The scientific label was critical because it suggested a neutral and value-free system that eliminated arbitrary and biased managerial practices. The rule of scientific law would replace the exercise of force and whim. This would benefit workers by establishing a more just and egalitarian system.

The second purpose of the "scientific" label was to denote the unbiased empirical basis for determining the most productive and efficient organizational system and division of labor. In short, it was claimed that "scientific management is thus at once scientific and democratic" (Hoxie 1966:9). In its defense, advocates of scientific management paid homage to the most sacred values of modern society and in this way sought its acceptance by those subjected to its dictates.

The defense of scientific management offered by its proponents points to an important fact regarding the relationship between organizational systems and the human factor of production. To gain the compliance of their employees, organizations must, at least in principle, adhere to certain normative values and ideals. Though science and democracy may not be the central objectives of industry, advocates of scientific management realize that these are widely held values. Ironically, in using these legitimating principles, scientific management provided criteria against which the organizational system could be measured, as well as an abstract vision of alternative organizational forms. The reference to notions of science and democracy sensitized humans to organizational possibilities unrealized under present systems claiming fidelity to both. This fact is reflected in trade union objections to scientific management (Hoxie 1915). On the question of the meaning of scientific management, labor took the following position:

> Organized labor makes a clear distinction between "scientific management" thus defined and "science in management." It does not oppose savings of waste and increase of output resulting from improved machinery and truly efficient management. It stands, therefore, definitely committed to "science in management" and its objections are directed solely against systems devised by the so-called scientific management cult (1915).

The statement affirmed labor's early devotion to the scientific ideal as a progressive force capable of advancing efficiency and output. Labor was not rejecting science per se but the particular scientific musings of the emerging managerial class. Thus, the scientific labeling strategy was strategically sound given the widespread attachment to the principle, but labor was not convinced that scientific management conformed to this scientific ideal. It would appear that the power of scientific ideology was less pervasive than often assumed and, as early as 1915, there was little confusion over the interests advanced by scientific management. Labor's position:

> "Scientific management" thus defined is a device employed for the purpose of increasing production and profits; and tends to eliminate consideration for the character, rights and welfare of employees.
>
> It looks upon the worker as a mere instrument of production and reduces him to a semiautomatic attachment to the machine or tool.
>
> It does not take all the elements into consideration but deals with human beings as it does with inanimate machines (Hoxie 1966:15, 18).

Just as labor rejected the scientific claims of scientific management, so too were the arguments concerning democracy.

> "Scientific management" is undemocratic, it is a reversion to industrial autonomy which forces the workers to depend upon the employers' conception of fairness and limits the democratic safeguards of the workers. . .
>
> It allows the worker ordinarily no voice in hiring or discharge, the setting of the task, the determination of the wage rate or the general conditions of employment (Hoxie 1966:17).

Again, labor defined the legitimating norm of democracy very differently. Scientific managers, on the other hand, saw a much stronger connection between science and democracy. The democratic nature of the production system stemmed from organizing tasks and routines on the basis of objective empirical analysis rather than personal authority. If the "one best way" could be determined scientifically, then presumably all parties would have an interest in following the procedures. The assumption of a common or general interest among organizational participants underlay the science-democracy linkage. Managers, given training and intellect, were best able to determine the means to increase productivity through the scientific method. If the organizational procedures were established through the neutral mode of scientific inquiry, the resulting scientific management system of organization would be fair, impersonal, and, ultimately, democratic. The scientific management view of democracy rested upon the value-neutrality of science and a "unitary" notion of a harmony of interest between workers and owners (Fox 1971).

The labor position of viewing scientific management as undemocratic was based on the assumption of antagonistic interests of workers and owners. Given these opposing interests, any organizational system proposed by managers—scientifically based or not—was suspect. Genuine organizational democracy required mechanisms allowing the participation and representation of workers as a protection from managerial intentions.

Hoxie's outline of the opposing positions of labor and scientific managers indicated the almost immediate resistance by labor to the scientific management system, and the effort by managers to justify the system by recourse to science, democracy, and a harmony of interests. The actual intention of scientific management, however, was not scientific accuracy or democratic work procedure but the simplification and routinization of the production process. Realization of these goals would represent a major accomplishment, though Hoxie suggested the system was only a partial success: "The most that can be said is that scientific management as such furthers a tendency to narrow the scope of the workers' industrial activity, and that it falls short of a compensatory equivalent in its ideals and actual methods of instruction and training" (Hoxie 1966:39).

However, as Hoxie's study made clear, the true failure of scientific management stemmed from its inaccurate conception of labor and the unanticipated reaction of workers to the system. The most compelling section of Hoxie's report is his discussion of the actual practice of scientific management and the inevitable slippage between theory and practice.

The practical deviations from theory are almost wholly the result of human factors operating on managers and workers alike. Managers failed to behave according to the scientific ideal, and workers could not be subjected to the precise measurement and control claimed by scientific management.

It is important to note that Hoxie's report is damaging to the arguments of scientific management on almost all counts. On the central questions of whether the principles of scientific management are actually implemented and, if so, whether they have the claimed effects on labor, the evidence is almost entirely negative; that is, there were virtually no instances in which the scientific management scheme was applied in its totality nor where, when applied, the effects were as beneficial and benevolent to labor as claimed. If one views Hoxie's study as a test of the opposing claims of labor and scientific management, it provides the greatest support for the labor position.

More important are the reasons for the failure of scientific management in practice. Hoxie suggested that there were certain practical limitations in applying the scientific management model. In addition, managers were torn by conflicting demands for quick results and continuous production. Thus, in almost all cases there was only a hodgepodge application of scientific management principles. The time required to reorganize the production process clashed with the pressures for short-term results. "Some particular aspect or feature of the system is not infrequently stressed out of all proportion and this is very apt to be task setting or some particular aspect of payment" (Hoxie 1966:29). Alongside the selective application of particular elements of the system, it is typically the case "that the spirit and principles are violated and discarded."

Apart from the question of whether the scientific management system can be fully implemented in letter or spirit, there is the more critical issue of whether there can be anything even approaching a "science" of human management. Hoxie repeatedly suggests that managers, like the workers they supervise, are influenced by subjective biases and irrational tendencies.

As noted, the legitimacy of the entire scientific management edifice rests on its scientific character. If the human factor at the managerial level prevents the realization of objective scientific inquiry, the whole system must be called into question. On some of the most critical scientific management methods—the selection of workers, time and motion study, and task setting—human subjectivity would seem to render their application unscientific:

> Far from being the invariable and purely objective matters that they are pictured, the methods and results of the time study and task setting are, in practice, the special sport of individual judgment, diversity, inaccuracy and injustice that arise from human ignorance and prejudice . . . (Hoxie 1966:40).

In opposition to the prevailing managerial ideology of the day—where managers presumably possess special qualities distinguishing them from the common laborer—Hoxie provided a truly sociological analysis that places managers in the same class of humanity as workers. As humans, managers are characterized by interests, emotions, and needs that both limit and extend the human potential. In this particular case the human factor at the managerial level undermines the scientific application of organizational methods. Nonetheless, there is still a system intended and a system imposed, albeit nonscientifically. The story of scientific management must also consider the human reaction to the elements of the system that were in fact instituted.

Hoxie's study does not document the forms of action workers took in opposition to the scientific management system. He does, however, confront the central issue of the theory's conception of labor as an object—scientifically measured, monitored, and rewarded. In a concluding section of the report titled "The Causes of the Shortcomings of Scientific Management in Practice," Hoxie identified what is essentially the major flaw of the system. He argued that the system assumed a technical approach to the problem of human management and neglected the complexities inherent in social organization. Scientific management experts only became aware of these shortcomings, according to Hoxie, when they were faced with widespread labor opposition.

The reaction of labor to the system of scientific management, manifested in turnover, absenteeism, sabotage, low levels of commitment, and collective resistance, prompted revisions in managerial strategies of control. As Hoxie indicated, these revisions required a different conceptualization and set of assumptions about the human factor. As we shall see in the next chapter, a different set of assumptions will generate a different set of strategies designed to control the human factor. However, the dynamic tension between human capacities and organizational systems of control, apparent from the earliest attempts to establish the factory system, is a constant force at every historical point. In his study of the origins of modern management, Pollard concluded that "it is doubtful whether, within the context of the present structure of society and industry, the dilemmas of its beginnings have been resolved even today" (1965:208).

Scientific Management: The Broader Context

It is important to place the discussion of scientific management in a broader context. While we have considered scientific management as a tactic used by capital in its struggle with labor, its application has extended beyond the capitalist factory. Specifically, the following points should be noted.

First, the obsession with the technical control of the production process was not confined to the capitalist class. In the early stages of the Russian Revolution, Bolshevik leaders were attracted by the promise of scientific management. Lenin himself wrote that "We must organize in Russia the study and teaching of the Taylor system and systematically try it out and adapt it to our needs" (Lenin 1965:259). What was called the "Stakhanovite" system was used to rationalize the work process using divisions of labor, quotas, and piece work in both the Soviet Union and China. This indicates that the drive for efficiency and the utilization of scientific management techniques transcends the labor-capital relationship and profit-based systems of organization.

Second, the principles of scientific management have both influenced and been employed in public administration. During the Progressive Era (ca. 1910) in the United States, the movement to separate politics from administration and eliminate the "boss" mode of municipal government, led reformers to embrace the spirit of objectivity and efficiency associated with scientific management (Schiesl 1977). This influenced hiring, budgeting, professionalization, specialization, and the delivery of services. The attraction of scientific management, in this case, was not its ability to socially control labor or advance productive efficiency but to establish procedures of public administration that would be divorced from purely political considerations.

Third, the narrow tasks and job assignments that we associate with scientific management have often been accepted and defended by industrial unions in the United States (Sullivan 1987). This seemingly paradoxical fact stems from the desire of trade unions to protect their workers by establishing work rules, job classifications, and seniority principles for each position. This prevents management from arbitrarily redefining responsibilities, shifting workers from one job to another at whim, or replacing skilled with unskilled workers. Thus, our emphasis on labor's historical opposition to scientific management and control strategies must be balanced with a recognition of the way workers may use these procedures to advance their own interests.

Summary

This chapter has introduced a variety of themes, based on the historical rise of the factory system, that are central to the development of organization theory and that continue to have an impact on contemporary organization. Each of these themes deserves further elaboration.

1. The historical analysis has employed a Marxian theoretical framework that highlights the effort by owners and managers to gain control over the organization of production and the activities of labor. Viewing organizations as *systems of control* is a pervasive theme in the literature of organization theory. A central point of the text is that the control of humans represents the most challenging aspect of organization. This fact is especially apparent as we review the struggles with labor during the rise and establishment of the factory system and the formulation and practice of scientific management.

   In contrast to some Marxist treatments of this subject, however, we have added the dimension of ongoing resistance and opposition to these managerial control initiatives. Rather than assuming the inevitable domination of one group or class over another, or that scientific management was smoothly imposed upon powerless workers, we have seen how both the practical difficulties of implementation and the resistance by labor complicates the picture. Our review of organization theories and developments acknowledges the wide variety of practical problems, contradictions, and paradoxical consequences associated with most organizational undertakings.

2. Scientific management principles continue to have a wide applicability to organizational theory, structure, and strategy. The differentiation of tasks and the separation of mental and manual labor represent fundamental features of most organizations. Organizational members occupy different positions and specialize in different activities. Conception is often separated from execution. These divisions are often defended on the basis of technical rationality and efficiency. They are also criticized for restricting the autonomy, skill, and discretion of workers. In either case, the structural differentiation of work, vertically and horizontally, can be expected to weaken the

attachment to the larger mission of the organization and generate conflict across departments and levels of authority. Frederick Taylor's system was designed to formally divide the workforce. However, workers were able to create their own forms of solidarity, largely in opposition to management. Thus, even though workers were divided by their tasks, they were united in their subjective reactions to the systems of scientific management. These reactions had an enormous impact on subsequent organization theory and management practice.

3. Many of the principles of scientific management have also become an integral part of what we call the bureaucratic organization. Formal structure, hierarchy, and divisions of labor are utilized in many organizations and remain successful models for certain organizations. Fast-food franchises, for example, have literally made a science out of the organization of tasks and the preparation and delivery of food. The automotive industry in the United States has long utilized fundamental precepts of scientific management in the organization of work around the assembly line.

THE HUMAN ORGANIZATION

4

The problems associated with defective communication are closely linked with the second weakness of formal organization: that by its very nature it tends to ignore certain emotional factors in human behavior. Designed precisely in order to be rational and logical and to keep the human factor at a minimum, it is liable to come to grief when faced with the irrational and emotional aspects of industrial life. Designed to deal with the predictable, the routine, and the typical, it is at a loss when confronted by the unforeseeable, the unusual, and the illogical. . . Since, as we have seen, these assumptions are false, any inferences based on them are also false and unlikely to work out in practice with any degree of success.

J.A.C. Brown, *The Social Psychology of Industry* (1954).

In the last chapter we reviewed the historical development of the factory system along with methods and techniques designed to control the human factor of production. Scientific management principles represented one of the leading strategies in this effort. However, as we emphasized in Chapter 2, the human factor of production possesses unique capacities that prohibit complete subordination. Through various actions of resistance and opposition, new organizational theories and management strategies must be devised. In this chapter we shall review the development of those theories of organization that recognize the centrality of the human equation.

The Hawthorne Revelations and Beyond

The Hawthorne Experiments: The Human Factor Observed

The Hawthorne experiments represent one of the most dramatic and well-known examples of the intricate relationship between management practices and the reformulation of organization theory. It is hard to imagine a single research project having as great an impact on a particular field as the Hawthorne experiments have had on organization theory. Like most great legends, there is also considerable debate about what really happened at Hawthorne and what it all means. There is a popular interpretation and a revisionist interpretation. Given the importance of Hawthorne, it is worth reviewing both interpretations though in the final analysis the consequences of the studies, whatever their validity, are not open to much question.

In the popular interpretation of Hawthorne, Elton Mayo is the central intellectual figure responsible for the research, interpretation, and insights. The standard tale is as follows. In the 1920s and 1930s, Mayo and his associates from the Department of Industrial Research at Harvard University conducted a series of experiments at the Western Electric Company plant outside of Chicago. The researchers were interested in the impact of physical conditions—lighting, work layout, work pace, and so forth—on output and productivity. The manipulation of physical working conditions was expected to have some kind of linear effect on the level of output; for example, the greater the illumination, the greater the expected output. As it turned out, however, productivity and output seemed to rise regardless of the direction in which the physical conditions were manipulated. No matter which way the physical conditions were altered—for better or for worse—output increased. The explanation for this paradoxical discovery is what is known as the "Hawthorne effect."

According to the standard accounts, the enhanced output during the various experiments were attributed to the interaction between researchers and workers. The communication and interaction during the course of the study, along with the interest shown by researchers in the workers' performance, presumably produced extra effort and commitment by the workers, who wanted to satisfy the researchers and demonstrate their ability. The Hawthorne effect—the sociopsychological process whereby behavior is altered and adjusted owing to the presence of and relationship with others—has implications for both methodological research and practical management.

Methodologically, the Hawthorne studies showed how the simple act of observation can influence the behavior of research subjects. For management, the

Hawthorne studies demonstrated how communication and interaction with workers can result in heightened levels of commitment and output. In the popular interpretation of Hawthorne, this latter "effect" was the most widely publicized finding.

Revisionist accounts of the Hawthorne studies tend to focus on the efforts of researchers other than Mayo, the distinct phases of the research project, and the absence of empirical support for the existence of a Hawthorne effect (see Whitsett and Yorks 1983).

The Hawthorne studies can be divided into three phases. The first phase was initiated in 1923 by the Committee on Industrial Lighting and funded by the General Electric Company under the supervision of Charles Snow. Snow conducted the illumination studies that yielded inconclusive results regarding the direct impact of factory lighting on output. However, during the illumination experiments the overall level of productivity seemed to increase. One of Snow's colleagues, Homer Hilbarger, who was to play a major role in subsequent phases of the research, suggested that the increase in productivity was attributable to the supervisory role played by the researchers. This was the first inference of a Hawthorne effect.

The second major phase of the research was the Relay Assembly Test Room Study conducted in 1927. Six women were chosen for the study, segregated from the rest of the workplace, and made responsible for assembling electrical relays under a set of unique conditions. For example, the women worked in a smaller room with better lighting, the layout operator serviced a smaller number of assemblers, a chute mechanism was used to count the output, the pay rate was altered, repair and quality assessment procedures were changed, the work group was smaller, the research observer played some role in task supervision, the women in the test room were given greater attention than the other workers, and the women were allowed to communicate with one another in the test room (Whitsett and Yorks 1983).

The last three social conditions of the Relay Assembly Room have been given the greatest weight in popular accounts of Hawthorne, particularly the supervisory role of the test observers. Recent quantitative analyses of the Hawthorne data fail to support the existence of a Hawthorne effect (Jones 1992). A number of revisionist accounts express similar skepticism regarding the research results and the empirical validity of the original claims (Kerr 1953; Carey 1967; Argyle 1953; Franke and Kaul 1978; Gillespie 1993).

The third and final phase of the research, begun in 1931 and known as the Bank Wiring Observation Room experiments, utilized more sophisticated research methods with the primary focus on small group dynamics. Fourteen men were selected for the observation room. They were responsible for wiring the components of electrical switches in a team effort of wiremen, soldermen, and inspectors. Methods of observation were intentionally less obtrusive than in the previous industrial illumination and test room experiments. Instead of an increase in efficiency and output, however, the results indicated that the work group was restricting output to some predetermined level.

Interpreting the Results

Together, the three major research experiments point to a mixed set of findings that are open to a variety of interpretations. The one finding that has not been challenged, however, and which was even supported in the final Bank Wiring Observation Room phase of the project, involved the informal social relationships that emerged within the work groups. Delbert Miller and William Form (1964:667) noted the most significant findings drawn from the bank and wiring room experiments. They are summarized as follows:

1. The output of industrial workers was determined by informal standards established by the work group.
2. The group standard reflected the impact of a larger set of norms involving customs, duties, routines, and rituals.
3. When there is a conflict between the standards of management and the standards of the work group, the work group is most likely to hold the greater sway.

From the perspective of sociology, the experimental results of Hawthorne point to some rather fundamental features of human association. The formation of informal groups is based on the human capacity to form a common spirit through face-to-face interaction, communication, and shared experience. What was a major discovery at Hawthorne has been analyzed in detail in studies on primary groups by the sociologist Charles Cooley. "They are primary in several senses but chiefly in that they are fundamental in forming the social nature and ideals of individuals. . . The individual will be ambitious but the chief object of his ambition will be some desired place in the thought of others" (1962:23–24). Individuals in primary work groups are able to interact, communicate, establish norms discursively, and coordinate behavior informally. In some cases, these bonds of solidarity may combine to generate a kind of "synergy" promoting higher than expected levels of output. In other cases, as the results from the bank wiring room suggest, these informal bonds can also form in opposition to the interests of management (Katz and Kahn 1966). Because these informal work groups form in all organizations, influence behavior, and are able to shape organizational performance, a vast literature has been produced on the dynamics and consequences of informal group activity and the potential of work teams (Dalton 1959; Bacharach and Lawler 1980; Guzzo and Dickson 1996; Cohen and Bailey 1997).

Recall that Frederick Taylor, in his formulation of scientific management, saw the restriction of output as the most likely result of primary group formation.

FIGURE 4–1

Hawthorne experiments and reformulation of organization theory

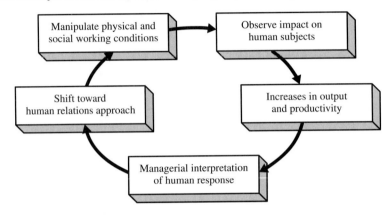

He advised managers to separate workers and deal with them one-on-one. He did not trust the outcome of informal group processes and assumed that they would only generate sentiments of the lowest common denominator. After Hawthorne, however, there was a wholesale reversal in this attitude toward informal groups. The informal primary group was viewed as a potentially positive force and one that managers could ignore only at their peril.

Further, on the question of the Hawthorne effect, it is largely irrelevant whether the behavior of researchers was actually responsible for the enhanced productivity of the workers. Clearly, patterns of worker-management interaction will have some impact on the way workers define and interpret their place within the organization. The theoretical logic underlying this assertion is that humans are able to consciously reflect, evaluate, and respond to their social environment and communicate these assessments among their co-workers.

The human factor dynamics documented in the Hawthorne experiments represent a concrete case that can be incorporated into the models of tension, paradox, and change presented in Chapter 2. More precisely, as outlined in Figures 4–1 and 4–2, the actions of the workers at Hawthorne (1) generated a revision of organization theory and management strategy emphasizing human social dynamics and relations (Figure 4–1); and (2) demonstrated an unintended consequence that had enormous influence on the larger organizational performance (Figure 4–2).

The results from Hawthorne clearly forced organization and management theorists to confront the complexity of the human factor and transcend the view of labor as merely an object inserted into a formal structure. The full significance of Hawthorne, however, awaited a series of interpretations provided by those who were not directly involved in the original experiments. The most notable contributions came from Fritz Roethlisberger and W. J. Dickson, and Elton Mayo.

FIGURE 4–2

Paradox and the Hawthorne experiments

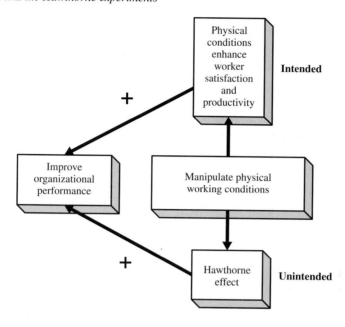

Hawthorne and the Revision of Organization Theory

Roethlisberger and Dickson

In *Management and the Worker* (1939), Roethlisberger and Dickson presented what is perhaps the most detailed and extensive account of the Relay Assembly Test Room and Bank Wiring Observation Room Experiments at the Hawthorne plant of Western Electric. In the final chapters of their book, they discussed the theoretical and practical implications of the Hawthorne study. Roethlisberger and Dickson, based on their thorough review of the Hawthorne data, advanced a model of the organization as a social system. In their conceptualization of the internal structure of industrial organization, they focused upon two major organizational functions that are carried out in response to the two major challenges facing the organization. The first function is the manufacture of the product under conditions of efficiency and cost effectiveness. This function addresses the problem of "external balance" between the organization and the market factors of supply, demand, and competition.

The second function involves "creating and distributing satisfactions among the individual members of the organization" (p. 552). This function addresses the problem of "internal equilibrium" between the needs of individuals and the needs of the organization. Roethlisberger and Dickson believed that insufficient attention had been given to the problems of internal balance. They noted that while a great deal of scientific and technological energy had been devoted to economic processes of efficiency, "Nothing comparable to this advance has gone on in the development of skills and techniques for securing cooperation. . ." (pp. 552–53).

To remedy this omission, Roethlisberger and Dickson placed heavy emphasis on social or internal factors and, in the process, developed a model for understanding individual behavior in the organization that revolves around the concept of "sentiments." Heavily influenced by the writings of Vilfredo Pareto, particularly *The Mind and Society: A Treatise on General Sociology* (1963), Roethlisberger and Dickson placed their analysis of organizational behavior in a framework that distinguishes between sentiments and logic. Sentiments refer to the subjective value-laden dispositions, formed from background experiences, that humans carry into the organization and that influence behavior. They argued that both meaning and behavior are determined by these sentiments.

The analysis of sentiments, however, was not confined to the individual level. Like other observers of Hawthorne, Roethlisberger and Dickson reserved space in their model for the operation of informal group processes. Sentiments may be carried into the organization, but they are also subject to significant modification as individuals engage in association with other workers. The "logic of sentiments" represents the "values residing in the interhuman relations of the different groups within the organization" (1939:564). Roethlisberger and Dickson recognized the emergent character of normative guidelines and felt that the ultimate impact of these group processes depended on whether the informal organization "facilitates the functioning" or "develops in opposition" to the formal organization.

The managerial implications of the transportation of sentiments from other social spheres, and the reinforcement of these sentiments through intergroup relations, were spelled out in later writings. Roethlisberger and Dickson (1966:133) referred to the "felt injustice syndrome" in their work on organizational leadership and counseling:

> Group norms develop around what is considered fair treatment . . . These are sentiments which are shared in common with the wider society and they constitute an important referent in terms of which the fairness of the distribution of rewards is gauged.

It is clear that Roethlisberger and Dickson were attempting to come to grips with the problems posed by the human factor of production. The focus on the distribution of satisfactions, internal equilibrium, sentiments, and group processes reflect an attempt to account for the social nature of organization. In discussing the human and social organization of the plant, Roethlisberger and Dickson pointed to the unique characteristics of the human factor that warrant special attention.

First, they highlighted what we have referred to as the "law of individual differences"—that individuals bring different backgrounds of personal and social experience to the work situation which influences worker sentiments and reactions to the organizational setting.

Second, they emphasized that the shaping of sentiments and orientations toward work is an ongoing social process involving interaction and conditioning that continues throughout the lifecourse (p. 554). These two points are a direct recognition of the distinctive and continuous shaping of human identity and orientation on the basis of experience, social action, and interaction. Humans enter an organization as a highly differentiated factor of production on the basis of past biography. The unstandardized nature of the human factor requires a system, in Roethlisberger and Dickson's terms, that can distribute appropriate satisfactions. It also militates against the implementation of universalistic incentive schemes that are insensitive to individual differences. In addition, as Roethlisberger and Dickson noted, the process of human identity formation is "never ending" so that sentiments and orientations may shift as a result of participation and interaction within the organization. These human processes pose a continual challenge for management because they disrupt the established "social equilibrium."

Third, Roethlisberger and Dickson delineated some rudimentary principles of an interpretive sociological perspective in their discussion of sentiments and meanings. While committed to a structural systems approach to organizations, their careful scrutiny of organizational behavior at Hawthorne led them to flirt with conclusions that highlight the subjective features of organizational life. The objects in the organization represent real structures, but the meaning workers gave to them is determined by the social situation and context and the assigned social value. As they struggled theoretically with the human factor, Roehlisberger and Dickson were compelled to make concessions to positions that are antithetical to their basic systems approach. In this way, a fundamental organizational tension is embedded in their theoretical framework.

Elton Mayo

Elton Mayo's analysis of the Hawthorne experiments has also been extremely influential. In many ways it complements the work of Roethlisberger and Dickson. Like them, Mayo used systems language to describe the "imbalances" and "disequilibrium" in the relationship between the human factor of production and the structural changes of industrial organization. He even used this language to explain the unexpected findings reported by the Hawthorne researchers: "Somehow or other that complex of mutually dependent factors, the human organism, shifted its equilibrium and unintentionally defeated the purpose of the experiment" (1933:54).

However, the scope of Mayo's analysis is broadened by his theoretical links to the Durkheimian concepts of anomie and social solidarity. In his books on industrial civilization (1933, 1945), Mayo argued that industrial society produces conflicts and disruptions that are manifested in an "increasing number of unhappy individuals" and the formation of groups that "are not eager to cooperate wholeheartedly with other groups." More specifically, he described the problem of industrial societies as an imbalance between social and technical skills, and went so far as to say "If our social skills had advanced step by step with our technical skills, there would not have been another European war: This is my recurrent theme" (1945:23).

The administrative or organizational implications of this thesis involve first a recognition that the human factor is not as logical or rational as the technological development of society would suggest. Therefore, organizations must pay attention to the social and psychological needs and sentiments of the workers. Mayo employed the term *sentiments* in the same manner as Roethlisberger and Dickson, denoting the existence of human emotions that are nonrational and nonlogical. These are manifested in what Mayo (1945:71) referred to as "pessimistic reveries," "whenever the conditions of work are unsuitable, physically or mentally, the immediate effect seems to be an increase of pessimism or bitter reflexion." Mayo also viewed the informal organization as a source for nonlogical sentiments, "The desire to stand well with one's fellow's, the so-called human instinct of association, easily outweighs the merely individual interest and the logical reasoning upon which so many spurious principles of management are based" (1945:43).

Mayo touched here on the recurring problem in organization theory that involves the disjunction between principles of organization that impose rational structures and processes, and a human factor of production that employs subjective and normative capacities. In Mayo's terms, the problem is presented in a somewhat elitist and ideological fashion; that is, average workers seem to possess sentiments and emotions that somehow lag behind the modern forces of technical and bureaucratic rationalization. He viewed managers, on the other hand, as more rational, logical, and able, through appropriate interventions, to satisfy the workers' needs and in turn elicit their cooperation.

Mayo's prescriptions for managerial intervention have had an enormous impact on management theory and foreshadowed the beginning of the "human relations approach." His analysis of the problems of industrial civilization and assessment of the human factor as nonlogical and emotional led him to view industry as a strategic integrating institution that could prevent social breakdown. Thus, management was given the enormous responsibility of implementing organizational arrangements that would nurture communication, interaction, and group affiliation. This would then satisfy the emotional yearnings of the workers and reestablish equilibrium. For Mayo, this was not only the key to organizational success but also to social stability. Mayo viewed informal group processes as a central mechanism promoting social integration.

It is significant to note here that the well-knit human groups that Taylor so vociferously opposed in developing scientific management play a redemptive role in Mayo's theory. Indeed, Mayo seemed to be responding directly to the failure of scientific management. He argued that a failure to allow informal groups to form would generate labor turnover, absenteeism, and discontent. This was based on Mayo's assumption that the desire for human association was a fundamental human impulse (1945:111).

The most notable feature of the organization theories of Mayo and Roethlisberger and Dickson was their heavy emphasis on the human factor which reflected the perceived omissions in earlier theories of organization. Prior theories tended to disregard the subjective and discursive elements of human existence which, especially after Hawthorne, were shown to have a significant impact on organization behavior.

Chester's World: Barnard's Theory of Organization and Management

Chester Barnard represents one of the most interesting, yet neglected, figures in the history of organization theory. Writing in the 1930s, Barnard was unique in combining practical experience in management and corporate affairs (president of New Jersey Bell Telephone Company) with a highly complex and sophisticated theory of organization and human behavior. In combining theory and practice, Barnard also offered more practical advice to executives and managers on matters of leadership and communication. What is most significant about Barnard, however, is his recognition of the problematic nature of human action within organizational systems. Unlike Frederick Taylor and the scientific managers, who assumed away the human factor or reduced it to a mass of interchangeable parts, Barnard clearly saw the inherent conflict between the character of the individual and the rigidities of formal organization. His theory of organization struggles with this tension in a philosophically and theoretically sophisticated fashion. While Barnard's resolution of the central organizational dilemmas may ultimately be unsatisfactory, he should be given credit for confronting an issue with which organization and management theory continues to struggle.

As noted, Barnard's work on organizations has not received much attention. Conventional management texts in organization theory tend to give it rather short shrift. Typical is the treatment by Hodge and Anthony (1984) who, in their review of the evolution of organization theory, lumped Barnard with a larger group of theorists making up the "behavioral school" of organization theory. Though they called Barnard's major work, *The Functions of the Executive* (1938), a classic in organization literature, there is only one substantive reference to the work in Hodge and Anthony's entire 600-page textbook. The general neglect may be due to the difficulty of penetrating Barnard's prose, to his highly abstract theory, and to his tendency toward philosophical musings. Barnard offered many concepts and connections but no single or straightforward theoretical sound bite that encapsulates his essential argument. In addition, the sociological literature on organizations also largely ignores Barnard's contribution, with one major exception (Perrow 1986).

The Organization and the Individual

The attention paid to Barnard's work in the present context stems from the central argument on the role of the human factor and Barnard's recognition of the fundamental dilemma facing all organizations—the effort to harness human energy. The break from the classical theory of the Taylorist school is based on the awareness that the human factor cannot be simply slotted into task assignments and motivated by external material reward. The normative elements of social existence must be included in any theory and strategy of human social control.

Barnard's theoretical model represents a shift from an emphasis on the organization of tasks to an analysis of the basic nature of the individual. As noted, the problems with scientific management were largely due to the primitive assumptions made about the human factor and, accordingly, the inability to effectively gain the compliance and cooperation of labor. This led Barnard to begin the formulation of his theory with some new and different assumptions about the human factor of production.

Barnard began *The Functions of the Executive* by emphasizing the tension between the individual and the organization. He noted that organizations are constructed for particular purposes, but they employ individuals who may have widely divergent objectives and desires. Any inquiry into organizations requires, according to Barnard, a set of theoretical postulates about individuals or persons.

He defined the individual as "a single, unique, independent, isolated, whole thing, embodying innumerable forces and materials past and present which are physical, biological, and social factors" (1938:12). This definition of the individual goes well beyond anything found in the classical theory of Taylor, suggesting instead that each individual is unique compared with others who make up the aggregate of employees or "participants" and is, therefore, different from other standard elements of the organization. Further, the definition points to the developmental nature of the individual and the multiple forces impacting this factor of production.

In addition, Barnard noted that among the properties of the individual were the power of choice and purpose. This further distinguishes the human

factor from the other organizational inputs and led Barnard to his major preoccupation with eliciting the support and cooperation of the individual and the
collective mass of labor.

According to Barnard, organizations, as "cooperative systems," emerge
when individuals have a purpose that they cannot realize individually because
of physical or biological limitations. At bottom, then, cooperation or organization is the necessary means for satisfying some individual purpose.

Dependence upon and participation in organizations, however, is only a
necessary condition for the realization of true cooperation among individuals
within an organization. After the individual chooses to participate and is recruited, trained, and assigned to a job, there is still a great deal of uncertainty
regarding human behavior. Barnard did not take compliance for granted. In
contrast to scientific management, selection, assignment, formal structure, and
reward are insufficient to guarantee organizational functioning or cooperative
effort. People can still exercise discretion and choose not to cooperate.

Common Moral Purpose

For Barnard, the essence of organization and one of the most important functions
of the executive was to influence individual choices as they relate to the purposes,
desires, and alternatives available to the individual. "Organization results from the
modification of the action of the individual through control of or influence upon
one of these categories" (1938:17). This ultimate form of social control is achieved
by instilling a *common moral purpose* among organizational participants.

In describing the manner by which the executive or the organization modifies individual action, elicits cooperation, and achieves a sense of common
moral purpose, Barnard made two very distinct arguments. The first is the
more sociological, or Durkheimian. Here Barnard argued that organized collective activity is by its very nature a moral undertaking. When individuals enter an organization to achieve some objective, there are "forces" that compel
individuals to put aside their personal interests and motives, and pursue the
larger organizational objectives.

This led Barnard to posit the existence of a "dual personality" divided between the "personal"—driven by "internal, personal, subjective" factors—and
the "nonpersonal"—driven by external, impersonal, objective factors (Barnard
1938; 77). He claimed that certain forces facilitate the rise of the latter personality, which contributes to organizational cooperation and the achievement of goals.
The forces that facilitate the pursuit of a common moral purpose over individual
self-interest emerge in a synergistic fashion—as emergent properties—and take
on the status of "social facts." In this particular argument, the spontaneous com-
bustion of common moral purpose requires minimal active intervention by the executive, except to encourage the continuation of these sentiments.

However, Barnard's theory of organization contains a second argument about organizational cooperation that suggests greater managerial intervention. While organizational activity is a moral undertaking by its very nature and it engenders the dominance of the "organizational personality" (in contrast to the "individual personality"), he also argued that sustained cooperation requires a consideration of incentives. This shifts the explanation for compliance and cooperation from one based on moral commitment to one based on the calculation of extrinsic rewards.

A large part of his book is devoted to a discussion of the relationship between incentives (or inducements) and contributions, and the need to establish some kind of equilibrium between the two. This shift from a moral to a calculated motivational scheme of social control reveals a major contradiction in Barnard's theoretical model. It clearly suggests that the forces promoting the common moral purpose have not sufficiently suppressed the individual personality. Thus, he advocated the implementation of incentive schemes that can satisfy individual needs and desires and elicit contributions from organizational participants.

For this satisfaction to occur, however, there must be an intervening process between the cooperative action and the satisfaction of personal purpose. He referred to this as "distribution." Distribution is a critical part of Barnard's model since its effectiveness will determine the likelihood that individuals will opt for cooperative activity within an organization. He also pointed to the problem, unique to the human factor, of shifting purposes, desires, and wants. This suggests that a form of distribution at one point in time may be insufficient at a later point; therefore, the stability of cooperative action may be threatened. Again, an important function of the executive involves dealing with changing conditions and purposes. In addition, Barnard also prescribed "methods of persuasion" that can change states of mind and promote the inculcation of motives. Together, the methods of incentives and the methods of persuasion form the central functions of the executive (1938:87).

Barnard also considered the social and psychological factors that affect the individual and come into play after they have entered into cooperative action. He was well aware of the social psychological dictum which provides the basis for human relations models: that social context shapes perceptions and motives; thus, individuals who may possess highly productive assets can, in the "wrong" social environment, be unproductive and unmotivated. "Hence, the group compels changes in the psychological character of the individual and, therefore, in the motives of individuals, which otherwise would not take place" (1938:42). These changes in character, Barnard pointed out, can have favorable or unfavorable effects depending on the extent to which they advance the cooperative systems.

It is important to emphasize that Barnard was explaining the problematic nature of the human factor *within* the organization. After the individual chooses to join an organization and is slotted into a position and role, uncertainty remains. Again, Barnard did not take compliance for granted, but seemed to view it as the single greatest challenge facing organizations. Selection, assignment, and formal structure are not sufficient to guarantee organizational functioning or the exertion of cooperative effort.

While Barnard was clearly most concerned with the viability and maintenance of cooperative systems or organizations, and the impact of forces on the organization, he never lost sight of the fact that organizations are "peopled." Therefore, his theoretical analysis constantly shifted between the aggregate and individual levels. In so doing, he produced a multitude of dichotomies distinguishing what happens at the individual compared with the organizational levels of analysis. In the case of sociopsychological group dynamics, there is the impact on the individual and the impact on the organization. The interplay and tension between these two units are the central issues Barnard addressed in his theoretical scheme.

The contradictions that emerged in Barnard's theory of organization and management reflect the larger tension involving the effort to subordinate the human factor. At the organizational level, Barnard struggled with the tension between the most efficient mode of accommodating the human factor, the ideal from his perspective as an owner and manager, and the reality based on his practical experience. Ideally, humans would be motivated to cooperate by a normative attachment to some organizational objective. This is the most efficient (cheapest) mode of compliance in the sense that it requires no coercion and minimal economic incentives (see Etzioni 1961). It is the form of compliance that was most conspicuously absent in the scientific management strategy. The inadequacies of a reinforcement model of compliance led Barnard to reject monetary and material incentives as insufficient for maintaining a cooperative system. To Barnard, social control from within—moral, normative, cognitive—rather than from without—utilitarian, material, reinforcement—represented the optimal organizational arrangement.

The reality of organizational life, on the other hand, involves a division of tasks, hierarchy, inequalities in prestige and income, repetitive manual labor, authority relations, and participants merely trying to make a living. Human experience in this structural context works against a purely moral attachment to the organization. Barnard was aware of this fact and this created the necessity for the additional methods of motivation oriented toward individual desires, self-interest, and socialization through persuasion. The same human capacities that thwarted the effort by scientific managers to reduce humans to machine objects also nullified the attempt to impose a moral imperative on organizational cooperation.

Humanistic Management Practice

Human Relations and Human Needs

The theoretical models of human relations, and Barnard's theory, reflect the attempt to develop organization theories that include the inherent complexities of human organization. In comparison with scientific management, these efforts represent a major theoretical advance. They recognize that humans are motivated by more than economic reward. They posit a *social* human.

However, these assumptions about the nature of organizations and the human factor still tend to result in essentialistic and reductionistic managerial practices. That is, they assume that human behavior can be explained by a single or narrow range of causes or motives. This is clearly seen in the central propositions of what is now known as the human relations approach. Human relations theory and strategy, most heavily influenced by Mayo's interpretation of the Hawthorne studies, is founded on a set of assumptions about essential human needs and the methods for and organizational consequences of need satisfaction.

Management texts provide the best examples of the application and assumptions underlying human relations theory. In the chapter titled "Satisfying Human Needs," Kae Chung and Leon Megginson outlined the organizational implications of need satisfaction:

> People have a multitude of needs, and satisfying those needs is their lifelong objective. Studying human needs is important for understanding organizational behavior, because it explains the internal causes of behavior.
> Why should managers study the needs theory of behavior?

The authors answered their question with a list of the following points:

1. To manage, direct, and coordinate human behavior in organizations, we need to predict it.

2. To predict behavior, we must understand the causal relationships involved.

3. To comprehend these relationships, we must undertake sufficient meaningful research to generate hypotheses that we can test under controlled conditions (Chung and Megginson 1981).

At the most general level, human relations theory views humans as social creatures who have a need and desire for communication and interaction. Based on the observation of informal groups and the presumed impact of investigator-worker interaction at Hawthorne, organization theorists and management widely believed that the key to promoting cooperation in the workplace involved providing opportunities for employees to interact with other workers and with managerial personnel. While they viewed employee interaction as primarily emergent and informal—as a means to satisfy basic needs for association and group membership—managerial interaction with employees was more strategic and purposive.

Another management text on organizations explains the "communication problem" (Scanlon and Keys 1979). The authors argue that communication plays a vital role in effective management. Managers must not only communicate basic instructions about job tasks and responsibilities but also more general information about the mission and goals of the organization.

> Information of this kind is being constantly generated and, if properly communicated, enables the employees to feel that they are integral parts of the organization; that is, that they are working *with* it, not just *for* it (1979:252).

From Human Relations to Human Resources

Maslow's Human Needs Hierarchy.   The relationship between human needs, organizational theory, and management strategy reached its peak with the application of Abraham Maslow's (1943) work on the human needs hierarchy. If the Hawthorne experiments can be viewed as the single most influential study for management practice, then Maslow's needs hierarchy represented the single most influential personality theory.

Maslow, a psychologist, developed a theoretical model independent of organizational concerns that posited a hierarchy of human needs that motivated human behavior. The needs hierarchy combines a theory of motivation with a model of human development. Over the life span, human behavior is directed first toward the satisfaction of simple, or lower-order, needs and later toward the more complex or higher-order needs.

The lower-order needs include *physiological and safety needs*—the need for food, shelter, and security. Once the lower-order needs are satisfied, humans are motivated to pursue the higher-order needs. They include *social needs* (the need for belonging, association, and acceptance) and *ego needs* (the need for self-esteem and recognition). The final, and ultimately most difficult, need to satisfy is the *need for self-actualization,* or the need to realize one's full potential and capacity as a human being.

Maslow's model of personality development and motivation brought a greater complexity to the standard assumptions regarding human behavior in organizations and also pointed to the potential tensions that may emerge in organizational contexts that are designed to control behavior, yet are negligent of the developmental nature of human needs.

McGregor's Theory X and Theory Y.   The full organizational implications of Maslow's model were perhaps best exemplified in Douglas McGregor's article, "The Human Side of Enterprise" (1966). The logic of McGregor's argument revealed the manner in which management theory and its assumptions created problems and unintended consequences when interfaced with human partici-pants, thus generating pressures for theoretical and practical revisions.

McGregor began by outlining the conventional managerial approach, which he labeled "Theory X." This theory contained a set of practical propositions—that management is responsible for organizing the factors of production; that managers must direct, control, motivate and modify the behavior of the human factor; and that without this managerial intervention people will be passive and potentially resistant to organizational goals and objectives. He then exposed the assumptions underlying this approach, including the assumption that the aver-age person is indolent, dislikes responsibility, is self-centered, is resistant to change, and is a gullible dupe. But McGregor viewed Theory X as unsatisfac-tory with regard to managerial practice, and noted that:

> Management often asks, "Why aren't people more productive? We pay good wages, provide good working conditions, have excellent fringe benefits and steady employment. Yet people do not seem to be willing to put forth more than minimum effort" (1966:12).

McGregor had a two-part answer to this perpetual managerial lament. First, he argued that the human factor assumptions of Theory X had the unintended consequence of serving as a self-fulfilling prophecy. The unproductive forms of human behavior observed in organizations "is *not* a consequence of man's inher-ent nature. It is a consequence rather of the nature of industrial organizations, of management philosophy, policy, and practice. The conventional approach of The-ory X is based on mistaken notions of what is cause and what is effect" (1966:7).

Second, he proposed that Theory X and its associated assumptions only focused on lower-level needs (physiological and security) and ignored the higher-level needs that now serve as the key to motivation. In this Maslowian context, unproductive organizational behaviors were "*symptoms* of illness—of deprivation of his social and egoistic needs." Thus, McGregor's observa-tions regarding the reaction of humans to Theory X styles of management, and the unique human capacity for developing new and different needs, led him to propose a "different theory of the task of managing people based on more adequate assumptions about human nature and human motivation" (1966:15).

Specifically, McGregor advanced "Theory Y," which retained managerial responsibility for organizing the workplace but allowed for a more expansive view of humans. He replaced the assumptions of intrinsic passivity and resist-ance with the potential for human development, a capacity for responsibility, and a desire to realize organizational goals. It was up to managers to enable peo-ple themselves to perceive and develop these human characteristics by creating an organizational environment that facilitates personal goal achievement while also advancing larger organizational objectives.

The implications for organizational structural changes, informed by Maslow's need hierarchy as the propositions of Theory Y suggested, were more far reaching than those imparted by the Hawthorne theorists. The managerial application of Maslow's theoretical ideas have involved the restructuring and redesign of job tasks and authority structures to enhance levels of variety, autonomy, and participation. McGregor, for example, suggested greater decentralization and delegation, job enlargement, consultative management, and employee-determined performance targets.

Pressures for Human Resource Reform.   The changing characteristics of the human factor entering organizations also fueled pressures for job design and human resource reform. During the 1960s and 1970s, it was widely assumed that younger workers entering the workforce were bringing a different orientation to the workplace. First, these workers would not be content with the old system that compensated meaningless work with material rewards. Instead, it was believed that young workers would only be motivated if jobs were intrinsically and qualitatively rewarding. Variously described as "post-materialists" (Inglehart 1977) and the "new working class" (Aronowitz 1973), these workers would reject an organization built on scientific management principles and demand a workplace that respected their mental skills and abilities. A second, and closely related, factor was the rising levels of educational attainment that raised the expectations of the new workforce. Better educated employees would expect jobs that were commensurate with their intellectual abilities. Again, this would place pressure on managers to redesign work tasks and organizational structures.

A distinction has been made between *human relations theory* which, at least in its initial form, retained the scientific management–based organization of production and tasks, and *human resources theory* which posits the necessity of certain structural reforms in order to tap into and satisfy the ego and self-actualization needs (Tausky 1970). Both perspectives are concerned with alleviating tensions, conflict, and recalcitrance stemming from the coordination of the human factor. They propose methods aimed at satisfying the various needs of workers while at the same time advancing administrative objectives in a predictable manner. Human relations theory assumes a human desire for association while human resources theory assumes a drive for self-actualization.

Both theories share the assumption that humans have some essential needs that motivate and drive behavior. The complexity of the human factor tends to be reduced to this or that need which, when given the opportunity for expression and satisfaction, will result in greater compliance, cooperation, and exertion. Thus, the human factor can be manipulated in a predictable and productive manner to the extent that management practices a particular leadership style, institutes a participation scheme, or enriches and expands the scope of work tasks (Likert 1961; Argyris 1964; McGregor 1960).

These methods of human administration are represented in hundreds of thousands of books, manuals, texts, videos, seminars, and workshops targeted for practicing managers. For their part, managers have proven to be a receptive and insatiable market for these packaged prescriptions. Nowhere is the link between organization theory and management practice stronger, prompting one writer to label human resource theorists "behavioral science entrepreneurs" (Watson 1980).

What began as human relations and resources theory has since become a widely accepted approach to understanding the important role of the human factor in organizations. The literature now linking social, psychological, and philosophical insights with management theories of organizational process and performance is vast and, for the most part, noncontroversial. Encouraging interaction, communication, and participation, and creating an organizational climate that values and invests in the human factor, is simply regarded as sound management.

Pfeffer (1994) presented a representative summary of the actual management practices implied by the abstract principles of human relations and resource theory. He labeled these the "Sixteen Practices for Managing People." The practices and a short rationale for each are presented in Table 4–1. It is worth noting, in reviewing the rationales, that the practices play as much a symbolic as substantive role in their impact on the human factor; that is, there is continuous reference to how the practices "signal," "send a message," and "provide a sense of" the values and priorities of the particular organization. How the practices will be interpreted by organizational members is a critical intervening process between initiating the practice and the ultimate impact on organizational behavior and organizational performance. We shall have more to say about these practices when we review the current and emerging organizational forms in chapters 6 and 7.

The various pressures for human relations and resource reform would scarcely exist, however, were it not for the continual challenge posed by organizational members. If human control and job satisfaction could be permanently achieved, there would be little need to continually revisit the latest management and administrative techniques. The tension produced by the human-organizational structure interface, however, prompts an ongoing adjustment and alteration in management and administrative practices and structures.

Leadership

A final topic that joins the concerns of organization theorists and management practitioners is leadership. The importance of leadership has already been suggested. Human relations theory places a great deal of emphasis on interaction

TABLE 4–1 Pfeffer's Sixteen Practices for People Management

Practices	Human Relations/Resources Rationale
Employment security	Signals a long standing commitment by the organization to its workforce.
Selectivity in recruiting	Security for employment and reliance on the workforce for competitive success mean that one must be careful to choose the right people.
High wages	Higher wages send a message that the organization values its people.
Incentive pay	If people are responsible for enhanced levels of performance and profitability, they will want to share in the benefits.
Employee ownership	Employees who have ownership interests in the organization for which they work have less conflict between labor and capital.
Information sharing	If people are to be a source of competitive advantage, clearly they must have the information necessary to do what is required to be successful.
Participation and empowerment	The evidence is that participation increases both satisfaction and productivity.
Teams and job redesign	Because most people are inherently social creatures, deriving pleasure from social interaction, groups exert a powerful influence on individuals. Positive results from group influences are more likely when there are rewards for group efforts, when groups have some control over the work environment.
Training and skill development	Worker autonomy, self-managed teams, and even a high-wage strategy depend on having people who not only are empowered to make changes and improvements in products and processes but also have the necessary skills to do so.
Cross-utilization and cross-training	Doing more things can make work more interesting—variety is one of the core job dimensions that affect how people respond to their work.
Symbolic egalitarianism	Ways of signaling to both insiders and outsiders that there is comparative equality and it is not the case that some think and others do.
Wage compression	Teamwork is fostered by common fate, and common fate is enhanced to the extent that people in an organization fare comparably in terms of the rewards they receive.
Promotion from within	Promotion from within . . . encourages training and skill development because the availability of promotion opportunities within the firm binds workers to employers and vice versa . . . it provides a sense of fairness and justice in the workplace.
Long-term perspective	The bad news about achieving competitive advantage through the workforce is that it inevitably takes time to accomplish . . . The good news is that once achieved, competitive advantage obtained through employment practices is likely to be substantially more difficult to duplicate.
Measurement of practice	Measurement assures that what is measured will be noticed . . . One of the most consistent findings in the organizational literature is [that] measures affect behavior.
Overarching philosophy	It provides a way of connecting the various individual practices into a coherent whole and also enables people in the organization to persist and experiment when things don't work out immediately.

Source: Jeffrey Pfeffer, *Competitive Advantage through People: Unleashing the Power of the Work Force* (Boston: Harvard Business School Press, 1994), pp. 31–57.

and communication as a means to motivate the human factor. Barnard included the inculcation of moral purpose as one of the burdens and functions of the executive. We shall consider the topic in the context of human motivation and social control. As Pfeffer (1997:42) noted: "Control in organizations is exercised through individual, interpersonal influence, in which those in roles of authority motivate and direct others to act as they would like. This interpersonal influence is often called leadership."

Beyond Legitimate Authority

Because the question of leadership is closely tied to authority, Weber's comments on this matter are worth considering. More specifically, Weber argued that the effective exercise of authority requires the authority figure to possess legitimacy. This can be based on (1) the particular characteristics of the authority figure, (2) the content of the authoritative commands, or (3) the occupation of positions of authority. That is, legitimate authority might be based on charisma, reputation, lineage, or the exceptional credentials of the authority figure. Alternatively, legitimacy might derive from the issued commands that are viewed as the best and most logical way to accomplish some goal. Legitimate authority can also stem from holding formal positions of power. Thus, one way to think about leadership is in the context of the various bases of legitimacy.

However, most work on leadership suggests that occupying formal positions of authority and issuing rational and logical commands is insufficient for effective legitimate leadership. If it were sufficient, we would not witness the infinite number of studies and handbooks on the secrets of successful leadership. This literature indicates that leadership is more than possessing particular characteristics, making good decisions, or occupying a position. Rather, it involves special actions designed to motivate and energize the human factor. Katz and Kahn (1966:300–2) put it this way:

> Difficult assignments are often awarded with the injunction to make it work; a kind of implicit recognition that something more than the formal prescriptions of organization is required for the system to function successfully. . . We consider the essence of organizational leadership to be the influential movement over and above mechanical compliance with the routine directives of the organization. Such an influential increment derives from the fact that human beings rather than computers are in positions of authority and power.

One of the central leadership challenges is to resolve the fundamental conflict, which Barnard emphasized earlier, between the individual and the organization. According to Henry Mintzberg (1973:62), all managers must adopt, among their many roles, the "leader role" which is designed to bring about the integration of individual needs and organizational goals. Managers need to promote efficient operation by concentrating their efforts on reconciling subordinate and organizational needs. Since subordinate and organizational needs will not converge automatically, this can only be accomplished, if at all, through largely informal and subjective leadership actions. The problem is now a familiar one. The effectiveness of leadership and authority depends on how it is evaluated and interpreted by subordinates, and whether it motivates action. Some methods, messages, and styles may be better received than others and, accordingly, have their intended effect.

The subjective informality of leadership makes it immune to easy formalization or codification. It is not mechanical but social. It involves style, symbols, culture, and attitude. Leadership is such an open-ended phenomenon that the thousands of studies and guides on the topic, taken together, produce a bewildering and contradictory assemblage of findings and advice.

Four Approaches to Leadership

Some of the confusion stems from the divergent focuses of the leadership studies. Bryman (1996) identified four approaches to leadership in his review of the literature. First, the *trait approach* emphasizes the relatively fixed physical and personality characteristics, such as physique, height, intelligence, sociability, and assertiveness, that are associated with effective leaders.

The second approach examines *leadership styles* that are less fixed and more malleable and pertain to the actual behaviors leaders employ. Together, the trait and style approaches have yielded a wide assortment of dualisms and typologies, along the lines of McGregor's Theory X versus Theory Y, which describe leaders as relationship-oriented or task-oriented, humanistic or authoritarian, people-concern or production-concern, participative or exploitative, reward-oriented or punishment-oriented, micromanagers or macromanagers, instrumental or supportive, participative-oriented or achievement-oriented, internal or external locus of control, and so forth (Likert 1961; Tannenbaum, Weschler, and Massarik 1961; Stodgill and Coons 1957).

Rather than define every trait, suffice it to say that leadership is assumed to be best if it includes a consideration of human needs for concern, expression, self-fulfillment, reward, and creativity. Because people seem to respond more readily to this consideration, leaders feel some obligation, whether they like it or not, to incorporate some aspects of human relations into their leadership style.

Some obvious problems can be pointed out in the theory and research that has generated leadership models based on traits and styles. First, these models reduce a person's organizational personality, in this case those in leadership positions, to a singular trait or style. However, leaders and authority figures, like everyone else, are likely to combine a variety of different operating styles in their organizational repertoire. There is no reason to assume that leadership behavior will conform with the idealized types invented by management specialists.

The issue of different styles raises a second problem that has been widely identified and partially addressed: the role of situational factors. That is, the style of leadership will likely be influenced by the type of organization, task, and employees. Since some of these situational factors can vary in a single working day, it is also likely that a range of leadership styles will also be employed.

This general criticism gave rise to the third approach to leadership: the *contingency model,* in which there is a shift from universal traits and styles of leadership to the relationship between traits or styles and the situation or context. The effectiveness of a leadership style or trait will depend on the particular situation, problem, or group of people that must be managed (Fiedler 1967; Hersey, Blanchard, and Johnson 1996).

The fourth approach—what Bryman (1996) called the *"New Leadership"* approach—represents a more general movement toward the creation of an organizational climate and culture that motivates, inspires, and stimulates constant quality improvements, self-initiative, and continuous learning among organizational members (Avolio and Bass 1994; Sims and Lorenzi 1992; Bass 1997).

The most widely used term to describe this style is *transformational leadership* (Bass 1997). Transformational leaders are change agents who are able to articulate and model a set of core values, are flexible and open to learning from experience and others, and are able to communicate a vision that inspires followers.

Theorists often contrast transformational leadership with *transactional leadership,* which is based on providing rewards for high performance and issuing penalties for substandard performance. Transformational leadership is viewed as the superior approach. Rather than simply eliciting conformity on the basis of external reward, transformation leadership presumably produces a change in the way organizational members think and approach their organizational roles.

Does Leadership Matter?

When all is said and done about leadership, a big question remains: Is there any evidence for a systematic relationship between leadership styles and organizational performance? Most studies and reviews of the literature conclude that the organizational-level effects of leadership are weak, small, nonexistent, or contradictory (Leiberson and O'Connor 1972; House and Baetz 1979). Many possible explanations exist for the null effects of leadership.

Pfeffer (1997) suggested that it is due to (1) low levels of variation in actual leadership behavior stemming from homogenous background and socialization, and (2) organizational constraints that limit leadership variation and channel leadership behavior in predictable directions.

There is, of course, another explanation: The theories about leadership effects are simply false. This is not to suggest that leadership behavior is meaningless or that it does not affect the organization; rather, leadership behavior is likely to have some influence on the organizational climate and the sentiments of workers but in a nonsystematic fashion that does not translate into any measurable impact on organizational outcome or performance. These outcomes are more likely to be influenced by organizational structure and environmental characteristics.

The accumulated inconclusive findings on leadership, however, have not stemmed the tide of organization and management theorizing on leadership. This state of affairs has been attributed to the "romance of leadership" that renders it immune from theoretical and empirical refutation (Meindl et al. 1985:99–100).

> When considering the "symbolic role" of management, the greater significance of leadership lies not in the direct impact on substantive matters but on the ability to exert control over the meanings and interpretations important constituencies give to whatever events and occurrences are considered relevant for the organization's functioning. . . One plausible hypothesis is that the development of a romanticized conception of leadership causes participants more readily to imbue the symbolic gestures of leaders with meaning and significance. Accordingly, the psychological readiness to comprehend things in terms of leadership, whatever dysfunctions it represents, may play an important role in determining the ultimate effectiveness of symbolism as a political tool, benefiting most those who are adept at its manipulation (Meindl et al. 1985:99–100).

This is an important observation about leadership. Clearly, how it is interpreted and the symbols it carries can be used politically as a means to manipulate the definition of the situation. In this sense, it is closely tied to the larger cultural terrain of organization reflected in the values of members and the common understandings of appropriate styles of conduct and interaction.

Summary

1. The rise of human relations theory and strategy is a powerful example of the relationship between organizational structures, the human response, and the revision and development of new organizational and management models. The reaction of labor to scientific management modes of control and the behavior by workers exhibited during the Hawthorne experiments prompted an expansion of models acknowledging the human dimension of organization.

2. Chester Barnard's model of organization also placed the human factor at the center. The fundamental problem of organization, according to Barnard, was to reconcile the diverse interests of organizational members with the objectives of larger organizations or

organization owners. The normative or moral dimension plays a major role in Barnard's theory and is seen as a more comprehensive form of social control.

3. Both human relations and the work of Barnard reflect the growing recognition that formal structures are necessary but insufficient conditions for the mobilization of the human factor of production.

4. Human relations and human resources theory each represent a significant shift in assumptions about sources of human motivation and behavior. While scientific management assumed an economic human motivated by the desire for a bonus, human relations emphasizes the social needs and human resources the need for self-actualization. When evaluating organizational theories, it is critical to determine the fundamental assumptions that are made about the motivating source of human behavior. These assumptions also have a direct relationship to associated managerial strategies. For human relations, this involves social interaction and communication, for human resources a reorganization of the labor process

5. Human relations theory also suggests a major role for organizational leadership. Energizing human effort beyond formal obligations may require particular leadership styles and traits. The literature on organizational leadership has identified many leadership types and authority strategies, but it has not been able to demonstrate a significant relationship between the types and larger organizational-level outcomes.

6. Most generally, the significance of the human relations and human resources approach to organizations is in its explicit acknowledgment—in theory and practice—of the tension between human capacities and organizational structure. As long as humans occupy organizations, there will forever be a need for extrastructural and informal modes of coordination and administration.

5 | BUREAUCRACY, RATIONALIZATION AND ORGANIZATION THEORY

If there has been a dominant perspective in organization theory, it is represented by the *rational-bureaucratic model of organization.* Human relations and resources initiatives have not eliminated this organizational form. The rational bureaucratic model is built on the machine metaphor of organization (Morgan 1997) that draws an analogy between the relationship among the parts of a mechanical device and the relationship among positions in an organization. The action of and relationship between parts and positions are designed to complete the job as efficiently as possible. The model prescribes explicit structural arrangements and administrative practices aimed at achieving specific goals and objectives. These include formal positions and procedures to coordinate and control human labor.

This mechanistic organizational image has been a constant feature of all organizational and management strategies. For many organizations, it continues to coexist with human relations and resources practices. In this chapter I will outline the central assumptions and guiding principles of the rational-bureaucratic model, as well as the relationship between bureaucratic theory and management practice. I shall also consider the inevitable tensions and contradictions inherent in this approach.

Weber and the Rational-Bureaucratic Model

We can begin with Max Weber's theory of bureaucracy, which has had an enormous influence on organization theory and management practice. Peter Blau and Marshall Meyer (1971) have outlined in great detail the specific elements

TABLE 5–1   Weber's Bureaucracy and the Organizational Implications

According to Weber	*Implications for Organizational Structure and Process*
The regular activities required for the purposes of the organization are distributed in a fixed way as official duties.	Formal job descriptions and job titles; specialization, horizontal division of labor
The organization of offices follows the principle of hierarchy; that is, each lower office is under the control and supervision of a higher one.	Hierarchical structure; authority resides in positions within the hierarchy; vertical division of labor
Operations are governed by a system of abstract rules [and] consist of the application of these rules to particular cases.	Universalism; rules and regulations that apply to all members of the organization; standardization and uniformity
The ideal official conducts his office [in] a spirit of formalistic impersonality without hatred or passion, and hence without affection or enthusiasm.	Impersonality; no favoritism; no nepotism; impartial decision making
It constitutes a career. There is a system of "promotions" according to seniority or to achievement, or both.	Recruitment, employment, and promotion based on qualifications and achievement; meritocracy; internal labor markets; professionalization
Experience tends universally to show that the purely bureaucratic type of administrative organization is, from a purely technical point of view, capable of attaining the highest degree of efficiency.	Means-ends structure of positions and tasks enhances efficiency; organizations interested in efficiency will model structures along ideal-type bureaucratic lines

of Weber's model and their implication for organizational practice. These are presented in Table 5–1.

Weber identified six central elements in a bureaucracy: (1) clearly defined division of labor and authority, (2) hierarchical structure of offices, (3) written guidelines prescribing performance criteria, (4) recruitment to offices based on specialization and expertise, (5) office holding as a career or vocation, and (6) duties and authority attached to positions, not persons.

These elements specify the manner in which humans are recruited, distributed, and controlled within a bureaucratic organization. More specifically, based on these elements, we would expect the organization to conduct its affairs as follows:

- Individuals are recruited on the basis of relevant qualifications for a particular task.
- They are assigned a position with fixed duties, responsibilities, and authority.
- The duties, responsibilities, and authority are tied to the assigned position and cannot be transported out of the organization or into other positions within the organization. The position or office is part of a larger hierarchical structure that defines superordinate and subordinate relations.

- Written "legal" documents represent the formalization of information prescribing task assignments and the rules and regulations of the larger organization.
- The tasks of a particular office are part of a larger vocation or career.
- Each of these elements is designed to guide and direct individual behavior toward the larger goals of the organization.

Weber's theory of rational bureaucracy suggests several organizational characteristics and processes:

- The organization will have clearly defined goals that are best achieved within a formal structure.
- Behavior within the organization is shaped by the formal structure and, therefore, is directed toward achieving these goals.
- Efficiency is enhanced to the extent that organizational members follow the formal rules and policies of the organization.
- Organizational decisions are based on a survey of relevant information and a calculation of costs and benefits.

Embedded in the above description of rational bureaucracy are the central principles: formalization, instrumentalism, and rational-legal authority. *Formalization* is the centerpiece of bureaucracy. It refers to the degree to which rules, procedures, regulations, and task assignments exist in written form. Written documentation indicating the procedures for acting, deciding, and communicating represent the formalization of organizational activity. These written directives exist prior to the entry of people into positions within the organization. They are designed to direct and regulate organizational behavior after one has been slotted into a formal position.

An organizational chart, outlining positions from the top down (vertical) and across (horizontal) the organization, and delineating the chain and channels of command and communication, is the graphic representation of formal structure. Each position in the organizational chart has predefined duties. These formal roles and duties determine the behavior of those who occupy the positions. When we say that "the role makes the person," we are speaking of the power of formal structure. This phrase implies that once a qualified person is selected for a position, his or her behavior will be determined by the formally stated job requirements. The converse phrase—"the person makes the role"—would suggest a very nonrational bureaucratic arrangement. This would imply that the personality characteristics and idiosyncratic behavior brought to the job will determine how it is carried out. This also would create a level of uncertainty that formalization is designed to extinguish.

The concept of *instrumentalism* conveys the notion that the organization is like a tool or machine designed to achieve a particular purpose. When we say that something is instrumental, we are viewing it as a means to an end. The rational bureaucratic organization is an instrument designed to achieve some objective. The formal internal structure—positions, procedures, rules, interaction patterns—are also regarded as instruments in the service of this larger organizational mission. It is the formal relationship between the structures and tasks of the organization (the means), and the goals or objectives of the organization (the ends), that makes bureaucracy a rational organizational instrument.

Weber emphasized that the third central piece of the model—*rational-legal authority*—was the most efficient and rational means to gain the compliance of human members. Rather than commanding authority on the basis of tradition (e.g., authority residing in a family name) or charisma (authority stemming from extraordinary personality or leadership traits), "legitimate authority" is based on the formal position (therefore legal) of the authority figure coupled with the belief by subordinates that these arrangements represent the best means to achieve organizational objectives (therefore rational). As noted, people in the bureaucratic organizational model will be recruited on the basis of ability and qualification—or "merit"—rather than personality, connections, or ascribed characteristics. This lends further legitimacy to the exercise of authority.

Weber outlined conditions that would constitute an ideal, perfectly functioning, bureaucracy. The model is often referred to as an "ideal type" because it represents the model or standard against which purportedly rational bureaucratic organizations can be evaluated. This suggests that we can assess existing organizations by their degree of conformity with the ideal-type characteristics. This also raises a number of questions: Is it possible for organizations to even approximate such a model of rationality? If an organization did conform closely to these characteristics, would it necessarily be more efficient? Are there aspects inherent in human organization that prevent the realization of the bureaucratic ideal? In striving for this ideal, are there unintended consequences that undermine the rational and efficient intentions of the model? Throughout this chapter, we shall address the relationship between rational-bureaucratic theory and the actual practices of organizations.

Weber and the Dilemma of Authority

A particularly interesting problem with Weber's formulation of bureaucracy pertains to his argument about authority. Weber contended that legitimate bureaucratic authority derived from formal positions filled on the basis of technical competence. However, as anyone who has worked in an organization is well aware, there is no reason to assume that those in formal positions of authority are necessarily the most technically competent. The sociologists Talcott Parsons

(1947) and Alvin Gouldner (1954) discussed some of the problems that stem from these potentially conflicting bases of authority.

Parsons (1947:58–61) raised the question of whether organizational members follow orders because the person in authority has *superior knowledge* or because the person occupies a *formal position* of authority. If the two characteristics are not joined and those in authority positions possess less technical competence than their subordinates, each group has a legitimate claim to exercise authority over the other. Weber emphasized repeatedly that the bureaucratic form of authority is stable, unambiguous, and clearly defined. However, if more than one basis for legitimate authority exists, instability and ambiguity could be generated.

In Parsons's example, if the less competent are making authoritative decisions, organizational efficiency could also be undermined because efficiency is driven by the merit-based allocation of positions. Gaining the willing compliance of workers may also be problematic because a normative foundation for the exercise of authority—superior knowledge—is being violated.

Gouldner (1954:22–23) pointed to a slightly different kind of confusion, one that stems from Weber's argument that bureaucratic authority is both legitimate because it is rational *and* based on formal position:

> In the first emphasis, obedience is invoked as a means to an end; an individual obeys because the rule or order is felt to be the best known method of realizing some goal. . . . In his second conception . . . the individual obeys the order . . . primarily because of the *position* occupied by the person commanding.

Gouldner highlighted the difference between compliance based on (1) the desire to achieve goals efficiently and (2) compliance based on an obligation to obey the commands of those in higher positions. In the first instance, compliance depends on the belief by subordinates that a command is relevant to the realization of organizational goals. The acceptance of commands and the system of compliance rest on an assessment of the methods, procedures, and directives as formally rational; that is, they are perceived as the best means to achieve a particular end. In the second case, compliance is unconditional. Here one is obligated to obey those in formal positions of power regardless of whether the command is perceived as a rational means to achieve particular objectives.

Parsons and Gouldner have identified an interesting contradiction in Weber's theory of bureaucracy that is endemic to all models of organization. On the one hand, organizations are made up of structures and positions that define the flow of tasks and authority. In the formal structure, authority stems from formal positions in the organizational hierarchy. This is the objective structural side of the organization. On the other hand, it seems clear that Weber, and almost every organizational theorist who followed, did not believe this was sufficient for gaining the compliance of human beings. He included other bases for the exercise of authority such as technical expertise or a collective appreciation for formal rationality. Thus, blind and mechanical obedience stemming from one's formal authority position is supplemented with *normatively legitimate forms of authority;* for example, that the more highly trained experts *should* make authoritative decisions, or that particular authority patterns are the *best* means to achieve some ends. Unlike the objectivity of positional authority, these bases of authority rest on normative assessments about the appropriateness of the exercise of authority and the particular decisions being made.

This as an example of how organization theories conceptualize humans as both objects and subjects. In Weber's description of the purely formal aspects of bureaucracy, people are recruited into positions that have predefined task assignments and authority relations. There is a clear division of labor— some command, others obey. In this formal conception of organization, humans are treated as *objects* controlled by written rules and regulations. However, in the process of exercising authority based on knowledge and position, humans are treated as *subjects*—possessing subjective consciousness and evaluative capacities—who are actually able to decide whether or not they will conform with the wishes of superiors. The notion of "legitimate authority" acknowledges human capacities that generate not only compliance but also potential opposition and resistance. For example, workers can decide that their bosses are not technically competent, that particular methods are not the best way to achieve some goal, or that the goals of the organization conflict with their goals. Weber's expansion of the bases of authority from the objective to the subjective opens the theoretical model to subjective human forces that threaten the machinelike rationality implied by the bureaucratic organizational model.

The analyses of Parson and Gouldner represent a sociological tradition in organization studies that reveals the less than rational and very human content of organizational life. As we review some additional contributions from the sociological literature, we should keep in mind the following critical theme: the manner in which the human factor shapes, modifies, and alters the operation of rational bureaucratic organization, and the associated unintended consequences that stem from the formal rational organization of human activity.

Bureaucratic Dysfunctions and Unintended Consequences

Robert Merton: The Bureaucratic Personality

There is a long tradition of sociological research that has grappled with and observed the dysfunctional and unanticipated consequences of rational bureaucratic organization. Much of this literature owes an intellectual debt to

Robert Merton (1957) who developed the concept of "unintended consequences" to describe the unplanned and paradoxical results of social action.

Merton's concept has special relevance for rational bureaucracy because there is supposed to be a clear and direct connection between the actions of organizational participants and the achievement of goals. Organizational behavior is viewed as the means to achieve the prescribed ends. If organizational behavior produces unexpected and unintended consequences, the rationality of the enterprise can be called into question.

Merton emphasized that unanticipated consequences might serve a "latent function" in actually preserving and reproducing the system; or the consequences may be "dysfunctional" and thus undermine the organizational purpose. These concepts came together in Merton's (1957) analysis of the dysfunctions of bureaucracy which referred to the negative consequences of structural and normative bureaucratic practices.

Merton's analysis of the "bureaucratic personality" stands as the classic statement on the dysfunctional consequences of bureaucracy. The normative attachment to formal rules and regulations, which bureaucratic organizations often encourage, can give rise to a rigid bureaucratic personality type that becomes obsessed with procedural compliance. The bureaucratic personality insists on the unconditional conformity to rules and procedures, regardless of whether they actually advance the goals of the organization or the efficiency of the enterprise. When rules become an end in themselves, rather than the means to an end, organizational behavior takes on a *ritualistic rather than rational character.* It encourages what Merton described as the "displacement of goals"—adherence to methods and procedures at the expense of the larger organizational purpose. People are so busy adhering to the official rules and procedures that they lose sight of the real purpose of the organization. The net result is dysfunctional and counterproductive organizational behavior.

Merton's analysis pointed to the way that bureaucratic structure influences (1) the individual's personality and (2) the ability of the organization to achieve its ultimate objectives. Thus, Merton revealed the key organizational paradox—strict and rigid conformity to formal methods can have the unintended consequence of displacing goals and undermining goal attainment.

It is important to note that much of the sociological research inspired by Merton's diagnosis of bureaucratic dysfunctions did not entirely confirm his argument about the personality-shaping power of bureaucracy. The classic and eternally valuable case studies carried out by Merton's students—Alvin Gouldner, Peter Blau, and Philip Selznick—discovered many dysfunctions, but these resulted as much from human resistance, conflict, opposition, and innovation as bureaucratic overconformity to prescribed norms.

Alvin Gouldner: Patterns of Industrial Bureaucracy

In the 1950s, Alvin Gouldner conducted a series of studies in a midwestern gypsum mining and manufacturing enterprise. This industrial complex combined a mining operation that extracted gypsum from the earth with a manufacturing operation that transformed the organic substance into wallboard. Gouldner's research was instigated by some unresolved tensions in Weber's theory of bureaucracy. In particular, Gouldner believed that Weber was unclear whether employee compliance was based on a consensual agreement about the value of rules and procedures or the authoritative command by superiors. This was an important matter for Gouldner's analysis of bureaucracy since he believed rule compliance would likely depend upon the way rules are formulated. As he noted, "our culture is not neutral but prefers agreed upon, rather than imposed rules" (1954:20).

The Patterns. Gouldner's analysis of bureaucratic rules was based on the assumption that not all organizational members had the same interests or goals. More specifically, workers were likely to have different interests than managers on many work-related issues. Therefore, bureaucratic rules and regulations should be examined to see whether they represented or conflicted with the interests of the different parties in the organization. This analytical framework yielded Gouldner's *patterns of industrial bureaucracy*: mock bureaucracy, representative bureaucracy, and punishment-centered bureaucracy.

Mock bureaucracy refers to the rules of which no party in the organization had a direct interest; therefore, these rules were rarely enforced and routinely violated. The no-smoking rule was one example of the mock bureaucracy. Neither managers nor workers had an interest in the prohibition against smoking. The rule was imposed to satisfy the interests of a third, external party—the insurance company.

Representative bureaucracy refers to rules in which all parties had an interest; therefore, these rules were followed closely and strongly enforced. In the mining facility, rules and regulations pertaining to safety practices inside the mine were followed to the letter. Both workers and managers had an interest in seeing that no one was injured on the job.

Punishment-centered bureaucracy denotes the rules that one group imposes on another. Gouldner mentioned rules that penalize workers for absenteeism and tardiness. These rules were imposed by management on the workers. Workers did not share a concern in these matters and believed they had the right to occasionally miss a day of work or arrive late for personal reasons. This form of bureaucracy, as might be expected, generated the greatest tension and conflict and was the most highly contested. It is also the form we most closely associate with the term *bureaucracy*.

Gouldner's analysis forces us to come to grips with one of the most critical organizational questions: Where do punishment-centered bureaucratic rules come from? Gouldner argued that these rules are created when people in organizations do not believe that those on whom they depend will fulfill their role obligations. The rules are generated by a lack of trust. If failure to meet organizational obligations is due simply to ignorance or carelessness, a representative pattern of bureaucracy can be developed. However, if failure is due to the intentional shirking by one party—because that party may not have a direct interest in following the rule—a punishment-centered bureaucratic pattern is imposed. Therefore, organizations plagued by conflicts of interest are likely to be the most bureaucratic.

Gouldner also argued that the stability of a bureaucratic rule depends upon the degree to which those subject to the rule willingly accept, rather than resist, the bureaucratic requirement. Resistance to bureaucratic procedures played a central role in Gouldner's analysis and enforced the view of bureaucracy as an emergent process—"the *degree* of bureaucratization is a function of human striving; it is the outcome of a contest between those who want it and those who do not" (1954:237). On this basis he concluded that "bureaucracy's march was not triumphant." In the end, humans are capable of enacting, reconstructing, and even eliminating bureaucratic constraints and guidelines.

Primary and Secondary Organizational Tensions.   Gouldner's analysis also pointed out that bureaucratic rules serve to obscure a more fundamental contradiction of organizational life. On the one hand, organizations are designed to control physical and human factors of production in order to achieve the goals of organizational owners. On the other hand, they depend on the cooperation and energy of organizational members who do not own the organization and who may have very different interests. Gouldner referred to this as the "primary tension." This tension is typically managed through various forms of supervision and coordination to ensure that organizational nonowners act in the interest of organizational owners. These supervisory processes generate a set of "secondary tensions." These tensions emerge in *managing* the primary tension; that is, trying to supervise, monitor, and control workers. The secondary tension, resulting from the supervisory process, is managed using written bureaucratic requirements and rules. In managing these secondary tensions through bureaucratic procedures, the primary tension is never addressed. In Gouldner's (1954:241) words:

> If bureaucratic rules reduce tensions that *emanate* from close supervision they make it less necessary to resolve, and thus safeguard, the tensions that *lead* to close supervision.

The issue of close supervision is critical here since it points to a managerial practice that is necessitated by the capacity of humans to act in ways that are contrary to and directly oppose the interests of organizational owners (the primary tension). Supervision, coordination, and the associated management practices, generate (secondary) tensions which in turn are managed bureaucratically through the development and implementation of bureaucratic rules and procedures.

The primary tension that Gouldner refers to is a special case of what is commonly called the *agency problem*. This problem stems from any transaction that involves a "principal" (e.g., an employer) who hires the services of "agents" (e.g., workers) to carry out actions on the principal's behalf. Agency theory assumes, as does Gouldner, that the agents will have different goals and interests than the principals. Therefore, there is no automatic guarantee that agents will do what principals wish. They may shirk their responsibilities and even act in opposition to the interests of the principal. There is no final solution to this fundamental organizational problem. The principal will typically attempt to monitor, control, or supervise agents in some fashion. In Gouldner's analysis, the control strategy generates the secondary tensions and, in turn, the bureaucratic rules.

Gouldner's explanation for the generation of bureaucracy in industrial organization can be extended to public sector organization where there is a parallel tension between agents and principals. In this case, the agents are public officials who have an obligation to uphold the public trust and conform with the wishes of the principals, who are citizens and taxpayers. The emergence of rational bureaucratic public administration was advanced by Progressive Era reformers interested in ensuring that public policy and expenditures would be based on public need rather than private political interests. Thus, distrust of those making public sector decisions prompted an expansion of rules, regulations, and bureaucracy.

This applies most clearly to the area of budget and public expenditure. Marshall Meyer's (1985) analysis of municipal finance illustrates the point. It is based on the two very general propositions: "First, that there is a preference for constructing formal organization as a solution to problems, and second, that increased formal organization yields bureaucratic growth" (1985:62). This "problem–organization–problem–more organization" cycle is demonstrated by examining the method used to gain control over the budget and spending priorities of major U.S. cities. Control produced greater levels of hierarchy and bureaucracy. Put another way, there were some significant unanticipated consequences of control and accountability. "Control is thus the antithesis of economy, and, under certain circumstances, efficiency" (Meyer 1985:68). A decentralized financial system was equated with the absence of control and the likelihood of corruption and fraud. Control therefore produced greater centralization and, presumably, accountability. To summarize Meyer's (1985:76) central finding:

> Each of the mechanisms of control . . . involved, in one way or another, the construction of categories of organization that had not existed absent the control mechanism. Some of the new categories were units of organization represented as such in tables of organization and in budgets. Other new categories were rules and work routines.

Bureaucratic Indulgency Patterns.   Not all organizational tensions necessitate bureaucratic rules. In his research, Gouldner observed some nonbureaucratic ways to manage human-generated tensions. Gouldner's notions of "structural adaptation" and "indulgency pattern" refer to both the selective exercise of supervisory authority as well as the nonenforcement of certain rules. He observed that supervisory personnel often allowed subordinates to bypass many rules and requirements. In the factory, workers would routinely punch in to work late, take coffee breaks, and socialize. While each of these actions violated a formal rule or procedure, supervisors permitted this behavior.

Gouldner believed that supervisors anticipate the consequences of stringent enforcement and settle instead on a posture of tolerance and indulgences because the ceaseless exercise of supervisory authority would produce resentment among the workers and a very unpleasant work environment. This would then make it difficult to gain worker cooperation if and when workers were needed to assist the supervisors with work tasks outside their immediate job responsibility. Supervisors had to exercise flexibility *with* workers if they were to expect flexibility *by* workers.

The importance of worker flexibility is powerfully demonstrated when workers employ a "work-to-rule" strategy against managers. Under a work-to-rule strategy, workers carry out only those tasks defined by their formal job description. That strict adherence to formal job requirements can be used as a weapon against management exposes the inadequacy of formalized procedure for the day-to-day functioning of the organization. All organizations, bureaucratic or otherwise, rely on organizational members to step out of their formal job descriptions and respond flexibly to unexpected demands. The work-to-rule strategy also reveals the creative capacity of humans to utilize formal structure as a resource to advance their particular interests.

Peter Blau: Dynamics of Bureaucracy

Peter Blau's (1955) study of federal and state bureaucratic agencies reported findings consistent with the patterns observed by Gouldner. Blau brought a "functional approach" to his analysis that focused upon the consequences of bureaucratic actions and routines. He was primarily concerned with determining whether bureaucratic procedures accomplished agency objectives and produced the expected organizational behavior. As a student of Merton, Blau suspected that bureaucratic procedures might generate various unanticipated consequences.

In the case study of a state unemployment agency, Blau reported various forms of innovation and adjustment that deviated from the prescribed rules and procedures. In this particular agency, job-seeking "clients" are screened by a receptionist who schedules appointments with "interviewers." The interviewers determine the job skills and prospects of the clients and assist in their job placement. An immediate appointment with an interviewer is granted only if clients have a high likelihood of finding employment. However, in the face-to-face interaction with the clients, receptionists did not feel comfortable delaying the appointment. This would send the wrong message to clients—that the agency was not interested in them or deemed them unemployable.

According to Blau, this pattern of receptionist behavior could be attributed to the design of the agency as a service organization for people in need of assistance. Further, face-to-face interaction made it difficult to apply impersonal scheduling rules. This is also a clear example of how organizational behavior, in violation of formal protocol, emerges out of the human interactions that take place in a context where actions are highly symbolic. In this particular case, the receptionist bypassed the official rules because they were perceived as symbolically inconsistent with the purpose of the agency and symbolically detrimental to a client's self-esteem. The alternative and unofficial course of action was considered more symbolically supportive of a client's needs. These kinds of dynamics are persistent aspects of organizational life.

The greater impact of the receptionists behavior, however, was to increase the interviewers' workload. This might have created some tension between receptionists and interviewers if it were not for the manner in which interviewers were evaluated. Evaluations of performance were based on the number of job placements, known as statistical performance records, that interviewers made. Therefore, even though the behavior of receptionists increased interviewer workload, it also improved the chances of an increased number of placements.

The method for evaluating the performance of the interviewers was a major focus of Blau's study. The evaluation procedure based on the number of placements was presumed to be the most objective and rational means to measure performance. In practice, however, it had numerous dysfunctional consequences. For example, the desire to maximize job placements and receive a favorable evaluation led interviewers to horde job information, compete directly with other interviewers, and falsify their records to indicate success. Since the statistical performance records were purely quantitative, many clients were placed in inappropriate positions. These counted as placements for the interviewers and thus enhanced their performance record. Interviewers even took credit for placements that involved the return of clients to their original job after a layoff period. According to Blau, all of these practices represented a "displacement of goals." Maximizing the statistical performance record took precedence over larger organizational objectives.

It should be noted that the statistical performance records were a managerial technique originally designed to motivate and ensure the accountability of the interviewers. Blau reported that the system was disliked by the interviewers because of the competition and lack of cooperation it tended to generate. These pressures eventually resulted in various revisions to the evaluation system.

Blau observed similar patterns of innovation and adaptation in the department of a federal agency responsible for enforcing laws regulating corporate financial transactions and accounting. The agents in this department were responsible for auditing the books and records of firms to determine the accuracy of information and compliance with legal regulations. According to the formal procedure, if agents had any doubt about how to rule on a financial entry or transaction, they were required to check with a supervisor. In practice, however, agents rarely consulted with supervisors.

Blau offered two reasons for this behavior. First, the complex nature of the task raised constant questions and doubts about various financial transactions and entries. Rather than take the time to consult with a supervisor, the agents found it more convenient to consult with fellow agents who may have had past experiences with similar problems. This action could be justified on efficiency grounds because other agents were in closer physical proximity than supervisors. Second, agents reasoned that constant consultation with supervisors regarding decisions and rulings would expose their ignorance and therefore have a negative impact on performance evaluations. And, if further justification was needed, the agents did not wish to disturb supervisors who obviously had other more important matters to deal with.

The emergent interaction and sharing of information and advice among the agents created a work environment characterized by collaboration and horizontal communication. It is interesting to note that what emerged informally and in violation of formal procedures is a widely prescribed and encouraged organizational arrangement in today's organizations.

The observations of agent behavior led Blau to the general conclusion that employees in bureaucratic organizations will avoid the unpleasant aspects of official procedures (e.g., consulting with supervisors) and will pursue instead alternative and available forms of behavior congenial with their interests (e.g., conferring with co-workers). The resulting behavior will then be justified in the context of larger organizational values. In this particular case, the innovative behavior of the agents was based largely on their perceived interests, but they explained and justified it in the name of efficiency and rationality.

Underlying this tendency to pursue alternative courses of action is the more fundamental reflexive capacity of employees to assess their behavior in terms of their values as well as how others will interpret that behavior. In the end, these deviations from prescribed procedure became the emergent norm. The informal relations that developed among the agents served a valuable solidarity function as well as a form of mutual information exchange. It also may have created a more efficient operation, as the agents claimed.

Blau's observations further reinforced the view that bureaucratic organizations did not necessarily produce mechanical followers of rules and regulations. Like Gouldner, he noted that many bureaucratic procedures and routines were seen by both subordinate and managerial employees as annoyances to be avoided rather than guidelines to be obeyed. Blau did not discover rigid and inflexible followers of bureaucratic rules, nor did he find support for the argument that bureaucratic structures produce overconformity, ritualism, or resistance to change.

This final point should be emphasized since the arguments about the negative human impact of bureaucracy play to a sympathetic audience and have become almost axiomatic. The criticisms of bureaucratic organization are based on the assumption that organizational systems have the power to dominate human beings, and that human beings lack the capacities to resist these powers. The studies of Blau and Gouldner point to a much more complicated picture that demonstrates the human capacities for innovation, resistance, and agency in bureaucratic organizations. Workers employ alternative means to achieve goals, they force supervisory personnel to revise strategies for compliance, and their actions generate tensions that result in the reformulation of bureaucratic procedures.

Philip Selznick: Bureaucracy as Institution

The final classic study of the unintended consequences of bureaucracy, Philip Selznick's (1949) analysis of the Tennessee Valley Authority, yields further evidence of the role of human action in producing deviations from formal rational goal attainment. In terms of the dynamic forces within the organization, Selznick identified the uniquely human elements that convert the organization from "a lean, no-nonsense system of consciously co-ordinated activities" to a "natural product of social needs and pressures" (1957:5). In Selznick's theory of organization, which he applied to his study of the TVA, he viewed "delegation as the primordial organizational act, a precarious venture which requires the continuous elaboration of formal mechanisms of coordination and control" (1948:25).

This is another example of the agency problem. The inherent contradictions involved in the act of delegating organizational responsibilities derive from, on the one hand, the desire for formal machinelike social control and, on the other hand, the inevitable delegation allowing for freedom and autonomy of action. Thus, as Selznick noted, the formal structures

> never succeed in conquering the nonrational dimensions of organizational behavior. The latter remain at once indispensable to the continued existence of the system of coordination and at the same time the source of friction, dilemma, doubt, and ruin. The fundamental paradox arises from the fact that rational action systems are inescapably imbedded in an *institutional* matrix (1948:25).

In terms of organizational members, they clearly fall into the category of what Selznick referred to as the "recalcitrant tools of action." Recalcitrant tools are influenced by larger commitments that prevent and constrain organizational rationality. Humans are recalcitrant tools to the extent that they transport and develop commitments that conflict with rational organizational purpose as defined by organizational owners. Selznick emphasized that humans operate as "wholes" rather than simply as the occupants of a formal role. This is an impediment to formal rationality because non-work-related roles and personality traits tend to deviate from those prescribed by the formal bureaucratic structure. As institutions, organizations must attend to the needs and commitments of these recalcitrant tools of action and, in the process, organizations adapt, evolve, and drift.

Robert Jackall: Bureaucracy as a Moral Maze

A more recent sociological analysis of how humans navigate their way through the bureaucratic morass is found in Robert Jackall's *Moral Mazes: The World of Corporate Managers* (1988). Jackall interviewed and observed corporate managers in a large textile firm, a chemical division of a large conglomerate, and a public relations agency. The purpose of his study was to gauge the way bureaucracy shapes moral consciousness and produces a bureaucratic ethic. Jackall reported a somewhat more powerful bureaucratic influence than Gouldner, Blau, or Selznick.

> [B]ureaucratic work causes people to bracket, while at work, the moralities that they might hold outside the workplace or that they might adhere to privately and to follow instead the prevailing morality of their particular organizational situation. . . what matters on a day-to-day basis are the moral rules-in-use fashioned within the personal and structural constraints of one's organization (1988:6).

Recall that Weber advanced a principle of rational legal authority based on formal positions of command and a belief by organizational members that this is a rationally superior arrangement. In the organizations studied by Jackall, authority is not a distant abstraction but one experienced in day-to-day personal relationships with bosses. These relationships and the actual rules-in-use that prescribe appropriate behavior take on the character of a *patrimonial bureaucracy.* Personal loyalty is the primary rule of behavior for managers. While this can be placed in an instrumental or rational context, it departs radically from Weberian notions of rational or instrumental action. Patrimonial bureaucracy supports behavior in which subordinates must symbolically reinforce at every turn their own subordination and willing acceptance of the obligations of fealty. In return, subordinates can hope for those perks that the boss can distribute: "the better, more attractive secretaries, or the nudging of a movable panel to enlarge [their] office, and perhaps a couch to fill the added space, one of the real distinctions in corporate bureaucracies" (1988:19).

There is a clear calculation here—of means and ends—but this is not quite what efficiency experts have in mind. In contrast to the rational bureaucratic principle that organizational behavior is directed toward the larger goals of the organization, or that rewards are allocated to those who advance these goals, Jackall's research supports the work of Offe (1976) who found that *symbolic substitutes* determine the allocation of rewards. Deferential forms of behavior are used as a substitute for other criteria, such as effectiveness, efficiency, and competence. This is not an uncommon practice given that it is difficult and costly to accurately or objectively measure one's contribution to an organization. Jackall (1988:64) noted that management evaluation criteria—"judgment and decision-making ability, creativeness, leadership, communication, working with others, and so on—is highly subjective and prone to a wide range of interpretation." Second, much of the symbolic behavior advances the interests of the immediate boss, who benefits from the patrimonial relationships that are so prevalent in the organizations studied by Jackall.

Alongside the personal, patron-client, relationships between corporate managers and their bosses are *circles of affiliation.* These alliances or networks within the firm do not correspond to the formal or rational-legal channels of communication that might be reflected in the organizational chart. Their crucial feature, according to Jackall (1988:39–41) is the use of informal criteria for admission, that are poorly defined and constantly changing. These informal criteria, that determine success and failure, have a weak relationship with one's personal accomplishments. Therefore, "The real task for the ambitious manager then becomes how to shape and keep shaping others' perceptions of oneself—that is, how to influence favorably or alter if necessary the cognitive maps of others in the central political networks of the organization—so that one becomes seen as 'promotable' " (1988:64). One's position and standing in this informal social structure both shape behavior and determine prospects for mobility. Symbolic interactions play a central role in this process.

If a single lesson is to be learned from Jackall's analysis, it is that the rationality assumed to operate at the level of the organization has been creatively adopted by organizational members. This does not mean they have been duped, brainwashed, or ideologically dominated. Rather, it signifies what the sociologist Karl Mannheim (1940) described as *self-rationalization.* As described by Jackall (1988:59), this involves "self-streamlining, that is, the systematic application of functional rationality to the self to attain certain individual ends" which he argued "is useful in understanding one of the central social psychological processes of organizational life. In a world where appearances—in the broadest sense—mean everything, the wise and ambitious manager learns to cultivate assiduously the proper, prescribed modes of appearing."

In this passage, Jackall viewed the presentation of self in the organization as a form of self-rationalization. If organizational rationalization is the construction of structures to achieve a particular goal, then self-rationalization is the creation of a persona, or image, as a means to achieve the goal of personal advancement.

Taken together, the case study literature on bureaucratic processes identifies the role of human action and interaction in reshaping, redirecting, and distorting the formal rationality of bureaucratic organization. W. Richard Scott (1981) referred to this literature as a "natural system approach" because the emphasis on the human factor makes organizations similar to other social groups and/or institutions.

The social and human aspects of organizational life also highlight the irrational, dysfunctional, and unpredictable character of organizations. This was clearly recognized by the human relations theorists who emphasized the emergence of emotions, sentiments, and informal group behavior in formal organizations. More generally, the commitments and orientations that workers carry into organizations can serve as impediments to administrative objectives and control; the reflexive interpretation of rules and procedures can result in innovation and adjustment; the development and revision of bureaucratic practices is the product of "human striving."

As Michael Crozier (1964:179) has commented, "In human relations terms, dysfunction appears to be the consequence of the resistance of the human factor to standardized behavior that is imposed upon it mechanically." These studies of bureaucracy confirm that humans are neither the receptacles of instrumental rationality nor the mindless followers of procedure. Rather, humans create the tensions, conflicts, and dynamism in bureaucratic structures and, through the exercise of their capacities, reshape the internal structures of organization.

Operationalizing the Rational Model: Administrative Science

The translation of the rational-bureaucratic logic into management and administrative principles represents the most direct relationship between organization theory and management practice. A number of organization and management theorists have attempted to apply the logic of rational bureaucracy to specific organizational structures and practices. The intended consequence is to enhance the rationality and efficiency of the operation.

Henri Fayol

Henri Fayol (1919: published in 1949) was perhaps the first to present some explicit guidelines on how to structure the organization. Best known for his definition of management—which he reduced to the five functions of planning, organizing, commanding, coordinating, and controlling—Fayol advanced a set of administrative principles that were based on his experience as an engineer and managing director of a mining-metallurgy enterprise. These principles included the division of work and specialization, the right to exercise authority and issue commands, discipline, the unity of command, the unity of direction, subordination of individual interest to organizational goals, remuneration, the scalar chain, achievement of material and social order, equity, stability of tenure, opportunities for the display of initiative, and esprit de corps. Each of these principles were further elaborated and refined by later management theorists (Gulick and Urwick 1937; Mooney and Reiley 1939) and remain an integral part of managerial training to the present day .

What is interesting about the principles, when taken as a whole, is the way they combine formal structural prescriptions (such as the unity of command in which each worker has only one boss) with informal nonstructural precepts (such as equity—a "combination of kindliness and justice"—and esprit de corps). While the former can be built into the organizational chart and be included as part of a job description, the latter cannot be formalized. Both the demand for and the implementation of the informal precepts reflect the uncertainty that characterizes formal organizational control and coordination. Further, the recourse to the informal precepts reflects a recognition that formal-rational structural principles are insufficient means for the generation of compliance and cooperation and that one must also pay attention to the noninstrumental side of human existence through the provision of equity and an esprit de corps.

James Mooney and Allen Reiley

The combination of rational administrative principles with less-formalized modes of human control exists as a constant tension in the administrative literature. In their influential work, *The Principles of Organization* (1939), Mooney and Reiley began with an elaboration of core management principles. These are the formal procedures for integrating and dividing the various tasks (functionalization) and implementing a system of hierarchical control (coordination and scalar principles).

The later chapters in their book are devoted to various problems that emerge in the practice of administration. In a chapter titled "Internal Problems of Modern Industrial Organization," Mooney and Reiley admitted that the application of these principles may be difficult because "the industrial engineer is faced with the proposition of determining how a common understanding, a full loyalty and a clear discharge of duty and responsibility can be achieved." This managerial dilemma has its source in the simultaneous need to coordinate, on the one hand, and allow for some freedom of action, on the other. To deal with this challenge, the manager

> must study human friction as well as the mechanical variety, and find out how to reduce it . . . Foremost in dealing with this problem is the vital matter of indoctrination . . . it seeks to establish a community of understanding . . . it brings into play the strongest disciplinary force evidenced in human history, the power of faith . . . when the laborer and the boss are bound by the same common understanding of some common purpose, the discipline is on a plane that no other form can reach (1939:173–78).

Again, we see that the formal structural prescriptions for the functioning of the organization are, by themselves, inadequate. The organization also requires an ideological or normative lubricant to reduce human friction and ensure the exercise of duty, responsibility, and discipline. This observation is based on practical managerial experience; both Mooney and Reiley gained their insights as executives for General Motors.

Herbert Simon

The work of Herbert Simon and his colleagues represents one of the most influential efforts to link the abstract principles of the rational model with concrete decision-making processes. This is clearly illustrated in Simon's analysis of the problems in applying the standard litany of administrative principles.

Contradictory Proverbs.   In his classic article, "The Proverbs of Administration" (1946), Simon noted that for almost every administrative principle "one can find an equally plausible and acceptable contradictory principle." For example, the unity of command principle recommends that each organizational member should have only one superior from whom he or she receives directives. However, this principle conflicts with the principle of specialization prescribing the authoritative input of specialists on decisions relevant to their particular area of expertise. The latter principle would suggest multiple directives from various specialists.

A second example is found in the span of control principle advising that the number of subordinates for each superior should be kept to a relatively small and manageable number. The implementation of this principle will result in an elongated hierarchical structure with an excessive number of levels through which communications would travel. Thus, the span of control principle would ultimately result in a potentially less efficient organizational structure. Simon provided numerous illustrations of this general problem with administrative theory. The internally contradictory nature of administrative principles are the result, according to Simon, of "superficiality, oversimplification, [and] lack of realism." Administrative theory "has confined itself too closely to the mechanism of authority and has failed to bring within its orbit the other equally important modes of influence on organizational behavior" (1946:64).

Simon's primary objection to administrative theory relates to the lack of sufficient attention to the human factor of production and, more specifically, the way humans go about making decisions in structured settings. A set of structural imperatives about the division of work and authority cannot be applied to organizations without a clearer sense of how these will affect organizational behavior. This general criticism could have led Simon in many different theoretical directions, but his devotion to rationality and the achievement of organizational goals led him to develop instead a model of humans that would be more realistic, on the one hand, and would contribute to rational control, on the other.

Bounded Rationality.   Simon is best known for developing, with James March, the concept of *bounded rationality*. Simon and March (1958) argued that the assumptions of human rationality had to be replaced by a more realistic conception of human capacities. With regard to decision making, humans are limited in (1) the amount of information they can access and process, (2) the number of possible alternatives they are able to entertain, and (3) their ability to predict the consequences of their actions. These human limitations create bounds on the capacity for rational decision making. Thus, March and Simon suggested that the rational economic human who made optimal decisions should be replaced with the administrative human who made satisfactory decisions. They believed that satisfactory decisions were, in most cases, enough for the efficient operation and realization of the goals of the firm.

The limitations on rational decision making has also been a major theme in the literature of public administration. In addition to the obstacles identified by March and Simon, Carl Lutrin and Allen Settle (1967:95) noted the following constraints:

- Unwillingness or inability to make decisions.
- Tendency to make snap decisions on the basis of incomplete information or superficial evidence.
- Acceptance of the most readily available short-range solutions.

- Making false analogies between old and new experiences or even relying on past experiences.
- Oversimplifying.
- Relying on preconceived assumptions.
- Group think.

Similarly, Harold Gortner's (1977:115–16) analysis of public-sector decision making led him to argue that:

> One of the most important factors that must be considered when discovering the limitations of rationality in decision making is that of the personal, or psychological, factors that influence the decision maker . . . The most common types of psychological barriers can be grouped into five general categories: (1) the determination of thought by position in social space; (2) the projection of values and attitudes; (3) oversimplification; (4) cognitive nearsightedness; and (5) identification with outside groups.

While the inability (or difficulty) to realize rational action might be viewed as a major organizational shortcoming, it can often permit an organization to exert greater control over the decisions and behavior of organizational members (Perrow 1986:121–22).

In Simon's model, organizations provide a context that is designed both to simplify and support the decision-making process of organizational participants. As with most rational models, goals play a central role. Here Simon viewed them as mechanisms that restrict the ends toward which activity is directed. More specifically, they supply what Simon referred to as "value premises" and "factual premises." *Value premises* pertain to the preferred or desired ends (sometimes termed "goal specificity"). *Factual premises* pertain to the means for achieving the desired ends (the formalized methods). The notion of premises is important because it suggests a set of accepted "givens" that people take for granted and carry in their heads, and which they access when a decision must be made. Establishing these premises contributes to the organizational control of the human factor:

> Given a complete set of value and factual premises, there is only one decision that is consistent with rationality. That is, with a given system of values, and a specified set of alternatives, there is one alternative that is preferable to the others.
>
> The behavior of a rational person can be controlled, therefore, if the value and factual premises upon which he bases his decision are specified for him (Simon 1976:223).

This particular model of decision making may be difficult to apply to decision making in the public sector. Organization theorists who study public administration are more likely to reject any assumption about rational decision making because public-sector policy decisions—both means and ends—are subject to enormous debate and difference of opinion. Thus, value and factual premises are constantly being contested. For this reason, decision making is described as a process of *incrementalism.* Compromises are made with the knowledge that there is no single or final solution (Lindblom 1959; Downs 1967). Rather, small steps are taken in agreed upon directions that do not pose any fundamental challenge to the status quo or entrenched interests. Gortner (1977:109) concluded: "[I]n making decisions dealing with public policy, there is seldom any agreement on the goals, nor is it possible to get much agreement; therefore, the incremental model of decision making is used."

The sense that decision making and problem solving are often more difficult in the public sector than in the private sector is captured in Horst Rittel and Melvin Webber's (1973) distinction between "tame" and "wicked" problems. *Tame problems* tend to be easily defined with the primary challenge involving the technical means to solve the problem and achieve success. *Wicked problems,* in contrast, are those for which it is difficult to establish an agreed-upon definition and for which it is equally difficult to determine whether a successful solution has been achieved. Government tends to take on and attempts to develop policies to solve wicked problems such as unequal opportunity and crime. Definitions, solutions, and measures of success for these kinds of problems are highly contested and subject to a wide range of interpretations.

Unobtrusive Control and Simplifying Assumptions.   In concluding this section, it is important to note that Simon's theory of administrative behavior, which has had an enormous influence on organization theory, developed as a corrective to the administrative principles that assumed structural arrangements would automatically generate the desired behavior from organizational members. Not only were the principles contradictory, but there was no clear specification about the actual process that results in the translation of formal structural constraints into rational organizational behavior ("the process of choice which leads to action"). Thus, Simon developed a model of bounded rationality that was supplemented by a more realistic theory of decision making. The use of value and factual premises is a powerful form of "unobtrusive control" (Perrow 1986) over human behavior. The organization provides the premises, the subgoals, the submeans, and the routine procedures which in turn impel organizational decisions.

Consistent with the view that organizations are rational instruments, however, Simon also regarded individuals as tools or objects and, accordingly, he constructed a model of human behavior that is limiting. "It calls for simplifying models of *individual* behavior in order to capture the complexities of *organizational* behavior" (Perrow 1986:122). While this is a standard and possibly unavoidable tendency of organization theory, it is especially applicable to individual-level decision theories. In the end, Simon's theory of administration and its assumptions about the human factor can be subjected to some of the same criticisms he himself leveled against the administrative proverbs and rational human principles.

Simon's subsequent theoretical work (1997) and, in particular, that of his associates, Richard Cyert and James March (1992), has attempted to deal with these problems by introducing the notion of organizations as coalitions made up of individuals and parties that have divergent interests and goals. Cyert and March have also considered the impact of new organizational members who transport interests and goals, formulated in other organizations and social spheres, into the organization. These revisions to the theory of organizational rationality serve to acknowledge the complexity of the human factor as well as the human forces that contribute to organizational dynamics.

Bureaucratic Rationalization and Domination

Arguments of Classical and Critical Social Theory

Bureaucracy is often accused of suffocating the human spirit and robbing organizational participants of their freedom and dignity. Many of the arguments about the dominating power of bureaucratic organization originated in the classical social theory of Weber, Marx, and Durkheim. For Weber, the modern forces of rationalization promoted the bureaucratic form that enhanced efficiency while stifling affective human relations. For Marx, the bureaucratic work organization of capitalism was the "hidden abode" in which humans were unable to realize their full potential as human species. For Durkheim, the rise of instrumental social relations and the division of labor raised the specter of disintegration, normlessness, and anomie. In all three cases, bureaucratic organization has negative human consequences.

Of the three theorists, it was Weber who directed the greatest attention to the relationship between capitalist modernization, rationalization, and bureaucracy. In spite of his ideal type construct of bureaucratic principles, Weber also took the most pessimistic view regarding the impact of bureaucratic modes of organization on the individual.

> Its specific nature, which is welcomed by capitalism, develops the more perfectly the more bureaucracy is "dehumanized," the more completely it succeeds in eliminating from official business love, hatred, and all purely personal, irrational, and emotional elements which escape calculation. This is the specific nature of bureaucracy and it is appraised as its special virtue (Weber 1946:215–16).

Weber's general assessment of bureaucratic organization has had a lasting impact on social theory in general and critical social theory in particular.

One of the central concerns of *critical social theory* has been the manner in which modern rational bureaucratic institutions attempt to gain mastery over the forces of nature through the application of the scientific method ("instrumental reason") and technology. Technology-based rationality was originally conceived as a way to liberate and emancipate humans from the problems of scarcity, ignorance, irrationality, and inefficiency. Critical social theorists (Horkheimer and Adorno 1976; Marcuse 1964), however, have argued that these instruments of human progress turn out to be the central sources of human oppression. The control of nature through science and technology extends to the domination of humans through bureaucratic forms of social organization. Technical rationality becomes a tool of organizational and ideological social control. Humans are socialized, or indoctrinated, to accept their own oppression as rational.

These linkages between the theory and practice of organizations, and the science and ideology of rationality, represent the central theme in Robert Denhardt's *In the Shadow of Organization* (1981). Denhardt argued that organizations, like science, "developed out of an interest in controlling nature, in conquering natural forces" and it is a short "transition from the domination of nature to the domination of other human beings" (p. 89). Technological rationality treats both natural and human entities as objects. As the logic of science spills over into the realm of administration, all human subjects are treated as manipulable objects.

In the rational-bureaucratic model of organization, the primary emphasis is placed on the means and methods to achieve particular ends. This feature of technological rationality is viewed favorably by administrators because it "can help eliminate those bothersome, inefficient, human qualities, such as feelings, that interfere with rational endeavor" (Denhardt 1981:28). Denhardt concluded that the impersonal treatment of humans in organizations ultimately affects the way we define our identities and results in "a life devoid of self-reflection" and a preoccupation with achievement and performance.

> The human characteristics and behaviors that deviate from the rational model of administration are eventually subjected to self-censorship.

In the tradition of critical theory, Denhardt attributed great power to the force of technical rationality. As an awesome form of domination, it squelches and suppresses those human characteristics and capacities that are at odds with the single-minded purpose of administration. In short, the rational-bureaucratic organization emerges victorious in the effort to control the human factor of production.

However, Denhardt left open the possibility of some form of resistance to the technically rational onslaught. In Denhardt's analysis, a glimmer of hope is found in the "shadow" of organization, which refers to Carl Jung's notion of the underutilized and neglected drives and desires of humans. While rational-bureaucratic organizations discourage and sublimate "irrational" drives and desires, they remain in the shadow as a form of potential opposition that can surface to challenge and negate instrumental rationality. Denhardt did not follow this line of reasoning to its logical conclusion, which would suggest a constant tension and conflict between human actions and organizational principles. This would also yield, in a dialectical manner, constant and subtle forms of opposition, accommodation, and the transformation of organizational arrangements.

Denhardt and the critical theorists tended to accept Weber's "iron cage" formulation while at the same time they minimized the human capacity for resistance and opposition. Gouldner (1955) referred to this tendency as the "metaphysical pathos" that pervaded theories of bureaucratic organization. It assumes an inevitable march toward a rigid division of labor, impersonal rules and regulations, an entrenched oligarchy, and effective control of subordinates.

There is a serious problem with this logic. It takes the purpose and intent of technical rationality, and the associated assumptions that humans can be treated as objects and means, as accomplished facts under modern capitalism. What might be wishful thinking among the dominant class and the managerial agents of social control—that humans can be molded, duped, and manipulated—is accepted as the defining characteristic of bureaucratic societies. This ignores the human capacity for reflexivity, transcendence, agency and, ultimately, opposition and resistance. These capacities do not automatically prevent or preclude the forms of structural control, class domination, or ideological inculcation that characterize all societies. They do, however, make their accomplishment much more difficult and eliminate the possibility that social control can be realized in a once-and-for-all manner.

Bureaucratic Domination and Marxist Theory

The profound impact of the bureaucratic domination perspective extends beyond the Weberian model of organization to Marxist theories of the labor process. The tendency to overestimate the ability of organizational forms to dominate and subordinate the human factor is found in some of the major Marxist works on organization (Clawson 1980; Marglin 1974). Most notable is Harry Braverman's *Labor and Monopoly Capital* (1974), which pointed to a fundamental aspect of all work organizations—the *control* of factors of production, generally, and the labor power of workers, specifically.

The emphasis on control and domination is consistent with the thrust of critical social theory. For Braverman, the application of science and technology to the labor process represented "weapons of domination in the creation, perpetuation and deepening of a gulf between classes in society" (1974:6). His insightful analysis of Taylorism and scientific management highlighted the role of management strategies designed to reduce the power and knowledge held by workers.

Braverman extended his analysis of scientific management and the division of the labor into the 20th century. He argued that there has been a ceaseless and progressive application of scientific management principles toward all forms of work. This has resulted, according to Braverman, in the continual *de-skilling* of all jobs and the continued separation of mental and manual labor. Thus, in this scheme all jobs, including white-collar and service occupations, are "proletarianized"; that is, they take on the character of blue-collar factory work that is repetitive, monotonous, and devoid of any opportunity to exercise mental conceptual skills in the labor process. The private ownership of the means of production and the ability of managers to organize the production process using rational bureaucratic principles are the central conditions allowing for the domination of the working class by the capitalist class. More specifically, the continued division and subdivision of the labor process into simple and highly specialized tasks serves to reduce skill requirements, reduce wages and salaries, increase productivity, and, most important, extend control over the working population. If you extend this argument to emerging organizational forms, you would conclude that all work will become more specialized and less skilled.

The accumulated evidence of trends in the organization of work and the task composition of jobs does not support this scenario (Form 1987; Howell and Wolff 1991). Studies of specific occupations that have undergone transformation point to a combination of de-skilling in some areas and re-skilling in others. Some jobs become more specialized and less skilled, while others expand their breadth of responsibilities both manually and mentally. One of the most rigorous empirical analyses of changing skill composition from 1960 to 1985 in the United States reported a *net increase* in the cognitive and interaction components of jobs (Howell and Wolff 1991). While there are a variety of possible explanations for this finding, nonetheless the progressive de-skilling and proletarianization of all jobs has not occurred. Thus, the thesis of the bureaucratic organization as an instrument advancing toward greater and more sophisticated forms of domination must look to other mechanisms of social control.

Consistent with our emphasis on tension, contradiction, and the perpetual problem of controlling the human factor, a number of further observations are in order. First, while de-skilling and specialization might be driven by an economic rationale from the perspective of the capitalist owner, they can also have a number of unintended consequences. The homogenization of labor can contribute to the development of a more cohesive common bond among a greater proportion of the workforce within and across organizations. This can enhance the likelihood of communication, organization, and collective action in opposition to the prerogatives of capital.

Second, there is evidence that some skill is relocated to other positions or sections of the organizational hierarchy; for example, to supervisory or middle management layers. This may hamper the efficiency and increase the cost structure of the firm. During the economic crises of the 1970s and 1980s, organizations expanded middle management forms of "guard labor" to control and supervise the labor force (Gordon 1996). This ultimately produced a costly layer of management fat that prolonged the crisis of productivity and profitability. This is a powerful illustration of the unintended consequences of seemingly economically rational decisions.

Third, as the example from David Gordon suggests and the human factor perspective argues, the subjective and behavioral response of workers to the strategies of de-skilling and proletarianization can nullify the anticipated economic gains. These can include declines in worker effort, commitment, and loyalty as well as increases in turnover and absenteeism. As we shall consider in Chapter 6, recent innovations and trends in management, while still designed to maximize productivity and profit, have employed strategies that expand, rather than restrict, the range of tasks and responsibilities.

Richard Edwards's neo-Marxist analysis of the labor process also centers on the concept of social class control but, unlike Braverman, Edwards recognized that the human factor of production cannot be easily dominated or subordinated.

> While the distinct and antagonistic interests of workers and employers necessitate strategies of managerial control, control is rendered problematic because, unlike the other commodities involved in production, labor power is always embodied in people, who have their own interests and needs and who retain their power to resist being treated like a commodity (Edwards 1979:12).

Edwards outlined the historical evolution of managerial control strategies shaped by "intensifying conflict" and "contradiction in the firm's operations" rather than a single instrument or logic of control. He analyzed three forms of control: direct, technical, and bureaucratic. *Direct control* involves the personal exercise of authority by bosses over their workers. *Technical control* refers to the application of technologies, such as the assembly line, that control the pace of the labor process. *Bureaucratic control,* which is of the greatest interest for our present purposes, ties the control of workers to the formal structure and social relations of the bureaucratic organization. Edwards (1979:21) wrote:

> The defining feature of bureaucratic control is the institutionalization of hierarchical power. "Rule of law"—the firm's law—replaces "rule by supervisory command" in the direction of work, the procedures for evaluating workers' performance, and the exercise of the firm's sanctions and rewards; supervisors and workers alike become subject to the dictate of "company policy." Work becomes highly stratified; each job is given its distinct title and description; and impersonal rules govern promotion. "Stick with the corporation," the worker is told, "and you can ascend up the ladder." The company promises the workers a career.

Bureaucracy's Other Face

Critical social theory and Marxist literature point to the way bureaucracy is used as an instrument of human control and manipulation. While not always successful, and often producing unintended consequences, bureaucracy can clearly be employed as a tool or strategy for domination. This is the dark side of bureaucracy that tends to receive the greatest attention. But is there another side to bureaucracy that can help explain why almost every organization employs some degree of formalized rules and procedures? Is it really the case that all forms of bureaucratic procedures are noxious and alienating? Recall that Gouldner (1954) made a distinction between mock, punishment-centered, and representative bureaucracy. These different forms indicate that some bureaucratic rules are irrelevant while others are supported by almost all members of the organization.

A similar distinction is noted by Paul Adler and Bryan Borys (1996) who identified two types of formalization: coercive and enabling. They challenged the widespread assumption that bureaucratic procedures are inevitably oppressive and antithetical to the interests of most organizational members. "Something is missing from these accounts: Surely employees' attitudes to formalization depend on the attributes of the type of formalization with which they are confronted." Adler and Borys wanted to "develop a way to distinguish good from bad rules." This led them to conclude that *enabling bureaucracy* is designed to enable employees to manage problems and make decisions. Enabling rules formalize the best and most effective practices and routines, and develop procedures that are responsive to practical work-related demands (1996:69–71). The enabling elements of bureaucracy are not only favorably received by employees, but they may often be demanded. It is not uncommon to find organizational members requesting or wishing there were some written instruction on how to solve a problem or navigate through the organization. Perrow (1986:26) wrote:

> "There ought to be a rule" is as valid as saying "there are too damn many rules around here." Rules do a lot of things in organizations: they protect as well as restrict; coordinate as well as block; channel effort as well as limit it . . . Social scientists, no less than the persons on the street, love to denounce them and propose ruleless organizations. But ruleless organizations are likely to be either completely automated . . . or completely professionalized . . . only a tiny fraction of organizations fit either case.

Bureaucratic rules and procedures are likely to persist in all organizations, so it is important to consider both their enabling and coercive features. They not only enable organizational actors to get certain things accomplished, but can also be used by subordinates as strategic weapons against superordinates. Gouldner's punishment-centered bureaucracy could be imposed from the bottom up in restricting the actions of superordinate managerial personnel. The work-to-rule strategy is used as a strategic weapon enabling workers to advance their interests. Greater attention needs to be devoted to these instances of "subversive rationalization" (Feenberg 1998) in which formal means are directed toward the realization of subordinate goals (see also Hodson 1995; Fantasia 1988).

McDonaldization: Diffusion of the Bureaucratic Ethos

If rational bureaucratic principles are a fundamental feature of all organizations and if we spend most of our lives either working for or being served by organizations, then the bureaucratic ethos will permeate almost every aspect of our lives. While such a rationalization of social life was posed by critical theorists in terms of domination, a more insidious form has been identified by George Ritzer in the guise of McDonaldization. In his now famous piece of popular sociology, *The McDonaldization of Society* (1993), Ritzer gave label and life to the "process by which the principles of the fast-food restaurant are coming to dominate more and more sectors of American society as well as the rest of the world." These include dieting, education, the family, health care, leisure, politics, travel, work, and nearly all aspects of society (1993:1).

The Principles of McDonaldization

McDonaldization is based on four interrelated principles that are closely associated with Weber's ideal type bureaucracy: efficiency, calculability, predictability, control. The fast-food industry is widely regarded as the one place where these organizational principles are employed appropriately and successfully (Morgan 1997: chap. 1). We can therefore discuss the principles in this context and then note their diffusion beyond the fast-food industry.

Efficiency is the more familiar term used to describe a formally rational process that employs the best and quickest means to achieve a particular goal. The provision of fast food can be regarded as efficient in that it is the best means of "getting from a state of being hungry to a state of being full." The various processes that enhance this efficiency include burgers cooked and produced on an assembly line, customers driving through or walking up to the counter, self-seating, no waiting for tables, cash on delivery of the food, no tipping, no bill paying, and self cleanup. It is important to note that this system is as dependent on well- trained customers as on well-trained employees.

Calculation, or calculability, is the attempt to measure, calculate, and quantify every aspect of the organizational process and product. In the fast-food restaurant, every element of food preparation is measured and timed. The 1.6 ounce precooked hamburger is exactly 3.875 inches in diameter, fitting on a bun that is 3.5 inches in diameter. Size and quantity are emphasized and reflected in the name of the menu items—Big Mac, Whopper, Whaler, Big Bite, and Super Big Gulp. Quantity takes precedence over quality or, to put it differently, the large quantity compensates for the low quality.

Predictability is built into the McDonaldization process in the way the food is prepared and delivered and in terms of the mutual expectations on both sides of the counter. The precisely timed, measured, and mass-produced fast food is based on the assumption that customers know what they want when they walk through the door and will limit their request to the narrow range of items on the menu. The transaction—from the insincere welcome to the disposal of one's garbage—is a highly predictable social ritual. The success of the McDonald's model is based precisely on people knowing what to expect and what they will get. For many consumers the best surprise is no surprise. When one is on the road and far from home, and in need of a quick lunch, the choice between McDonald's or Floyd's Take-Out is really no choice at all.

Control, as we already know, is a fundamental feature of all organizations. Formal control is the particular characteristic of McDonaldization. Control is exercised over the production of food—measured, timed, technologically controlled—as well as the behavior of employees and customers. Because the leading source of unpredictability and uncertainty resides in the human factor, the labor process is designed to minimize employee discretion. Scanners and automated soda dispensers eliminate further human control. Even the verbal exchange with customers is pre-scripted. Innovation is discouraged.

Ritzer's primary thesis is that the principles of McDonaldization are applicable to almost every sphere of life. In the media we have CNN, and *USA Today* with its "news nuggets" (McNews). Banking is done through ATM machines (McMoney). Health care is dispensed through walk-in/walk-out medical centers (McHealth). Management practices are reduced to the "one-minute manager" (McManagement). College courses can be taken online in the comfort of one's home (McCollege).

Application to Higher Education

The principles of McDonaldization, as rational bureaucratic practices, are also widely employed in higher education. Taking the principle of calculation first, students are admitted on the basis of their high school averages and their SAT scores. As one proceeds through the university, your academic ability and whether you can stay or must leave, is based on your grade point average (GPA). To graduate you must have a certain *number of credits.* Faculty are required to teach a certain *number of courses* per semester, meet with class *twice* a week for *one* hour, and post *six* office hours per week.

Efficiency is reflected in the design of the curriculum that indicates how one gets from a high school degree to a college degree by following a general education and major plan. Walk-in, telephone, and online registration make it quick, easy, and convenient to sign up for classes.

Predictability is built into the standard organization of majors; the three and four credit courses; the distribution of the syllabus on the first day of class; the reading list; the midterm and the final; and the standard course operating procedures of walk in, sit down, listen to a lecture, take notes, memorize material, and take the exam.

Control is also built into the system through the designated time when classes can be taken, the choice of courses, the requirements and prerequisites, the dispensing of grades, and the physical design and normative order of the classroom.

The power of Ritzer's analysis lies in its ability to present the often abstract principles of rationality through the familiar and widely shared fast-food experience and apply it to a vast assortment of other organizational and social practices. He also identified a number of tensions that emerge from the diffusion of McDonaldization. First, there is the "irrationality of rationality." This means that the organization of society around rational principles (efficiency, calculability, predictability, control), which are designed to achieve particular goals, actually undermine the ability to realize other objectives such as freedom, creativity, contemplation, quality, and individuality.

Second, Ritzer noted and even encouraged methods and movements designed explicitly to counter and resist the McDonaldization temptations. These include countercultural trends toward quality over quantity, health food over fast food, soliciting local independent businesses rather than franchises, and seeking out alternative, less commercialized, services and businesses. In short, one can observe the emergence of a lifestyle that revolves around an explicit opposition to everything McDonaldization represents. This development in turn provides an opportunity for other organizations to appeal to the growing segment of the population looking for alternative modes of product and service delivery. We now find many "noncommercial" businesses that project a counter-McDonaldization identity such as The Body Shop (dedicated to "the pursuit of social and environmental change") or Starbucks (where "coffee and community go hand-in-hand"). Resistance to McDonaldization is thus co-opted by other commercial profit-making establishments.

The Charges against Bureaucracy

I have attempted to present a balanced view of the rational bureaucratic model, noting the strengths, weaknesses, and contradictions that emerge out of this organizational arrangement. Most of the contemporary literature on bureaucracy is highly critical. Management and organizational theorists now devote much of their energy documenting the shortcomings of bureaucracy and celebrating the new, less bureaucratic, organizational systems. Chapters 6 and 7 will take up the issue of alternative organizational forms that include postbureaucratic organization. In this section, we will simply consider some of the common but important charges made against the rational bureaucratic model. These charges are based primarily on the assumption that the bureaucratic model is either inherently less efficient and productive (in retrospect) than alternative, less bureaucratic, forms, or it is no longer an effective organizational form because of changing economic conditions. In almost every case, the negative assessments of bureaucracy can be classified under the more general organizational paradox of unintended consequences. Bureaucracies are designed to be efficient and productive, but it turns out that either in practice, or over time, many of the very structural characteristics intended to advance these goals yield perverse and self-defeating consequences. Much of the literature reviewed here confirms this paradoxical pattern of organizational life.

The first charge against bureaucracy concerns its inability to adapt in a timely fashion to changing conditions. Recall that a central principle, formalization, is intended to establish a fixed and systematic set of positions and processes. These are the means to achieve organizational goals. If the organization is suddenly or even gradually faced with different goals, conditions, or demands, the formal structure can become a rigid obstacle rather than a well-oiled machine.

The bureaucratic solution to this problem involves reorganizing the formal structure, or "restructuring." However, this is typically a long and drawn out task because the formal structure—be it coercive or enabling—was designed to regularize and institutionalize behaviors and processes. The greater the success of the organization in establishing this tight connection between formal structure and organizational behavior, the more difficult is the transition toward an alternative structure. In short, the rational bureaucratic organization is by its very nature inflexible, and thus unable to rapidly shift its structure and purpose. As we shall see in considering emerging organizations, rather than "restructure" it is preferable to develop an organizational system that can adapt flexibly to changing conditions.

A second related problem is the formal structure of specialized positions and departments. Again, such differentiation of job tasks is intended to be the most rational way to organize work. However, it turns out to have some debilitating effects. Bureaucratic segmentation can create a mind-set that fixes the attention of workers only on their particular job. This produces a kind of parochialism that generates subgoals, conflicting interests, and restricted loyalties in place of a universal attachment to the larger organizational mission.

The differentiation of tasks and functions, widely embraced by most organizations, inevitably produces conflicting interests. This necessitates the equally ubiquitous integration mechanisms such as mission statements, corporate cultures, and normative appeals.

Bureaucratic segmentation also restricts the mobilization and application of knowledge in the organization (Heckscher 1994). When people are responsible only for their particular job, they will be less likely to extend their knowledge toward other "independent" organizational tasks or processes. Restricted job assignments "systematically limit the use of intelligence by employees: the system uses only a fraction of the capacities of its members" (Heckscher 1994:20). Employee knowledge is applied to a narrow range of activities rather than exchanged or shared across positions and among employees. This limits the "mobilization of multiple intelligence." The bureaucratic organization cannot compete with a new conception of work based on collective efforts, teamwork, multiple skills, increasing autonomy, and evaluations on results and outcomes (Powell forthcoming).

The neglect of informal organizational behavior represents a fourth widely cited shortcoming of the rational bureaucratic model. The Hawthorne discoveries, and the subsequent research by Gouldner, Blau, and Jackall, confirm what is now a widely accepted premise: Without the informal organizational processes there would be no organization. Put another way, the routine deviation of organizational behavior and interaction from formally prescribed patterns is the rule rather than the exception. The inherent limits on the ability to formally control human behavior and the enhancement of organizational functioning through informal behavior undermine a defining principle of the rational bureaucratic model—that behavior is formally determined and that adherence to formal directives constitute the most efficient means to achieve ends.

The many problems of bureaucracy can be linked to a more fundamental paradox noted by Max Weber. It is fitting that we conclude our critique of bureaucracies by consulting the social theorist who is both its principal defender as well as it leading critic. The paradox centers on Weber's (1946) distinction between formal rationality and substantive rationality.

Formal rationality refers to the development and implementation of methods designed to facilitate the efficient realization of organizational goals. The bureaucratic organization and its elements of formalization represent a formally rational system. *Substantive rationality,* on the other hand, involves the degree to which the social organization allows the realization of "ultimate values." These might include freedom, creativity, individualism, autonomy, and democracy. The great paradox of bureaucratic organization lies in the way it structurally embodies formal rationality while at the same time defeating substantive rationality; that is, the methods of bureaucratic administration that constitute formal rationality—specialization, authority, and formalization—work against the realization of creativity, freedom, and democracy. This paradox generates tension and change. Systems employing formally rational principles generate critical reactions from the human factor that is capable of evaluating organizational conditions on the basis of ultimate values. The substantive irrationality of the formally rational bureaucratic system galvanizes individual and collective forms of opposition and resistance.

Another way to pose the issue is to consider the dual challenge facing all organizations. This can be thought of as developing an objective structure of coordination (formal rationality) that can also accommodate subjective reactions of labor (based on substantive rationality). The pressure to rationalize as much of the production process as possible is often frustrated by the equally pressing need to elicit human cooperation. The uneasy joining of rational and normative management strategies reflect this basic dilemma.

One version of this dilemma is outlined by Evan (1976) in an essay on the effects of organizational hierarchy. Most large complex organizations that produce goods and services hierarchically stratify formal positions. This hierarchical arrangement has usually been regarded as either indispensable for a rational bureaucratic system of administration or inevitable in all large organizations. In both cases, the long-standing assumption has been that hierarchical structure advances organizational efficiency.

The hierarchical and formal structure of coordination is prescribed with the corollary assumption that humans cannot be left entirely to their own devices because they might engage in counterproductive behavior. This represents an assumption about subjective preferences—employees may prefer to engage in alternative, or informal, activities. Thus, bureaucratic structures of control and coordination must be erected. But humans do not mechanically adhere to formal directives. They retain their subjective and reflective capacities. This then poses the problem of how to manage the *subjective reaction* to the structures of control. Evan pointed to the inequality in the distribution of resources that stem from the hierarchical structure—inequality in skills and knowledge, inequality in rewards, and inequality in authority. He argued that these tend to be cumulative, resulting in alienation, disaffection, and weak commitment among those who lack some or all of these resources. These subjective reactions to hierarchical arrangements can, therefore, counter the intended positive effect of hierarchy on organizational effectiveness.

Rational methods involving differentiations, specialization, chains of command, and evaluation/accounting systems limit the freedom and autonomy of employees. Where the subjective response counteracts the potential advances in efficiency and productivity, efforts must be made to develop systems that placate workers and facilitate their attachment to the enterprise. This requires symbolic rewards, ideological appeals, human relations strategies, or systems of worker control. As Stephen Barley and Gideon Kunda (1992:386) put it, "For those who run corporations, this dualism often evinces itself in the practical issue of how to prevent anomie, construed as lack of commitment, while reaping the benefits of the very rationalization that exacerbates anomie." The normative "requirements" do not always fit comfortably in a model of organization built on the machine metaphor of exclusively formal rationality. However, as long as the organization is peopled with human capacities, extra-rational mechanisms will be imperative for organizational functioning.

Summary

1. The rational bureaucratic model of organization is based heavily upon Max Weber's delineation of the ideal-type bureaucracy. Three principles are central to this model: formalization, instrumentalism, and rational-legal authority.

2. There is a rich tradition in sociology aimed at examining the relationship between the theoretical precepts of bureaucracy and the actual day-to-day operation and unanticipated consequences of this organizational model. The classic works of Merton, Gouldner, Blau, and Selznick remain relevant for organizational analysis of bureaucratic organizations.

3. The rational bureaucratic model has had an enormous influence on management and administrative practice. This is especially apparent in administrative science which proposes a host of formal organizational principles, including delegation, hierarchy of command, specialization, and differentiation. We continually note the practical problems of applying these abstract theoretical principles. Simon's notion of bounded rationality is a powerful acknowledgment of the limits of the rational model.

4. A large portion of the literature on bureaucracy is devoted to the issue of domination. Weber and Marx viewed bureaucracy as an instrument of oppression and exploitation. This is consistent with the view of organizations as instruments of social control. The important role of human resistance and struggle is emphasized in limiting the dominating influence of bureaucratic organization.

5. The rational bureaucratic model, while a central feature of the McDonaldization of society, is increasingly regarded as an inadequate organizational form. Changing economic conditions, and the

increasing importance of knowledge and collaboration, make the
rigid bureaucratic structure less effective. Some of the emerging
contradictions of bureaucracy can be framed in the context of Weber's
distinction between formal and substantive rationality.

6. Today, bureaucracy is viewed as an increasingly ineffective
organizational form because it is unable to respond flexibly to
changing conditions and demands, divides the workforce into
segmented activities, restricts the mobilization of knowledge, and
disregards the vital role of informal behaviors and structures.

6 EMERGING ORGANIZATIONAL FORMS: BEYOND FORDISM

Managers and academics spent the majority of this century building and perfecting the hierarchical organization. If we are to believe the press, however, they are now busily destroying it, proposing in its stead networked, process-oriented, shamrock, learning, team-based and fast cycle organizational models.

Lynda Applegate, *The New American Workplace* (1995), p. 33.

The previous chapter focused attention on the most prevalent organizational structure designed to control the factors of production: the rational bureaucratic model. The next three chapters will consider alternative and emerging organizational systems and paradigms. While there has always been some variation in organizational forms, recent theorizing on organizations posits a general trend toward qualitatively different organizational forms among a wide range of organizations. Indeed, most organization and management theorists now believe that bureaucracy is no longer the most widely accepted or effective way to organize purposive activities. But what kinds of organization will replace the traditional bureaucratic structure? What kinds of organization can more effectively achieve the goals and objectives of organizational owners? What kinds of tensions, contradictions, and unintended consequences are generated in the transformation of organizational forms? This chapter will address these questions primarily as they apply to the transformation of industrial organization.

Fordism

In discussing new organizational forms and methods, it is common to construct a departure point for comparative purposes. The rational bureaucratic model, with its formalized procedures and hierarchical structure, is one such point of comparison. Another comparative case is the Fordist model which pertains to a very specific historical phase and national system of workplace organization. It is important to outline the key features of the Fordist system because it represents a significant and effective organizational model and also serves as the standard against which emerging organizational forms can be measured and compared.

Features of the Fordist Model

The term "Fordism" (Aglietta 1979) describes a particular industrial organization system typified by U.S. automobile manufacturing and is associated with the early innovations of the Ford Motor Company. This system has a number of widely recognized features. First, there is a rigid division of labor both vertically and horizontally. Horizontally, workers are separated into specialized, sequentially interdependent, tasks occupying positions on an assembly line. Tasks are highly specialized and repetitive. Vertically, there is a sharp distinction between the manual and mental, or production and managerial, responsibilities. Consistent with the principles of scientific management, conception is the province of the managerial strata while assembly line workers execute physical tasks. The use of the assembly line reduces the need for direct supervision and conforms to the model of *technical control* (Edwards 1982). The pace and intensity of work is determined by the speed of the automated assembly line.

Under Fordism, the assembly line system reflects and embodies a particular orientation toward the organization of production and a particular conception of cost-effective manufacturing. The technical organization of the line represents fixed capital and dedicated machines devoted to the sequential assembly and production of a single product or model. Given the significant capital invested in technology and the time expended in perfecting and standardizing the production process, cost effectiveness is realized through *economies of scale.* This requires long production runs, the maximization of output, and the continuous and intensive use of line technology. All this is done to drive down the cost of production per unit. It is sometimes referred to as a *push production system;* the objective is to push as much product off the line and into the market as quickly as possible. When the line is down, capital is not "performing." Therefore, every effort is made to squeeze as much product out of the fixed capital in the shortest amount of time.

To avoid any line stoppages, buffer stocks of parts and components are accumulated. The fear of a supply shortage and a temporary line shutdown drives the inventory system. Fordism is also a *"just in case"* system of production (Sayer and Walker 1992). Material inventories are stockpiled just in case requisite supplies cannot be obtained or just in case there are defects that require reworking. The pressure to push as much product out the door, and to avoid downtime, produces a managerial mind-set that emphasizes quantity rather than quality, and mass production for a mass market.

Fordism has also been associated with a particular labor-management relationship. Historically, this has involved union representation for workers and collective bargaining agreements that cover the terms of employment. While the conditions of work were characterized by principles of scientific management, high wages and generous benefits compensated for this work arrangement. The wage gains were linked to and contingent on increases in productivity. During the heyday of this industrial model, productivity gains resulted in steadily rising wages for production workers. The connection between productivity and wages also contributed to positive macroeconomic conditions. As productivity increased and greater quantities of products were pushed into the market, rising wages supported demand for the products.

A further aspect of the employment relationship was the tacit compromise between labor and management. Under this "capital-labor accord" (Bowles and Gintis 1982), labor was willing to cede control of the workplace to management if resulting productivity increases were matched with rising compensation levels. Similarly, employers were willing to tolerate increasing monetary compensation as long as productivity increased, and the rising wages stimulated demand for the large quantity of products pushed into the market.

The Demise of Fordism

The demise of the Fordist system in the 1970s and 1980s is linked to a variety of factors. Generally, managers and owners assumed that the system had become uncompetitive and unprofitable and, therefore, they were required to develop and implement alternative arrangements of industrial organization. More specifically, the literature points to changing external conditions that could not be adequately addressed with Fordist techniques. Manuel Castells (1996:154) summarized the typical argument: "When demand became unpredictable, in quantity and quality, when markets were diversified worldwide and thereby difficult to control, and when the pace of technological change made obsolete single purpose production equipment, the mass production system became too rigid and too costly."

Eileen Appelbaum and Rosemary Batt provided a more detailed assessment (1994:15):

> Here we simply note two important contributing factors: (1) the ability of the newly industrialized countries (NICs) and even the less developed countries (LDCs), with their much lower wages, to compete successfully in price conscious markets for standardized products has undermined both the rise in real wages that drove the consumption dynamic in the industrialized countries and the high capacity utilization that supported investment and (2) the increased capacity for customization and diversity inherent in micro-processor-based process technologies has reduced the cost advantages of mass production and increased competition in quality-conscious markets.

These two accounts touch on a number of points worth elaborating. First, increased competition—from smaller domestic firms, low-cost firms in the NICs and LDCs, and larger firms in Germany and Japan—challenged the position of U.S. producers who had dominated product markets during much of the period following World War II. Thus, there was a two-pronged competitive assault—from *low wage producers* who could manufacture products in a Fordist fashion at a significantly lower cost, and from *higher-quality producers* who developed superior production processes. It is important to distinguish these competitive challenges because they suggest distinct organizational responses by the established Fordist firms; that is, to reestablish competitive prowess a firm might either (1) seek out lower wage production sites or (2) develop higher quality production processes. Firms might also combine these two strategies.

A second important issue raised by Castells and Appelbaum and Batt concerns "single-purpose equipment" and "customization and diversity." One of the central features of the Fordist model—considered one of its strengths—was the ability to develop and fine-tune a production process to the point where a standardized item can be mass produced at low cost, thus yielding significant economics of scale. The great contradiction in this model, noted by Appelbaum and Batt (1994:15–18), is that the perfection of the system and the achievement of cost reduction are based on establishing a standardized process and specialized division of labor which in turn locks firms into a single production process and makes it difficult, if not impossible, to innovate or shift into new product markets. Many key features of cost effective mass production—sunk costs in "single-purpose" technologies, large inventories, and standardized procedures—are the same factors that militate against quality improvement, innovation, and flexibility.

References to single-purpose technology and product diversity also suggest the growing importance of emerging *economies of scope*. This refers to the competitive advantages based on an ability to produce a range of products for diverse market segments and niches, along with the capacity to organize production for these markets in a timely fashion. Sunk costs in an expensive production complex, geared toward a single product, obviously works against the realization of scope economies. The emphasis on "scope" has been linked to a wider social and cultural transition related to narrow rather than mass market categories, increasingly specialized tastes and fashions, and a diversity of social identities that translate into different consumption patterns for different groups.

The Transition from Fordism to New Forms

While each of these factors—competition, rapid innovations, product diversity—contributed to the crisis of Fordist organizations, there is no reason to expect a singular organizational response or shift to some coherent post-Fordist organizational arrangement. Before considering the variety of alternative organizational forms, it is important to note an analytical caution (Sayer and Walker 1992; Vallas 1999). Much of the literature on newly emerging organizational forms reduces the analysis to nothing more than dualistic or binary comparisons between old Fordist and new post-Fordist organizational characteristics. This usually appears as a listing of polar opposite characteristics that conform more to conceptual elegance than empirical reality. To avoid this tendency, a few qualifiers are in order.

First, organizations do not convert themselves overnight from one form to another. An organization possessing all the features of Fordism would have to go through a long and extended transition to even partially approximate the kinds of alternative organizational structures currently in vogue. Many obstacles and contradictions would emerge. For example, the enormous investment in assembly line technology represents a significant financial constraint limiting the ability to totally transform the production process. Thus, one often finds second-, third-, or fourth-best alternatives that retain the technology while attempting to cut other costs, such as labor or inventory. Similarly, the very rigid division of labor, horizontally and vertically, on which the efficiency of the Fordist system is based, may have produced a labor force that is reluctant to adopt alternative collaborative systems of production. Relatedly, the labor-management collective bargaining process, institutionalized under Fordism, reinforced both rigid work rules and an adversarial climate that may have precluded any attempt to implement a flexible organizational structure. Finally, the firm may decide to shift capital resources to lower-wage or nonunion locations to regain the competitive edge through lower costs and an intensified labor process. In each of these hypothetical examples, the crisis of Fordism yields varied organizational outcomes which have little relationship to the neat conceptual models of post-Fordism, flexible manufacturing, or high-performance systems.

Second, as Andrew Sayer and Richard Walker (1992) emphasized, there are considerable sectoral, spatial, and temporal variations in the existence, adoption, and abandonment of Fordist and alternative organizational systems. Sectorally, there may be some industries in stable and predictable markets that continue to successfully employ the Fordist model of mass production. Spatially, not all nations or regions have an established Fordist tradition and, therefore, the Fordist/non-Fordist dichotomy is of little explanatory value. Historically, it is difficult to pinpoint the crisis of Fordism or when the failings of the system were actually realized, and whether there has been any real, widespread, genuine transformation to a qualitatively different system. While most observers identify the mid- to late-1970s as the major period of crisis for advanced capitalist societies and their industrial organizational systems, major industrial corporations continue to struggle with the reorganization of production.

The transformation of organizational forms from the mass production Fordist model has taken a wide variety of forms and has proceeded in an uneven fashion. This results in a combination of pieces of the old system with qualitatively different organizational processes and practices that we associate with the "new" organization. Major industrial organizations continue to experiment with the new methods and techniques (Vallas 1999). This reality is reflected in the numerous reports found in the business press and research literature.

For example, while the crisis of Fordist-style production began in the late 1970s, only in the last few years have German automakers, among the most successful and innovative in the world, institutionalized significant workplace reforms:

> Germany's carmakers have been in the forefront of Germany Inc's effort to circumvent the country's high wage costs, rigid work rules, and heavy tax burdens. They have adopted Japanese-style lean production techniques, hammered through more flexible work rules, and slashed costs by trimming employees and simplifying the design of their cars. ("Germany: Carmakers Show the Way," *Business Week, Int'l Edition,* September 15, 1997, p. 51.)

In another case, Toshiba, a Japanese firm and a world leader in digital electronics, was unable to institute the necessary organizational changes because of a variety of constraints. A report on the challenges facing its chief executive Taizo Nishimuro explains:

> Radical surgery, however, isn't an option for Nishimuro. He has eliminated one managerial layer and plans to trim the parent company's 63,400-strong workforce by 5,000 by the year 2000. . . But Nishimuro can't follow his Western instincts and ax masses of workers. Radical restructuring to achieve the returns typical of U.S.

companies might "ruin our whole culture," he concedes. "The easiest thing to do is to eliminate aged middle managers to create a very lean and flat organization," he adds. "But if we did so, we'd eliminate a very essential source of knowledge." ("Toshiba: Digital Dreams: Can the High Tech Giant Come Up with the Goods and Rearrange Its Bureaucracy?" *Business Week, Int'l Edition,* October 13, 1997, p. 33.)

Finally, Lynda Applegate's survey of corporate managers in the early 1990s, confirmed the pattern of slow progress in transforming the organization.

[M]ost managers stated that their firms were still organized and operated in very traditional ways. Standardized jobs, rigid procedures and policies, and the hierarchical chain of command continued to be managed by current supervisors. . . Finally, in most firms, mass customization was far from the norm; product and market strategies continued to emphasize mass production and mass markets, and operations continued to be designed to achieve economies of scale (1995:34).

The difficulties that managers cited were directly related to the contradictory objectives pursued by the various firms studied. Most were trying to combine the global competitive reach of a large business with the nimble agility of a small firm; decentralized operating units with centralized reporting and control; the management of complexity with the realization of speed. The central challenge, according to Applegate (1995), has been to implement alternative organizational designs that retain the necessary degree of hierarchical control to manage complexity, while at the same time allowing the entrepreneurial autonomy necessary in a rapidly changing competitive environment.

These cases indicate that world-class corporations face considerable obstacles in their effort to transform their organizational systems. Even when there is widespread awareness of the limitations of the existing system and a set of blueprints for establishing a flexible and presumably more competitive organizational structure, human, financial, political, and cultural constraints also shape the possible managerial strategies. These factors must always be considered in models of organizational transition and change.

Toward Alternative Manufacturing Models

In this section, the wide assortment of organizational theories and models that have been offered as alternatives to Fordist arrangements will be reviewed. Keep in mind that many of these new organizational models are derived from the actual experience of a single or restricted set of organizations. The success of these organizations, representing alternatives to the mass production Fordist approach, makes them models for other organizations to emulate.

Toyotaism

While U.S. automakers were struggling with low profits, declining sales, and foreign competition in the 1970s and 1980s, Japanese automakers were conquering the world with high-quality, affordable automobiles. The success of Japanese firms, highly productive and competitive, was largely attributed to the management methods used by Japanese corporations. If Ford was once the model for mass production, Toyota became the model for quality and productivity. Toyotaism (Dohse, Jurgens, and Malsch 1985) therefore became the logical alternative to Fordism (Boswell 1987).

The most notable elements of Toyotaism pertain to the organization of the labor process and the nature of labor-management relations. Numerous studies have indicated that Japanese workers have a greater affective emotional attachment to their work organization, higher levels of commitment and loyalty, and greater identification with the firm than Western workers. Though often assumed to be a cultural phenomenon, it became increasingly clear that Japanese managerial practices contributed to the positive orientation of employees. The most notable practices are human relations strategies designed to engender the creative involvement of workers in the tasks of production and quality control. Production workers are integrated into areas of managerial concern, and responsibility for productivity and quality is spread among a broader cross-section of the workforce. Bonuses, guarantees of lifetime employment, and long-term career ladders further serve to attach employees to their place of work. Under this general system, there is a greater likelihood that workers will view their interests as consonant with those of managers, and thus comply with managerial efforts to promote greater productivity and efficiency.

James Lincoln and Arne Kalleberg (1985) summarized the key structural components of the Toyotaist model. First, *structures facilitating participation* involve expanded opportunities for input in the decision-making process to gain consensus on the goals and methods of production. Second, workers are integrated into the organization through *cross-cutting divisions and hierarchies* that tend to cut across class and status lines, thus defusing potential worker solidarity and class polarization. Third, an elaborate *constellation of mobility and career ladders* are used as bureaucratic control techniques engendering long-term organizational attachment, motivation, and loyalty. Finally, there is a broad sense of all organizational members as *"corporate citizens"* with legal rights and obligations within the organization, as well as social and recreational ties outside the factory. Together, these structures foster employee attachment to and support for the organization and, in turn, make for a highly efficient and productive workforce.

Managing Tensions: Fordism versus Toyotaism.   It is important to consider how these organizational and managerial methods represent an improvement over Fordism, and address some of the tensions inherent in it. We can consider the familiar organizational tension between differentiation and integration. Fordism places a great emphasis on differentiation, or a rigid division of labor, extending horizontally across positions in the production process and vertically between production workers and managers. This produces a relatively alienating work environment based on specialization, repetition of work tasks, and a manual-mental labor divide. It also reinforces class and occupational identity above attachment to the organization. This work environment becomes problematic from the perspective of owners when human labor collectively organizes in opposition to the system of production. Acts of resistance, such as the labor uprising at the General Motors plant in Lordstown, Ohio, were few and far between, though they received an enormous amount of attention in the literature (e.g., Aronowitz 1973). Much of the simmering discontent was quelled and worker attachment facilitated by the relatively generous economic benefits and perceived job security accruing to workers under collective bargaining agreements negotiated by the union. Thus, the less than humanized workplace and the stultifying aspects of the labor process were compensated for by material rewards.

One of the problems with this form of "worker attachment," if it can be called that, is its contingency on the continuous flow of material incentives—wage increases, bonuses, and extended benefits. This represents a form of *specific attachment;* that is, compliance and identification with the objectives of the organization are based on a specific and calculative quid pro quo. An employee is loyal and committed so long as the company continues to provide material rewards. When profit rates decline, markets dry up, and the firm is no longer competitive and thus less able to continue high levels of remuneration, support and compliance of workers are likely to be withdrawn. This creates a serious human motivation problem for the organization and, in the case of Fordist firms, difficulty gaining the support for alternative or more flexible work arrangements (see Gordon 1996). Here the Toyotaist model demonstrates its superiority—in the area of integrating the worker into the larger objectives, mission, and identity of the organization. In contrast to the exclusively specific attachment of Fordism, Toyotaism establishes *diffuse attachment* that provides a source of identity and motivation that is not entirely contingent on the flow of extrinsic rewards.

The reaction of the human factor under Fordism takes a number of further forms that point to the advantages of the Toyotaist alternative. Rather than overt acts of resistance chronicled in the highly celebrated but isolated case of Lordstown, there are many more serious, subtle, and covert human reactions. These take the form of undetected sabotage, absenteeism, turnover, burnout, and the withdrawal of commitment and effort. These less dramatic reactions can have a much more insidious influence on quality and productivity (Hodson 1995). One of the important features of the Toyotaist system involves the communication, interaction, and exchange of ideas between workers and managers. In contrast to U.S. human relations techniques—whose objective is limited largely to massaging the subjective sentiments of workers—interaction in this model has wider consequences for the labor process. The objective is the improvement of the production process, the elimination of wasteful work practices, and the establishment of total quality.

As conceptualized in the work of Ikujiro Nonaka and Hirotaka Takeuchi (1995), the systematic and regularly scheduled communication between workers and managers allows management access to a valuable form of information termed *tacit knowledge* (Polanyi 1967). All workers in all organizations possess this unique and privileged understanding of the aspects of their work tasks, but these are typically beyond the comprehension or easy formalization of management. However, if managers are able to gain access to these intricacies of the labor process—those aspects of the work process that are problematic, cumbersome, or time consuming—they can take this information and convert it into *explicit knowledge* that informs the reorganization of production and further rationalizes and streamlines the production system. In this way, Toyotaism creates what Nonaka and Takeuchi described as the "knowledge creating company."

There is an interesting irony here. If we think back to the principles underlying scientific management, one of the purposes of the vertical division of labor between management and workers, and the time and motion studies, was to place knowledge about the "one best way" in the sole possession of managers. Workers would simply execute the predesigned work tasks. Toyotaism turns this system on its head while also revealing a fundamental fact of organizational life. Humans accumulate valuable knowledge in the process of carrying out even the most manual of labor tasks. This craft knowledge, as it is sometimes called, can either be hoarded and used as a weapon *against* management, or it can be shared with and used *by* management. Under the Fordist system, there was plenty of implicit knowledge but few mechanisms for converting it into explicit knowledge. Toyotaism addresses this shortcoming through structures that facilitate vertical integration and communication between workers and managers.

A final aspect of the social integration of workers under Toyotaism involves the organizational or corporate culture. More will be said later about the role of culture, but for the moment it is important to note that the ideology and practice of Toyotaism are designed to promote a cooperative culture and strong identification with the corporation. Social events, picnics, and recreational activities are designed to advance a communal familylike atmosphere that further cements attachment and identity. This is a critical, sociologically relevant, component of all emerging organizational models. It reflects the need to integrate differentiated and increasingly autonomous positions and units while also generating the diffuse attachment that can translate into higher levels of motivation and work effort. These aspects of what we have called Toyotaism are now widely practiced management techniques in almost all large organizations.

Lean Production: "The Machine That Changed the World"

Thus far, the focus has been primarily on the social or human relations aspects of emerging organizational forms. However, Toyotaism, and Japanese firms generally, are closely associated with another list of practices that come under the heading of *lean production.*

Features of the Model.   Lean production (Womack, Jones, and Roos 1990) refers to a wide array of organizational techniques designed to minimize waste, continually improve the efficiency and quality of the production process, and eliminate bottlenecks and slack in the production system. As it relates to what has already been said about Toyotaism, lean production requires job switching, cross-training, multiple skills, and teamwork. Hence, it is antithetical to the rigid division of labor that characterizes the Fordist model. Production is carried out in functional work teams with all members of each team rotating through and mastering the complexities of each task. This process enhances communication among team members and also contributes to the diffusion of knowledge and information that can be used for problem solving.

Interaction and communication across work teams is carried out through the *kanban system.* This is a horizontal communication system that uses circulating cards or tags requesting parts and components when they are needed for production. Parts are produced and delivered only when needed. Lean production is also referred to as the *just-in-time (JIT)* production system. As it applies to the organization of the labor process and the relationship among work teams, JIT is designed to minimize inventories of raw materials and parts. Raw materials and components are requested, produced, and delivered as needed. This reflects the lean zero-inventory nature of the production process. Fordism was described in these pages as a just-in-case system that stockpiles supplies and "pushes" production into the market. In contrast, lean production is a just-in-time system with output "pulled" by product orders and market demand (Sayer and Walker 1992).

> The objective of the JIT system is to increase productivity not through the super-exploitation of labor but through increased technological efficiency, heightened utilization of equipment, minimal scrappage or rework, decreased inventory, and high quality. It thus increases "value" extracted in production, decreases materials consumed per unit output, and minimizes circulation time, making the actual production process much more efficient (Kenney and Florida 1988:136).

Another element of the Japanese lean production model involves the process of continuous improvement, or *kaizen* ("kai" meaning change, "zen" meaning good). Unlike the Fordist model which seeks to establish a fixed production process directed toward economies of scale, the kaizen system emphasizes the notion of "learning by doing." Therefore, the production process is continuously, or incrementally, changed and improved to reduce materials waste and production errors. This system requires employee training in quality assessment, quality standards, and problem solving. It also requires a labor-management communication system that provides formal channels for raising, discussing, and acting upon production-related issues. There is a vital connection between the kanban and kaizen components of the lean production system. The latter is driven by the former:

> [K]ey targets of management are to reduce buffer stocks towards zero and to eliminate errors and rejects in each task. In fact these targets are related. The smaller the buffer, the more sensitive the system is to error, and hence the more visible the source of error and the greater the incentive to remedy it and ensure that it does not happen again. . . The reduction of buffers therefore not only keeps capital more active, but also stimulates a continual learning process. . . when the learning curve of Western firms in consumer electronics, air conditioners, cars, and office machinery were thought to have reached a plateau, those of the Japanese continued to improve (Sayer and Walker 1992:192–75).

Organizational Implications.   The just-in-time system is built on its own particular paradox that joins mutually competing demands and objectives (Eisenhardt and Westcott 1988). Consistent with Eastern philosophy, the contradictory demands are not viewed as irreconcilable trade-offs but as a "harmony of competing values." The explicit combination of what are seemingly mutually exclusive objectives can serve as a powerful force for change, transformation, and creativity (Eisenhardt and Westcott 1988). It is difficult to combine demands for low cost *and* high quality or to insist on perfection when operating in a highly unstable and uncertain manufacturing environment. Yet these conflicting objectives are pursued under the just-in-time system. This results in an examination and reassessment of assumptions about quality versus cost tradeoffs and a renewed effort to achieve each without compromising the other. In an industrial organizational context, this might mean exploring alternative production processes or forming new supplier relationships. "The major effect of the paradox of ultimate goals is creativity" (Eisenhardt and Westcott 1988:175).

This is an interesting way to think about organizational paradox. Thus far, paradox has been viewed as an inherent organizational feature associated with the conflict between differentiation and integration, and the effort to control the human factor of production and the more general unintended consequences of organization. In the just-in-time system, paradox is explicitly created to force organizational members to rethink their premises and operate in a more creative and innovative fashion. This managerial strategy, like all others, is likely to produce unintended consequences and further paradox. We shall see some of these as we review how the human factor has responded to lean production techniques.

A widely heralded U.S. application of lean production principles took place at the New United Motor Manufacturing, Inc. (NUMMI) plant in California (Kenney and Florida 1993). Initiated as a joint venture between General Motors and Toyota, NUMMI employs a *Kaizen teian* suggestion system intent on "maximizing ongoing frontline involvement in continuously upgrading production processes and working conditions." In the words of a NUMMI human resource specialist, "We strongly believe in the philosophy of Kaizen and feel that employees know their jobs better than anyone else, so their ideas about how to make a job better are usually the best" (Productivity Consulting Group, 1998).

The primary areas for employee suggestions are: improvements in manufacturing methods; tangible saving of labor, material or supplies; and intangible upgrades of productivity, quality, safety, or the work environment. In 1995 there were 13,815 suggestions at the NUMMI facility, an average of 3.1 suggestions for each employee. In terms of assessing and implementing the suggestions, "the real action, most of the time, takes place at the team member/team group leader level. Team members do most of the work of conceiving, developing, and refining an action plan for an idea, including doing a cost/benefit analysis" (Productivity Consulting Group 1998).

Martin Kenney and Richard Florida's (1993) analysis of the Japanese-style production system combines elements of Toyotaism and lean production into what they call *innovation-mediated production*. An important component of this model is the effort to integrate what were previously, under Fordism, differentiated processes and activities. The five dimensions of innovation-mediated production are:

1. A transition from physical skill and manual labor to intellectual capabilities or mental labor.
2. The increasing importance of social or collective intelligence as opposed to individual knowledge and skill.
3. An acceleration of the pace of technological innovation.
4. The increasing importance of continuous process improvement on the factory floor and constant revolutions in production.
5. The blurring of the lines between the R&D lab and the factory (Kenney and Florida 1993:14).

Notice that the system rests upon joining individual skill and knowledge into collective intelligence, and integrating research and development with manufacturing. The perceived disadvantages of specialization and differentiation give way to a holistic integrated organizational unit. The objective is to generate and share as much knowledge and information as possible and direct it toward continuous improvement.

Lean Production in Practice

Incomplete Transitions to Lean Production.   While the key features and relative advantages of Toyotaism and the lean production system are highlighted, a number of additional points must be added. First, many U.S. Fordist firms took a number of detours before embracing the principles of the Japanese-style lean production model. One initial response to the crisis of Fordism was not the restructuring and redesigning of the production process, but an effort simply to cut production costs. This led many U.S. firms to retain Fordist organizational practices while shifting production to low-cost locations. While more will be said about the globalization of production in Chapter 9, it is important to emphasize that many firms pursued a "global Fordist" strategy through the 1970s and 1980s (Dicken 1998; Dassbach 1994). This involved relocating segments of production to unregulated, low-wage, cheap labor, regions and nations. However, this did not entirely solve the productivity and quality problems plaguing U.S. manufacturers. Eventually, U.S. automakers began to explore Japanese-style lean production techniques. In his analysis of the automobile industry, Carl Dassbach concluded that future strategies might logically combine "low road" and "high road" elements or *"low-wage lean production."* Mexico is a prime location for this form of production.

> The most important reason for this growth in Mexican production is the lure of low wages. . . labor costs still represent 20 percent of total costs. . . automakers have found that Mexican workers are highly motivated and capable of learning advanced production techniques. . . if high wage lean production can be profitable, "low wage lean production" can be even more profitable (Dassbach 1994).

Another adaptation strategy, which falls far short of the lean production model, is represented by *flexible mass production* (Appelbaum and Batt 1994).

> This approach. . . retains hierarchical management structures, old-style power relations between supervisors and workers, the separation between conception and execution, the relatively high use of low-skilled workers, and the routinization of work. It also includes, however, the use of less dedicated, more flexible technology. . . cross-training of skilled workers. . . and subcontracting, outsourcing, and contingent employment contracts to achieve flexibility in responding to market turbulence and variations in demand (Appelbaum and Batt 1994:21–22).

The authors regarded this as a highly incomplete effort to build a high-quality competitive operation because it retains the "basic organization or power structure of the firms."

Both the low-wage lean manufacturing model and the flexible mass production model illustrate how an abstract conceptual model suggesting a smooth and seemingly obvious transition from one organizational form to another oversimplifies and fails to recognize the constraints and contradiction that produce hybrid and amalgamated organizational structures.

Work under Lean Production. A second point to consider is the actual impact of the lean production model on workers. We have reviewed the basic principles, the theoretical and practical advantages over the Fordist system, and the public relations pronouncements of firms that employ lean production techniques. But how are workers affected by this system? On this question there is considerable debate. There are those—many of whose work we have already reviewed—who emphasize the greater levels of participation, involvement, input, control, and cooperation characterizing working conditions and labor management relations (Womack, Jones, and Roos 1990; Kenney and Florida 1988; Dore 1973). On the other side are a range of theorists and observers who view both Toyotaism and lean production as sophisticated managerial methods designed to undermine organized labor, extract greater work effort from employees, intensify the pace of work and the level of exploitation, and gain greater control over all aspects of a worker's time on the job (Dohse, Jurgens, and Malsch 1985; Fantasia, Clawson, and Graham 1988; Milkman 1991; Parker and Slaughter 1988).

Laurie Graham's (1995) participant observation study of the Suburu-Isuzu automotive plant in Indiana provides some relevant data on which to evaluate the divergent claims. Her analysis revealed a number of interesting findings about the lean production system. It is important to begin with the employee selection process. To obtain employment in this Japanese transplant, applicants had to submit to a multiphase preselection screening process involving aptitude tests, attitude questionnaires, and team and individual problem-solving exercises. Applicant performance on the general aptitude test determined entry into Phase I; success in Phase I permitted entry into Phase II; satisfactory performance in Phase II qualified an applicant for employment, but only after a physical exam and a final set of face-to-face interviews.

As Graham noted, this intensive selection process differs dramatically from personnel decisions made in U.S. auto plants, which are based on formal qualifications and past experience. In contrast, the Japanese-style selection process combines socialization with an effort to identify particular personality characteristics—the most important being a willingness to work with others, share information, participate in suggestion schemes, and work under pressure. Given what has already been said about Toyotaism and lean production, these are obviously relevant qualifications for this organizational model. However, some applicants felt that the highly competitive selection process was antithetical to the espoused principles of cooperation and team play. Graham also reported that many of the applicants knew exactly what the recruiters were looking for and adjusted their attitudes and behaviors accordingly. Graham repeatedly described the process as a "charade." One applicant put it this way, "I wanted the job and I was not going to blow my chances by really letting the company know how I felt" (1995:32). Graham defined the ability of applicants to readily interpret the normative expectations of superordinate personnel, and to exhibit the desired behavior, as one form of "resistance."

There is a more general theoretical explanation for the intense preselection screening process and the emphasis on particular personality and behavioral characteristics. In an organization that operates with a highly formalized and rigid division of labor, with strict job classifications and task specifications, human control is shaped by the formal structure. Failure to perform is more easily detected; it can be linked to the successful completion of assigned tasks. In contrast, under the lean production model, workers are not tied to a single task; they exercise more discretion and initiative, and their potential range of job behavior is more variable. Therefore, the work orientation and personality of workers has a greater opportunity to impact the production process. Under these conditions, the selection process should logically be more intensive and focused. Diffuse forms of attachment and commitment, based on normative and corporate cultural appeals, should play a greater role.

If Durkheim's insights on the relationship between the division of labor (differentiation) and social integration are applied, one might also say that as rigid differentiation decreases—as it presumably does in the shift from Fordism to Toyotaism—integration is based less on formal directives and more on common sentiments and values. The worker selection process at Suburu-Isuzu, though relatively superficial and transparent from the perspective of applicants, served to recruit a fairly homogeneous collection of workers who appear to share particular personality and behavioral traits.

After being selected, but prior to the start of production, Graham and her co-workers were also given formal orientation and training. Consistent with the preselection process, this further reinforced the company's philosophy about teamwork, communication, and work. This included instruction on the principles of Kaizen, and its objective of eliminating *muda,* or waste, which was defined as overproduction, inventory, waiting, conveyance (movement of parts), defective products, and motion (personal motion) (Graham 1995:46). The 10 principles of SIA management philosophy were also presented and distributed in document form (see Table 6–1).

Once production commenced, Graham's observations support the critics of the lean production system, who have emphasized the rapid intensive pace of production and its negative impact on workers. Worker safety was an immediate issue: ". . . the overriding discrepancy between shop floor reality and company

TABLE 6–1   **Philosophy of Management at Suburu-Isuzu (SIA)**

1. SIA is made up of its people—We are the corporation.
2. Together, we must beat the competition.
3. Job security is important to all of us.
4. Quality is the top priority.
5. We must eliminate *muda* (waste) throughout the company.
6. Kaizen means searching for a better way.
7. Each of us should strive to be a multitalented person.
8. The spirit of SIA is enthusiastic involvement.
9. Open communications build mutual trust.
10. We build Hoosier pride into every vehicle.

Source: Laurie Graham, *On the Line at Suburu-Isuzu: The Japanese Model and the American Worker* (Ithaca, NY: Cornell University ILR Press, 1995), p. 53.

philosophy involved injuries. Immediately after official start of production, there was an outbreak of hand and wrist injuries" (Graham, 1995:86). The injuries were caused by the repetition and physical stress of the assembly line work.

It is important to emphasize that the lean production system does not do away with the assembly line. Rather, it eliminates rigid divisions of labor and single-task specialization in favor of multiskilled teams. Thus, technical control is still a key feature of the system. Graham claimed that it is reinforced by the teams that "chain us psychologically to the line." The just-in-time system also serves as a form of technical control. "It had the effect of directly intensifying and speeding up team members' work. . . Just-in-time production often forced speedup when workers were forced to work down the line to install parts that arrived late or when they were forced to modify a part before it could be installed" (Graham 1995:114).

Graham's observations about the condition of work at the SIA plant are confirmed in another study of a Japanese transplant in Canada (Rinehart, Huxley, and Robertson 1997). CAMI Automotive, a joint venture of General Motors and Suzuki, also implemented a lean production system. In the study, the job tasks and skill requirements of production team members were carefully examined. Instead of multiskilling, meaning a variety of skill levels utilized by a single team member, *multitasking* was the more common practice. The training for different jobs and job rotation meant that the workforce had to take responsibility for multiple tasks at any given time. The net result was an increased workload for all team members.

In thinking about skill level, the authors employed three criteria widely used in sociological studies of work: the substantive complexity, diversity, and autonomy of a job. "*Substantive complexity* refers to the degree, scope, and integration of mental, interpersonal, and manipulative tasks. *Diversity* refers to the range of tasks and responsibilities required by a job. *Autonomy* involves the extent to which the job permits or demands self-direction and individual discretion over, for example, how, when, and at what pace work is performed" (Rinehart, Huxley, and Robertson 1997:59–60). As it turned out, most of the jobs analyzed were standardized, short-cycled, and repetitive. The learning of and training for different jobs did produce job diversity, but the authors concluded that job diversity did not increase workers' discretion or make the work more complex. Consequently, they believed that multitasking was a more appropriate label than multiskilling (1997:62).

Another study, based on a comprehensive survey of more than 1,600 workers employed in automotive components firms in Canada, confirmed the single-factory findings.

> Workers are employed in jobs which offer them little real control over working conditions and at tasks which can be learned in a very short period of time. Most workers lack any real control over how they work, how fast they work, or when they work. Workloads are high and increasing, health risks are high and increasing, work is stressful and becoming more stressful. . . Compared with workers in traditional Fordist-style plants, those at lean companies reported their workload was heavier and faster (Lewchuk and Robertson 1996:79).

These studies suggest a conflict between the theory and the practice of lean production. According to these studies, workers did not exercise wide latitude or autonomy, nor did they engage in substantively complex tasks. The objective of producing automobiles for a segmented but mass market—without slack, buffers, waste, reflection, contemplation, or deliberation—would appear to preclude the theoretically more attractive workplace features of lean production. Once the production process starts, the constraints kick in. The researchers at CAMI Automotive (Rinehart, Huxley, and Robertson 1997:60) wrote, "Standardization, the tight schedules and low buffers associated with JIT procedures, and precise time limits to complete a set of tasks leave little room for workers to exercise discretion over what to do, how to do it, and when to do it." Graham's (1995:114–15) experience at SIA led her to conclude that "the Fordist thrust of technically advanced work processes, such as the computer controlled assembly line and just-in-time production, were direct barriers to instituting a company philosophy of fairness, cooperation, and egalitarianism."

Social Control and Resistance.   The conclusions above suggest two points. First, many theories about organizational process—how it will work, what the outcomes will be—are unlikely to be realized in practice. Once the job or process begins, principles and philosophies that seem attainable in the abstract are shoved aside or given a lower priority. Enormous constraints operate in a system that is, first and foremost, lean, and in which the ultimate objective is production for profit, not production to satisfy or meet the needs of workers.

Second, it is equally plausible that many of the claims made about meaningful skilled work and a cooperative egalitarian work environment under lean production are nothing more than forms of managerial ideology. They are designed to manipulate, motivate, and mobilize workers. As a form of control aimed at the human factor of production, lean production techniques seem to combine both social (that is, cultural, ideological, normative) and technical methods in a much more comprehensive fashion than Fordism. This may be one of the major reasons for the success of this model. The lean techniques are combined with philosophical principles, practices formalizing worker participation and input, a team approach, and strong peer pressure. None of these would be needed if human compliance was unnecessary, if the plant was run exclusively by machines, or if workers could be programmed. But, the unique nature and capacity of the human factor prompts this incredibly comprehensive, systematic, and elaborate managerial system—of selection, training, socialization, philosophy, and participatory practices—as a way to tap both the compliance and the knowledge of workers.

Kenney and Florida (1993:164–71) described the tension in their extensive analysis of the Japanese organizational model:

> This is a tension between the model's powerful ability to unleash human creative and intellectual capabilities and the use of forms of corporate control which differ from those used by U.S. corporations. . . A key element of this form of corporate control involves establishing an identity between workers and the corporation—creating what might be termed "corporatist hegemony" over work life.

For many organizational analysts, the team-based work groups associated with lean production are simply sophisticated and insidious forms of labor control (Jermier 1998; Barker 1993; Ezzamel and Willmott 1998; Sewell 1998). More specifically, James Barker (1993) labeled as *concertive control* the team-based norms of social control that prescribe procedures for task performance, evaluation, and discipline. Concertive control replaces the more bureaucratic techniques of Fordism while still directing organizational behavior toward managerial objectives through small group norms and work group peer pressure shaped by an organizational culture and philosophy. It has already been noted that management has presented these work groups as opportunities for worker collaboration and task variety intended to generate worker enthusiasm and commitment. Like most managerial initiatives, however, this one also has some unintended consequences. Reporting on one group-based scheme initiated in a manufacturing enterprise, Mahmoud Ezzamel and Hugh Willmott (1998:362) wrote, "Instead of employees embracing teamwork as an opportunity to become self-determining, they experienced teamwork as an intrusion and divisive form of control that sets machinist against machinist as each was required to become the others' supervisor and controller." A report in *The Wall Street Journal* on a team-based empowerment model implemented by a steel manufacturer indicated a great deal of worker ambivalence regarding these programs.

> "They say there are no bosses here," says Randy Savage, a longtime, devoted employee, "but if you screw up, you find one pretty fast." Indeed, with everyone watching everyone else, it can feel like having a hundred bosses (Aeppel 1997:A10).

More generally, in spite of the comprehensive effort at human control under lean production, resistance remains widespread and is manifested in a variety of actions. Graham, as already noted, observed considerable cynicism among U.S. workers toward Japanese principles and philosophy. Many workers played along with the "charade" during the selection and orientation processes. Over time, as the contradictions between the claims and actual workplace experiences become increasingly evident, other expressions of resistance emerged. Individual resistance took the form of withdrawal from and nonparticipation in various company rituals, and anonymous suggestion letters complaining about working conditions. Collectively, Graham observed sabotage, line stoppages, and walkout threats.

In the case of CAMI, which happened to be a *unionized* Japanese transplant, workers elected to strike the plant in "the strike that was not supposed to happen" (Rinehart, Huxley, and Robertson 1997). During the five-week strike, workers burned company T-shirts and carried banners that crossed out the company slogans of "open communication, empowerment, Kaizen, and team spirit" and replaced them with "dignity, respect, fairness, and solidarity." One worker, quoted by a local paper, summarized the sentiments of many: "CAMI was a great place to work until we started making cars. It seems that once we started production, all the values got tossed out" (Rinehart, Huxley, and Robertson 1997:4). The strike ended with a new agreement that covered wage and benefit issues as well as changes in lean production working conditions. What was once viewed as the ideal optimal organizational system, and one which seemed to accomplish the objective of technical and social control, is gradually being transformed in the face of worker resistance.

Cracks in the System.   In concluding this extended discussion of the lean production model, it is important to add that Japan's economy and lean production manufacturing firms have experienced a severe downturn since the early 1990s. Much of the success of the Japanese economy during the 1970s and 1980s was credited to management techniques and lean production principles. It is now clearer than ever that other features of the Japanese corporation, such as interfirm relations and access to finance capital (see Chapter 8), and the larger domestic and global economic environment, were equally important in fueling the growth of the Japanese economy and the competitive prowess of Japanese corporations. As conditions have changed, the lean manufacturing system has been unable to single-handedly sustain the economic expansion (Stewart 1996; Kochan, Lansbury, and MacDuffie 1997).

This points to a general principle that will be further elaborated in the discussion of the environment: The viability and success of organizational arrangements are heavily influenced by external conditions. When these conditions change or organizations find themselves operating in a different environment, the formerly successful organization may perform very differently. One version of this perspective argues that:

> [T]he evidence—both *before* and *after* the serious downturn in the Japanese economy around 1991—suggests that much more weight needs to be given to the particular structural factors within which Japanese industry operated. Attention is thus drawn to the extent to which Japanese manufacturers operated in a domestic environment where the social settlement was favorable to them (especially in terms of wages, hours worked, and managerial control over the labor process), and then the products were sold in markets where quite different social settlements set prices at levels which guaranteed a great deal of cash for Japanese producers. . . the erosion, if not the disappearance, of these favorable conditions from the mid-1980s onward has contributed substantially to the recent difficulties of Japanese producers (Haslam et al. 1996:21–22).

Further support for the general principle can be found in reports from lean manufacturers who suddenly face surging demand for their products. The original movement to lean production was based on an environment of unstable demand that resulted in excess capacity and sunk costs in "just-in-case" supplies and inventory. The lean production system eliminated much if not all of the slack. While this reduced costs under those economic conditions, the more recent phase of rapid growth and demand has revealed the system's vulnerability. As reported in *Business Week:*

> The surprising demand leaves companies in a bind. They must spend to fill orders and keep customers happy, but they can't raise prices because competition won't allow it. So, unless they can keep ahead with productivity improvements, they eat the extra costs from overtime, expensive overnight shipments, melted-down assembly lines, and high worker turnover rates. . . . Now, lean operations may have come back to haunt them. "We leaned things so much, got rid of so many people that you just don't have the capacity anymore." ("Just-in-Time Manufacturing Is Working Overtime," *Business Week,* November 8, 1999, p. 36.)

The second analytical principle that can be deduced from this case is that the *agency* of managerial intervention and techniques is constrained by the *structural* conditions in which organizations operate. Management theory tends to assume considerable managerial discretion and control over the strategy and performance of the organization. In this particular scenario, structural conditions beyond the control of management intervention have proven the more powerful force.

There is a third principle that is confirmed and reinforced in our analysis of lean production—that is, there is no final solution to the managerial challenge to control the human factor of production or the external conditions that have an impact on the organization. Human resistance, internal contradictions, and unintended consequences plague all human organizations and stimulate organizational change. Thus, we now find an emerging literature that documents the radical transformation of the formerly celebrated Japanese lean production model (Stewart 1996; Kochan, Lansbury, and MacDuffie, 1997).

Two concrete examples point to some interesting and unexpected trends. First, Japanese industry, once the envy of the industrialized world, is undergoing a formal reassessment of its organization model. This is reflected in the Japanese Confederation of Management Organizations' publication in May 1995 of a proposed agenda for fundamental reform of the prevailing management system (Ogasawara and Veda 1996). The two primary areas for reform are working conditions and the application of automation technology. The relationship between these two areas is a major focus of organizational restructuring as a study of changes in Toyota's Japanese auto plants noted:

> The parent company believes that its previous approaches to automation carried many negative features. Operators experienced stress, feelings of estrangement and a stagnation of work motivation (and decline in *Kaizen* activities). . . In response to these problems, the parent company took the path of ensuring that the automation facilities would both coexist and be controlled by workers. . . that there should be sufficient room for *Kaizen* activities (Ogasawara and Veda 1996:52).

Back in the United States, there are reports of Japanese-style lean management principles translated into actual and meaningful work practices (Babson 1996). In Wayne, Michigan, Ford's Integrated Stamping and Assembly (ISA) plant produces bodies for the Ford Escort. Using lean production technology and layout practices learned from its close association with Mazda, this Ford plant employs 1,200 United Auto Workers who perform their jobs in worker-centered teams that "wield routine authority over specified areas of their work environment." In contrast to the Suburu and Suzuki lean production plants, where work tasks were heavily monitored and controlled by unit leader supervisors, the work teams at the Ford plant manage scheduling of job rotation, training, vacation, and personal leaves. They also decide on safety and quality improvements, the rebalancing of workloads, and how to implement engineering changes (Babson 1996:85). In comparing the Wayne ISA facility with the Mazda-run plant in Flat Rock, Michigan, Steve Babson (1996:87) concluded that "while 'teamwork' exists at Flat Rock primarily as a rhetorical device to obscure the dominant role of supervision, at Wayne ISA teams are worker-centered groups that wield genuine authority." Thus, in this case lean production is taken a step further and approximates what is described as an *American high performance work system.* As Appelbaum and Batt (1994:126) defined it, "The American team production approach relies heavily on decentralized decision-making through collaborative teamwork and on joint labor-management structures that allow workers to be represented at every level of the company—operational, tactical, and strategic." It is also worth noting that while Japanese transplants have deliberately avoided organized unions, the existence of labor unions appears to be a factor and potential asset in developing a better-coordinated and more participatory, team-based structure (Appelbaum and Batt 1994; Babson 1996).

The Flexibility Paradigm

Flexible Specialization

A more abstract and neo romantic perspective on organizational change is presented by Michael Piore and Charles Sabel in their highly influential manifesto, *The Second Industrial Divide* (1984). Like most arguments about emerging organizations, Piore and Sabel chronicled the various shortcomings and inevitable demise of the Fordist mass production system. Their image of the brave new world of organization was shaped by a particular case—the industrial districts of northeastern Italy and the system of *flexible specialization* (Clegg 1990: 120–25; Harrison 1994: chap. 4). In this region, Piore and Sabel studied the organizational arrangements employed by apparel producers such as Benetton. They associated the innovative practices of these firms with the broader market changes in consumer demand, fashions, and tastes. Under these new market conditions, long production runs must give way to production systems that can respond quickly to rapidly changing fashions and consumer demands (flexibility) while also being able to target products for narrow niche markets (specialization).

Presenting this as a type of craft alternative to the Fordist model, Piore and Sabel highlighted (1) the existence of small- and medium-sized firms, (2) the application of highly skilled labor exercising considerable control and discretion over the labor process, (3) the use of process and information technology, (4) interfirm cooperation, and (5) the production of a wide range of products for differentiated markets. These organizational features appear particularly functional in an era that emphasizes shortened product life cycles, rapid innovation, quality over quantity, greater worker involvement, flatter organizational hierarchies, and responsiveness to consumer needs. Appelbaum and Batt (1994:37) identified the following characteristics of the flexible specialization model:

1. Small-scale production of a large variety of goods, a strategy whose viability has been increased in recent decades by the introduction of informative technologies that improve the cost competitiveness of small-batch production.
2. Strong networks of small producers that achieve efficiency through specialization, and achieve flexibility through collaboration.
3. Representation of workers' interests through strong unions that bargain over wage norms at the national level and seek cooperative solutions to work organization and the flexible deployment of labor locally.
4. Municipal governments that provide collective goods and services, thereby reducing costs and encouraging cooperation.

The small-firm, short production-run, character of the early theorizing on flexible specialization suggested the importance of economies of scope for these enterprises. However, Appelbaum and Batt did not believe that flexible specialization is exclusively the affair of small- or medium-sized enterprises. Large firms can also achieve some of the advantages of flexible specialization by establishing alliances and networks (see Chapter 8) and by developing the technological means to achieve scope along with scale. Honda's effort to produce multiple models of a car for the global market is one example of the latter.

> Executives at Honda Motor Company knew they had a problem on their hands the moment they launched the sporty, restyled Accord four years ago. It was too cramped for U.S. drivers, but not stylish enough for the Japanese. . . For most of the Accord's 21-year history, Honda has been frustrated in its struggles to popularize its biggest seller in all the world's major markets. . . The obvious solution to the Accord's woes—designing a different model for each market—was out of the question. . .
>
> Honda may have found a way to customize the Accord. . . The American Accord will be a big, stout family car. . . The jazzy Japanese car will be a smaller, sportier compact, aimed at young professionals. The European version will be short and narrow and is expected to feature the stiff and sporty ride Old World drivers prefer. . .
>
> Honda's secret lies in an ingenious frame that allows the auto maker to shrink or expand the overlying car without starting from the ground up. By coming up with a platform. . . that can be bent and stretched into markedly different vehicles— Honda might have cracked the code for developing a global car. ("Can Honda Build a World Car," *Business Week,* September 8, 1997, p. 72.)

This is just one example of how flexibility and specialization can be realized in an organizational structure that does not possess the romantic characteristics of the small craftlike firm. It also points to what is now the obvious problem with Piore and Sabel's prognostication that rapid innovation and shifting market tastes would give rise to a singular organizational form. There are many ways for a company to become flexible, and large powerful organizations can pursue a variety of strategies to get there.

Lean and Mean, or Fat and Mean?

The debate over leanness, meanness, flexibility, and firm size is nicely captured in a comparative review of two books published in the mid-1990s—David Gordon's *Fat and Mean* (1996) and Bennett Harrison's *Lean and Mean* (1994). The titles suggest contradictory assessments. One might ask which is it, fat or lean? The answer depends on where and when you look.

Harrison's work has two major objectives: first, to describe and analyze the methods used by large corporations to reduce their girth and establish leanness; and second, to debunk the argument that big corporations are losing out to smaller innovative firms. In essence, these two issues are intimately related. The process of creating a leaner organizational structure has provided niche opportunities for smaller firms that can specialize in the activities that are being eliminated, downsized, or outsourced by the large corporations. Thus, counter to Piore and Sabel's claims about the rise of the small firm, Harrison argued that market power is still concentrated in the hands of the largest corporations while economic activities are decentralized. This observation yields the central conceptual framework—*concentration without centralization.*

The creation of the lean organization, according to Harrison, is based on (1) reducing the number of activities deemed vital to a firm's survival and focusing resources on core competencies, (2) using computerized manufacturing methods to coordinate decentralized activities and relations with other firms, (3) constructing strategic alliances with smaller firms that can supply services, parts, and components formerly supplied within the corporation, and (4) eliciting the active collaboration of the most highly paid and skilled employees.

The net result of all of these strategies is to reduce the size of the organization's workforce and the number of in-house activities. As single organizations become leaner in this fashion, they also become more involved in networks and alliances with other, much smaller, firms. Power and control remain concentrated to the extent that the smaller firms react to and depend upon the larger corporations.

In contrast, David Gordon contended that the leanness thesis is overstated and historically inaccurate. He based this point on his analysis of corporate strategies over a longer time period and his focus on internal labor management relations. Gordon also confirmed the important point that organizations do not move smoothly and quickly from one conceptual model to another. Instead there are extended transitions, trials and failures, and unintended consequences. In the case of the transformation from Fordism to the present, Gordon saw no direct shift from fat to lean but rather a transition from chunky to fatter to (eventually) slim.

Gordon's analysis rests on the fundamental conflict between labor and capital and the strategies used by capital to control labor. During the Fordist period, labor discipline and compliance rested heavily upon the flow of economic rewards in the form of wages, benefits, and job security. As U.S. corporations faced increasing international competition and declining profit rates, these economic incentives were cut back or eliminated. Thus, the initial response to crisis was a cost-cutting strategy. The resulting wage moderation and income stagnation eliminated the monetary incentives used to motivate workers. The growing absence of "the carrot" gave rise to the increasing prominence of "the stick." The stick was used to maintain levels of work effort in an organizational climate of economic deprivation. However, the stick involved an increase in middle and supervisory management who were hired to monitor the work effort of employees. Gordon referred to these managerial tasks as "guard labor." As the managerial proportion of the labor force increased, the organization became fatter, not leaner, and definitely meaner. As organizations become saturated with managerial fat, bureaucracy expanded, costs increased, efficiency suffered, and workers were increasingly distrustful. These unintended consequences extended and prolonged the crises of productivity and competitiveness. Eventually, many companies reassessed this self-defeating strategy and pursued counterstrategies.

One example: at the Lubbock, Texas, Frito-Lay plant, the number of managers fell from 38 to 13 since 1990, while the hourly workforce grew by more than 20 percent to about 220. Despite less worker supervision, the plant logged double-digit cost cuts and saw its quality climb into the top 6 of Frito-Lay's 48 U.S. factories. ("Team Player: No More 'Same-ol'-same-ol'," *Business Week,* October 17, 1994, p. 51.)

Despite the contradictory titles of Gordon's and Harrison's books, each revealed important patterns of organizational change. Harrison examined the most recent phase of corporate restructuring that produced the rise of production networks while Gordon chronicled the road taken from Fordist to fat to leaner organizations. Both writers documented the dark side of the restructuring process involving rising income inequality and economic dualism between large and small firms. They both made a clear distinction between low road strategies—cost cutting based on reduced labor costs—and high road strategies—innovation, worker training, and adequate compensation—with a decided preference for the latter.

Forms of Flexibility

Flexibility is now the single most popular trait of the new organizational form. New organizations are praised for being more flexible than old organizations. Almost all of the positive changes attributed to new organizations are couched in the language of flexibility. The assumption that flexible is good and rigidity is bad is based on the belief that organizations must be malleable in an environment characterized by rapid change, innovation, and emerging markets. Flexible implies the ability to restructure, reengineer, learn more quickly, and adapt to changing circumstances. "Managers everywhere have responded since the 1970s in various ways—all of which can be characterized as a search within large and small firms alike for greater flexibility" (Harrison 1994:127).

Like the shift from Fordism to non-Fordism, the shift from rigid to flexible, or less flexible to more flexible, can take a wide variety of trajectories. Given the centrality of the concept in the literature of contemporary management and organizations, it is worth examining the various organizational forms and practices associated with flexibility.

Harrison identified three distinct types of flexibility. First, *functional flexibility* involves the "efforts of managers to redefine work tasks, redeploy resources, and reconfigure relationships with suppliers." (1994:129–33). Instituting lean production and just-in-time practices constitute a form of functional flexibility. A primary purpose is to achieve economies of scope and enhance the ability of the firm to shift production toward different products, designs, and markets.

Wage flexibility, a second form, entails the termination of long-term job security, greater wage competition among workers, and a greater reliance on the external forces of the labor market. These pressures weaken the bargaining power of workers and have resulted in wage and salary givebacks, and multitiered wage structures.

The third form is *numerical flexibility,* which is also aimed at labor costs and the employment relationship. Numerical flexibility is achieved through the use of substitute part-time, contract, and other "contingent" labor. It is also realized through the outsourcing of various functions (maintenance, clerical, and accounting) formerly carried out within the firm. Temporary workers receive lower compensation and fewer, if any, benefits than permanent full-time workers. Numerical flexibility represents the application of just-in-time principles to the deployment of the human resource. Workers are hired and services are subcontracted when they are needed.

Sayer and Walker (1992) also "unpacked" the concept of flexibility. They argued that firms have always combined flexible and inflexible practices and processes, and that one cannot group these varied combinations according to the inflexible dualistic frameworks that contrast "the old as inflexible and the new as flexible. . . What is therefore needed is . . . a broader awareness of new forms of the division of labor and new ways of organizing these divisions" (1992:199). Sayer and Walker (1992:199) listed the following varieties of flexibility: flexibility in output volume, product flexibility, flexible employment, flexible working practice, flexible machinery, flexibility in restructuring, and flexible organizational forms.

Flexibility in output volume and *product flexibility* relate directly to the issues of economies of scale and economies of scope, respectively. Greater organizational flexibility might be signaled by calibrating output volume with market demand. This is consistent with a pull, not push, approach to production. Similarly, it might be reflected in rapidly shifting product designs and models to meet changing or diverse market demands. The example of Honda's world car strategy is an attempt to combine these two forms of flexibility—the appropriate volume (scale) directed toward diverse market segments (scope).

Flexible employment, like numerical flexibility, involves a smaller full-time workforce and the capacity to use temporary or subcontracted labor services.

Flexible working practices are associated with lean production systems. These include multiskilling and multitasking, which break down rigid job classification and allow workers more job variety and managers greater flexibility in the deployment of workers.

Flexible machinery is the use of microelectronics-based automation that, instead of being devoted to a single task or process, can be reprogrammed and integrated with multiple production processes and platforms. Computer integrated manufacturing (CIM) and flexible manufacturing systems (FMS) are based on these technologies which are still in their infant stages. "Compared to human labor, even the most flexible machine is crude and rigid, and unintelligent when it comes to handling the unexpected . . . No matter how flexible technology may be, it is still fixed capital and shares the inherent problems of that status" (1992:200–01).

Finally, *flexible organizational forms* move us from the intraorganizational to the interorganizational level. Flexibilities can be achieved when networks of firms come together to jointly research, design, and manufacture a product. This is an important feature of the flexible specialization model. Interorganizational arrangements will be discussed in greater detail in Chapter 10.

The various forms of flexibility reviewed above can be seen as pieces and fragments of organizational *restructuring.* While the concept of flexibility gives one the impression that there is a single underlying logic directing this organizational shift, it is more accurately a piecemeal, trial-and-error process. Most firms are under pressure to restructure some or all aspects of their operation as a way to remain productive and competitive. The language of flexibility suggests a rational direction and defined objective. Some of the elements of organizational restructuring include the elimination of product lines, early retirement, combining internal units, selling nonessential units, closing plants and downsizing the full-time labor force, outsourcing, reallocating or relocating employees, changing top executives, and shifting facilities to cheaper geographic locations (Usui and Colignon 1996; Castells 1996). Some of these actions may contribute to flexibility; others are simply designed to cut costs, which has always been a fundamental organizational objective.

These methods of restructuring obviously have differential effects depending on one's organizational location. Wage and employment "flexibilities" are likely to contribute to less secure employment, lower wages, and heavier workloads for many organizational members. As one labor economist has explained, "Almost every employment relationship is contingent on the employer being able to continue in the same business with the same product and the same technology with the same quiescent competition. Now, who's in that position?" ("Rethinking Work," *Business Week,* October 17, 1994, p. 77). The answer is no one. Therefore, employment relationships tend to be altered in the direction of greater job insecurity.

Flexibility and restructuring strategies are also ways to reconfigure the divisions of labor (Sayer and Walker 1992; Castells 1996). If new forms of differentiation in work tasks, decision-making authority, or the supply and distribution chain are implemented, new mechanisms for socially and functionally integrating people and production processes will be required. Under the Fordist division of labor, functional integration or coordination was accomplished largely by technical control of the assembly line and managerial supervision. Social integration was achieved through union-based representation, generous compensation, and relative job security. With a more flexible organizational model, work tasks may be reorganized to allow greater levels of discretion and decision making, compensation levels may be lower, job security tenuous, the number of part-time temporary workers greater, and the organizational climate less stable. Under these conditions, organizations face a significant challenge coordinating the different members and activities functionally and socially. It will be more difficult and require qualitatively different methods than existed under a more tightly controlled system. One of the unintended consequences of organizational change toward greater flexibility is the unraveling of traditional forms of integration. These problems might nullify the expected positive consequences of new flexibility strategies.

Herbert Kaufman (1985) has argued that flexibility should never be regarded as a costless organizational strategy. While designing an organization for flexibility theoretically allows the rapid shifting of gears, resources, and commitments, he noted that "under certain conditions concentration of resources and wholehearted commitment to a single option may be advantageous." There is also the inherent paradox that "maintaining flexibility can itself shut off options and impose limits on flexibility. . . it cannot do all sorts of things because they would be commitments and therefore would reduce its freedom of action" (Kaufman 1985:73). Thus, long-term contracts, employment guarantees, or capital investments—all of which have potentially positive organizational consequences—cannot be pursued if the primary objective is flexibility.

Kaufman also referred to the "costs of disunity" which is related to social integration. Flexibility "can weaken the internal unity of organizations that is sometimes a key factor in triumphs over environmental adversity. . . it can weaken unity because it clashes with the cathexis strong bonds require. . . to preserve flexibility, an organization dare not let attachments grow too strong. . . So if an organization strives for flexibility, it frequently must eschew unifying devices that might otherwise be employed" (1985:74–75).

The paradox of flexibility expressed by Kaufman was also addressed by Dore (1986) in his analysis of the textile industry in Japan. He used the term *flexible rigidities* to describe the paradoxical joining of "flexible" production processes and organizational practices with "rigid" constraints based on trust, obligations, and long-term commitments in Japanese industry. The success of these Japanese organizations has been based on combining or balancing organizational traits regarded as contradictory (Kenney and Florida 1988; Sayer and Walker 1992:212–21). In the Japanese case, much of this flexible rigidity finds its source in the distinct interorganizational alliances that will be the subject of Chapter 10. Within the firm, the system hinges on multiskilling and task flexibility alongside lifetime employment and seniority-based reward systems.

Summary

This chapter has reviewed a wide assortment of new organizational forms and processes that have emerged over the past 20 years. The key points are as follows:

1. In their analyses of emerging organizational forms, organizational theorists have tended to use the Fordist industrial model as the basis for comparison. New organizational forms are said to depart from the Fordist reliance on a rigid division of labor and standardized job tasks because this form of organization can no longer meet the demands of a rapidly changing economy and market.

2. We have cautioned against the widespread tendency to conceptualize organizational change as a smooth transition from one ideal-type model to another. The standard Fordist/post-Fordist comparison obscures the fact that the shift from one organizational form to another is fraught with dilemmas, contradictions, compromises, and constraints. Organizational transformations are most likely to produce some amalgamated or hybrid structure that combines pieces of the old with elements of the new.

3. Toyotaism and lean manufacturing have represented two major models for organizational transformation. Based on a significant transformation of labor-management relations, quality, and the organization of the production process, many elements of these

Japanese-inspired systems have been incorporated into industrial organizations. Studies of the lean production system in the automobile industry indicate that the impact on workers is not unambiguously positive. It represents an intensification of work and a more comprehensive system of social control.

4. *Flexibility* is the term most often used to describe the direction of organizational change. The centrality of this concept is consistent with the assumption that the key to organizational success is the ability to adapt quickly to changing circumstances and demands. Flexibility applies to a wide range of current organizational practices ranging from just-in-time supply chains to the use of temporary workers.

7

EMERGING ORGANIZATIONAL PARADIGMS: POSTBUREAUCRACY, CULTURE, AND KNOWLEDGE

This chapter continues the discussion of emerging developments in organization theory and practice. However, the terrain will shift from industrial organizational structures to several broader paradigmatic approaches that inform thinking about organizational processes. These include the postbureaucratic model, the cultural component of organizations, and the idea of a learning or knowledge organization.

Postbureaucratic Organization

The Postbureaucratic Organization in Theory

If the organizational mantra of the 1990s was flexibility, the bogeyman was bureaucracy. No one seemed to be advocating, or discovering a shift toward, greater bureaucratic structure or formalization. Instead, the desire to transcend bureaucracy translated into the rise of the postbureaucratic organization. Since bureaucracy and organization have long been joined synonymously, postbureaucratic organization suggests an oxymoron. However, postbureaucracy is clearly the trend in both the practical world of management theory and the theoretical world of organizational studies (Clegg 1990; Heckscher and Donnelon 1994; Barzelay 1992). Behind discussions of post-Fordism, lean production, and flexible specialization is the implicit assumption that organizations will be more effective if they debureaucratize. What does this mean for organizational structure and process?

Max Weber provided the ideal-type conceptualization of bureaucracy. Charles Heckscher (1994) attempted the same task for the postbureaucratic

TABLE 7–1   Ideal-Type Features of the Postbureaucratic Organization

1. Consensus through *institutionalized dialogue* rather than acquiescence to authority and rules.
2. Influence by *persuasion* rather than official position.
3. Influence based on *mutual trust* and *interdependence* rather than narrow self or departmental interest.
4. Integration through a strong emphasis on *organizational mission* rather than formal job definitions and rules.
5. *Sharing of information* rather than hoarding and hiding information.
6. Organizational behavior and action based on *principles* rather than formal rules.
7. Consultation and communication based on the *problem* or *project* rather than a formal chain of command.
8. Verification of qualifications and expertise through open processes of *association* and *peer evaluation* rather than formal credentials and official position.
9. *Looser organizational boundaries* that tolerate outsiders coming in and insiders going out rather than the insular organization man/women emphasis.
10. Evaluation, compensation, and promotion based on *public and negotiated standards of performance* rather than rigid objective criteria.
11. Expectations of *constant change based on continual assessment* rather than expectations of permanence based on the assumption of a fixed set of appropriate procedures.

Source: Charles Heckscher, "Defining the Post-Bureaucratic Type," in Charles Heckscher and Anne Donnelon, eds., *The Post Bureaucratic Organization* (Thousand Oaks, CA: Sage, 1994), pp. 25–28.

organization. Table 7-1 outlines the central conceptual characteristics according to Heckscher. These ideal-type features reveal a number of postbureaucratic patterns. First, the formalization associated with an organizational chart, outlining the appropriate chain of command and channels of communication, is deliberately eliminated. Instead, command is replaced by *dialogue, persuasion,* and *trust* which allow a wider range of opinion and influence across the organization, flowing from the bottom up, rather than from the top down. The role of trust and the larger organizational mission also play a large role since organizational members should not believe that persuasion is designed to advance particularist interests or the "hidden agenda." Receptivity to the claims and arguments of other organizational members requires such trust and a widely internalized attachment to the larger organizational mission. Consensual decision making will be more likely under such conditions.

Second, the postbureaucratic organization will be an *information-sharing and disseminating organization.* The effectiveness of dialogue, mutual influence, and persuasion depends on the equal access to and wide distribution of information about organizational resources and performance. Hoarding and monopolizing information and knowledge in order to gain advantage and exercise power is antithetical to the postbureaucratic model.

Third, organizational behavior and action are dictated not by formal roles and job descriptions but by *general principles* that allow greater discretion, flexibility, and adaptation. This will encourage greater reflection about the relationship between organizational actions and broader organizational objectives. If an organizational principle is "the prompt delivery of services to customers," organizational members should abandon or revise formal procedures that hinder the realization of this objective. The emphasis on *principles* rather than *methods* addresses the classic bureaucratic problem of obsessive attachment to rules and the displacement of organizational goals. If procedures are assessed in relation to the organizational mission and principles, there will also be greater receptivity toward organizational change.

Fourth, interaction, communication, and decision making will be driven by *problems and projects* rather than a hierarchical chain of command. Cross-functional teams of employees from different departments and strata within the organization will meet to solve problems and work on projects.

The fifth and final feature of Heckscher's conceptualization of postbureaucracy pertains to the assessment and evaluation of personnel. Instead of seniority or formal credentials—or the immediate supervisor as the evaluator—as the criteria for performance evaluations and promotion, there will be greater reliance on *peer evaluation and negotiated standards of performance.* Given the greater levels of horizontal and vertical interaction and the use of teams, there will be wider knowledge about the strengths and weaknesses of various organizational members. Effective communication and consultation depend on the diffusion of such information. In this fluid environment, it is also likely that members can develop certain skills and competencies that extend beyond a formal job description. Therefore, employees can negotiate and demonstrate their particular organizational assets.

Taken together, Heckscher's ideal type features rest on what he called the "master concept" which is

> *"an organization in which everyone takes responsibility for the success of the whole.* If that happens, then the basic notion of regulating relations among people by *separating* them into specific predefined functions must be abandoned . . . organizational control must center not on the management of tasks, but the management of relationships . . . they are essentially structures that develop *informed consensus* rather than relying on hierarchy and authority" (italics in original 1994:24).

The postbureaucratic organization faces the challenge of replacing one method of control, formal structural differentiation of functions and authority, with another, structures that develop "informed consent." Again a central organizational tension emerges. In the absence of formal bureaucratic control and coordination, organizational members are given wide latitude to pursue a variety of goals. Under these conditions, organizational "mission plays a crucial integrating role in an organization that relies less heavily on job definitions and rules. Employees need to understand the key objectives in depth in order to coordinate their actions intelligently 'on the fly' " (1994:25).

As with Weber's ideal-type bureaucracy, it is difficult to find an existing postbureaucratic organization but there are a number of telltale signs of infiltration. According to Heckscher, when key elements of the postbureaucratic form are introduced, they "mix poorly, producing conflict and resistance." This may happen because organizational members have developed an attachment to standard operating procedures or because postbureaucratic practices threaten the established authority structure. Second, evidence for the new form may be found in the introduction of elements that "will be rejected as 'foreign,' or they will so infect the organization that other aspects will change as well." The power of the new postbureaucratic paradigm is presumably measured by its degree of influence in prompting either resistance or a wider reassessment of all organizational practices. Third, the new type should eventually impact on larger institutional processes that are separate from, but support, existing organizations. Heckscher cited socialization, careers, classes, and the work ethic:

> Career systems, for example, are being severely shaken by the need for flexibility . . . this in turn affects residential patterns (when is one secure enough to buy a house?), socialization (what expectations should one have in entering the labor force?), and class relations (how can one anchor one's identification in an insecure world?) (Heckscher 1994:27).

Evidence for various aspects of postbureaucracy have been reported widely. As students of organizations, we can find this kind of evidence in media coverage such as *Business Week*'s report on "rethinking work," which highlighted the tensions, questions, and uncertainties that accompany the rise of the new paradigm:

> We confront a workplace that will evolve year after year. Many will find the result both enervating and rewarding. In companies that are flattening hierarchies and, bit by bit, decentralizing decision making, workers are gaining greater control over what they do; self-direction has superseded the doctrine that workers do only what they are told . . . The question: How many losers will have to rethink traditional roles and relationships. Even as both sides look each other up and down, they'll be confronted with the need to act fast, to transform new competitive pressures into mutual gains. ("Rethinking Work: Special Report," *Business Week,* October 17, 1994, p. 77.)

Business Week's summary editorial used even starker language:

> It's getting positively Darwinian. The American workplace, once a protected habitat offering a measure of prosperity in exchange for a lifetime of dedicated work, is now a dangerous place. Like it or not, Americans are being forced to give up security for opportunity and stability for mobility (down as well as up). ("Editorials: Rethinking Work," *Business Week,* October 17, 1994, p. 252.)

And from the trenches, workers shared the following:

> Years ago, we had one guy who told us what to do and we did it. He made all the de-
> cisions. We never really had any input. Now, you have to listen to your men. They
> have empowered us so much that we don't have to do a job if we think it's unsafe. If
> I tell one of the men to do a job and he thinks it's unsafe, we sit down and talk about
> it. ("Rethinking Work: Special Report," *Business Week,* October 17, 1994, p. 80.)

This last item is certainly consistent with a central component of the postbureaucratic organization. "Because of the crucial role of back-and-forth dialogue rather than one-way communication, or command, I will call it the *interactive* type" (Heckscher 1994:24). The superiority of this model, according
to Heckscher, is not the increased satisfaction and commitment but the way
commitment is translated into better organizational outcomes in the areas of
innovation and decision making.

The Postbureaucratic Organization in Practice

While there may be few existing postbureaucratic organizations of any size
and significance, Heckscher mentioned the Shell-Sarnia plant in Ontario,
Canada, as the "most advanced exemplar" of this organizational type. Let's
look at some of the actual workplace practices in this organization (the following account is based on information from Sirianni 1995 and Wells 1993).

Shell-Sarnia.   The Shell-Sarnia facility is a $200 million plant that produces
alcohol and polypropylene using continuous process technology. The plant
employs 130 workers all of whom are members of the Energy and Chemical
Workers Union (ECWU). The physical layout and social organization of the
plant were designed by a team with representatives from Shell management
and the ECWU.

   The social organization of the plant is based on semiautonomous
teams—six 18-member process teams, each with a coordinator, and one 14-
member craft team. The process teams carry out all process operations,
which range from lab work to janitorial tasks, during their rotating shifts.
Teams decide work assignments, scheduling, vacations, overtime, and
training. The other team of craft personnel (e.g., electricians, pipefitters)
perform their functional specialties while also instructing process team
members in basic craft techniques. This is designed to reduce excessive reliance on craft specialists. Unrestricted learning in a supportive team environment allows all operators to learn every task necessary to run the plant.
Strict job classification and seniority-based promotions are eliminated in
order to facilitate the acquisition of progress- and performance-based skills.
Carmen Sirianni reported that "skill levels in the plant are so impressive
that managers visiting from a Shell petrochemical complex in western

Canada remarked to the plant superintendent that they could not distinguish the operators from the engineers" (Sirianni 1995).

The physical layout of the plant is also designed to reduce divisions and increase mutual access to administrative offices, labs, and information technology. The latter entails computer software and online information available to all employees. The information and data are subject to changes and revisions based on the suggestions and experiences of the employees. Reflecting Heckscher's interactive form:

> Discussion and dialogue revolve around "what it means for employees to be considered responsible and trustworthy, and for work organization to encourage initiative and the development of skills to their fullest capacity." Labor has a voice on all issues other than strategic business policy and workers meet formally and informally within and across work teams. Because the organizational design at Sarnia directly empowers workers, provides them with access to information and open discussion, and makes them much less dependent on managers in their everyday activities, the internal culture of the union as well as the plant has been considerably democratized (Sirianni 1995).

As an example of a potentially postbureaucratic organization, the social and physical organization of the plant is informed by both sociotechnical systems theory and psychoanalytically oriented group process theory. These combine to produce an organizational model that uses autonomous team collaboration, group activity, and attention to self-development and reflection. These theories about work organization have been around for a long time, but they may be especially relevant for organizations that are trying to restructure away from the bureaucratic model while at the same time introducing new forms of process and information technology.

Oticon Holding. An even more striking example of postbureaucracy is found in the renovated factory facility of Denmark's Oticon Holding A/S (Labarre 1996). A global leader in the production of hearing aids, Oticon decided in the late 1980s to reinvent the company. Rather than incremental changes and improvements, the firm's leader, Lars Kolind, decided to *dis-organize* the operation. The first thing to go was the formal organizational chart with its specialized positions and hierarchical relationships. In its place Kolind set up an entirely structureless organization best reflected in the concept of the mobile office. Each employee was given a standard-issue office on wheels. The office "caddies" contained the bare essentials—room for hanging folders and binders, desk space to work, no drawers, and a networked computer. Because the defining work unit was the *project* rather than the department or the function, workers physically moved, with their mobile offices, from one project team to another. The employee's office was "parked" for the duration of the project, which might last from a few weeks to several months.

Employees were not separated by partitions, walls, or secretaries. The objective was to maximize walking, talking, and acting. Many of the different project teams worked side-by-side, which also enhanced the sharing of information and served to socially integrate the 150-person workforce. Two forms of technology played a key role in the dis-organization. All employees were issued a mobile phone that facilitated the footloose work environment. Groupware software systems were also used to conduct electronic brainstorming sessions and collectively compose technical documents and manuals. Oticon also sought to establish a paperless organization, so the company now has a "paper room" where employees review mail, scan important documents, and then shred all originals.

The postbureaucratic scheme, and the cases of Shell-Sarnia and Oticon, direct us toward an organizational trend that is redefining the parameters and meaning of formal structure. One of the key elements of the postbureaucratic organization is the elimination of obstacles—both formal roles and physical structures—that prevent the flow of information and communication. This suggests the greater use of process and project teams that exchange knowledge and information and define their own parameters for completing a task. Organizational roles emerge from the interaction with team members. Control is also generated through collective peer pressure and obligations stemming from team membership. In the postbureaucratic organization, social and functional integration takes precedence over differentiation and specialization.

Postbureaucracy and Physical Space

The cases of Shell-Sarnia and especially Oticon point to the routinely ignored but increasingly important issue of physical space. It is a given that organizational structure and bureaucracy are embodied in organizational charts, formal rules and regulations, and other paper directives. Is bureaucracy also embodied in the physical layout of the organization? The answer is clearly yes. Many organizations even reproduce the pyramid-shaped organizational chart in the design of buildings and the assignment of space. The president occupies the top floor with the best view and the greatest space. The subordinate organization literally rests underneath the office of the president. It is common for the next highest executive positions to be physically located on the floors immediately below the president, with the remainder of the hierarchy arranged from the upper to lower floors, even down to the basement, in descending order of authority and status. Physical divisions by floors, buildings, walls, and partitions are typically employed to separate workers by function, department, and status. Given these fundamental facts about most organizations, any effort to develop nonbureaucratic forms must consider the physical work environment.

Organizational ecology considers the broader physical workplace environment that shapes subjective feelings about work and the objective patterns of behavior, interaction, and process.

> It includes the ways in which organizational leaders consciously and deliberately make decisions about the form of their buildings: the choice of furnishings; the arrangements of office and work stations; the layout of circulation; the number and location and character of conference and meeting rooms, stairwells, elevators, cafeterias and break areas; choices about how and to whom space is allocated; and the nature of the processes used to plan design and manage all these workplace elements over time. In short, organizational ecology is about how an organization's leaders choose to convene their employees in space and time in pursuit of a long-term competitive edge (Becker and Steele 1995:11–12).

Organizational ecology suggests that emerging organizational forms, and the specific kinds of activities and processes they are designed to engender, must include the physical restructuring of the work space. If an organization is committed to teamwork and cross-functional interaction, people cannot be physically separated but must be provided with the physical layout and space that allows and encourages interaction and exchange. If the emphasis is on a learning organization, the facility must be designed to provide settings and materials for organizational members to access and use the information resources. If the objective is to encourage "serendipitous communication and interaction," "magnet centers" must be created to draw people together in an area conducive to conversation and extended contact (Becker and Steele 1995:40–41).

One organizational process that has undergone significant change is product development. Franz Becker and Fritz Steele (1995) conceptualized the transition from the old to new product development technique as the shift from a "relay race" to a "rugby" model. In the *relay race model,* product development proceeds as a series of sequential activities by different functional departments. Engineering hands off a plan to design, who then hands it off to manufacturing, who then turns the responsibility over to marketing. As each department completes its job, it is passed on to the next department and so on down the line. In the *rugby model,* players from all departments rub elbows (and throw an occasional forearm). The constant interchange inherent in this model, which brings all the departments together from start to finish, is viewed as a more productive arrangement that can enhance innovation and a rapid development cycle. Is there an organizational ecology consonant with the rugby model?

Steelcase, Inc., a manufacturer of office furniture based in Grand Rapids, Michigan, constructed a Corporate Development Center designed to encourage and realize the rugby-style model of product development. Steelcase management was interested in maximizing informal contacts across departments and project teams, and breaking down organizational divisions based on the different cultural work styles of the various departments and disciplines. These objectives translated into physical work spaces that included (1) multiple work areas for private, project, and shared purposes; (2) "mixed neighborhoods" combining clusters of personnel from different functional departments; (3) a cluster of senior management directors located in the middle of the building and easily accessible; (4) "activity generators" such as a town square, cafeteria, and break areas that allow informal and serendipitous contact; (5) "corners commons" containing movable furniture and walls allowing for the creation of partitioned or open areas for private work tasks or miniconferences; (6) escalators that increase visibility and contact; (7) "functionally inconvenient" meetings rooms and labs that require people to walk through different areas of the organization to reach their destination and, as a consequence, come into contact with organizational strangers.

Steelcase represents just one powerful example (see Becker and Steele 1995 for others) of how the physical design of buildings and work spaces can be informed by social principles and can in turn advance organizational change. This adds an additional dimension to restructuring that goes beyond mission statements and written documents that proclaim a new organizational model. The philosophy is literally built into the physical structure in which people work.

Postbureaucracy in Government

Postbureaucracy is also an emerging trend in the public sector. Widespread calls for reinventing, streamlining, and privatizing governmental operations are all based on the assumption that public-sector bureaucracy is especially inefficient and unproductive and unresponsive to citizen needs (Schacter 1997; Osborne and Gaebler 1992). One notable example comes from the state of Minnesota which in the 1980s initiated the Striving Toward Excellence in Performance (STEP) program. Michael Barzelay studied the reorganization effort in *Breaking through Bureaucracy* (1992). In his analysis he compared the old bureaucratic with the emerging postbureaucratic paradigm. The key elements of this are shown in Table 7–2. A number of points are worth noting in this comparison. First, the notion of the "public interest" as defined by government officials is replaced with the term "results citizens value." The emphasis has shifted from the abstract to the more concrete objectives of "results" that the customers, or citizens, can evaluate for quality and value. This is consistent with the belief by many critics of government that public-sector orientations should be more closely aligned with the private-sector philosophy of producing goods and services that consumers value. Thus, the shift from "administration" to "production." As a way to avoid the displacement of goals, functional authority and structure is replaced by mission, services, and customers. What is critical for the postbureaucratic government organization is not the bureaucratic means but the agency

TABLE 7–2   Bureaucracy and Postbureaucracy in Government

Bureaucratic Elements	Postbureaucratic Elements
Public interest	Results citizens value
Efficiency	Quality and value
Administration	Production
Control	Winning adherence to norms
Specify function, authority, and structure	Identify mission, service, and customers
Justify costs	Deliver value
Responsibility	Accountability
Follow rules and procedures	Understand and apply norms, solve problems, improve processes
Operate administrative systems	Expand customer choice, provide incentives, measure and analyze results

Source: Adapted from Table 3 in Michael Barzelay, *Breaking through Bureaucracy* (Berkeley: University of California Press, 1992), p. 118.

"products" and their conformity with the agency's mission and the needs of citizens. A final element that is taking on increasing importance is "norms." Behavior, action, and policy should be based on a normative foundation of values and principles rather than mechanical rules and procedures.

At the federal government level there is the National Partnership for Reinventing (NPR) Government, an initiative driven by the same kind of postbureaucratic principles outlined above. In terms of organizational restructuring designed to achieve these principles, STEP and NPR have attempted to decentralize decision making and allow line agencies greater control over policies and expenditures, reduce administrative oversight and approval, increase incentives for agencies and employees that develop quality schemes, and measure success by customer satisfaction. In comparing the postbureaucratic efforts of the private and public sectors, it is important to keep in mind the broader range of legal and regulatory constraints operating in the public sector which limit the latitude of reform.

Organizational Culture

Levels of Culture

In Chapter 1 organizational culture was discussed as one of the metaphors used for organizational analysis (Morgan 1997). In this metaphor, the essence of organization revolves around the development of shared meanings, beliefs, values, and assumptions that guide and are reinforced by organizational behavior.

To this can be added the three levels of culture identified in the work of Edgar Schein (1992) presented in Table 7–3. The first level shows the *artifacts*

TABLE 7–3   **Levels of Organizational Culture**

Level	Definition	Example
Artifacts	Tangible and observable aspects of organization	Written documents, physical layout, dress, behavioral rituals
Espoused values	Beliefs about what should happen in the organization	Organizational philosophy vision and mission
Basic assumptions	Taken-for-granted ways of doing and thinking and achieving goals	Standard operating procedures, presumed methods of efficiency

Source: Edgar H. Schein, *Organizational Culture and Leadership* (San Francisco: Jossey-Bass, 1992), p. 17.

that are subject to sensory perception; this is, they can be seen, heard, and felt. These include the organizational architecture, the physical and material elements of the organization, and the language, technology, and observable rituals of the organization. Schein noted that artifacts represent the easiest level of culture to observe but the most difficult to decipher. The precise meaning that organizational members attach to artifacts can be ambiguous and unclear. Consider the mobile office caddy used by Oticon employees. This object might communicate an unwillingness by the organization to invest in a comfortable and stable work environment for its employees. Alternatively, it can represent the symbolic trappings of a high-energy organization that encourages continuous movement and team interaction.

The second level of culture, according to Schein, are the *espoused values.* This is the normative side of the organization that communicates what ought to be rather than what is. The espoused values represent what the organizational members believe they should be doing and how they should be acting. Public statements and pronouncements often reveal the espoused values of an organization. A firm may claim that it is devoted to continuous innovation and lifelong learning. There is no reason to assume, however, that such espoused values are actually translated into organizational behavior and processes.

The third level of culture is the *basic assumptions* of the organization. These assumptions are manifested in behavior and action—the taken-for-granted premises that guide behavior and determine how people will respond to organizational stimuli and problems. The standard operating procedures of an organization are built on a set of assumptions that are rarely scrutinized or challenged. In higher education, for example, a basic assumption is that the classroom is the best place for students to learn and instructors to teach. The whole mental model of a teaching and learning process revolves around this assumption. It shapes how we plan, schedule, and organize learning time.

One kind of organizational analysis, using these three levels, would involve examining the correspondence or consistency between the three levels. Do artifacts reinforce the values that are then affirmed by the basic operating assumptions? Or, does the organization have a physical architecture and set of operating assumptions that are inconsistent with the espoused values? How does the organization reconcile this inconsistency or tension?

Is Culture an Emerging Form?

It would be incorrect to argue that normative strategies of social control, of which organizational culture is a major component, are new organizational phenomena. As noted in Chapter 2, managerial ideologies (Bendix 1956) have been a constant source of social control since the rise of the factory system. Stephen Barley and Gideon Kunda (1992) pointed out that "managerial discourse" has historically alternated between rational and normative rhetoric. While these are often viewed as alternative strategies of control, the argument in this book is that a central tension in all organizations is generated by the attempt to balance objective rational structural with subjective normative modes of control.

Barley and Kunda argued that different historical periods are characterized by particular surges of managerial theorizing. Rational modes of theorizing surged under the ideologies of scientific management (1900–1923) and systems rationalization (1955–1980), while normative modes of theorizing swelled under the ideologies of industrial betterment (1870–1900), welfare capitalism/human relations (1923–1955), and organizational culture (1980–present). More generally, "one might argue that rational rhetoric should surge when profitability seems most tightly linked to the management of capital. Conversely, normative rhetoric should surge when profitability seems to depend more on the management of labor" (1992:389). Again, because each is a fundamental and necessary feature of organization, Barley and Kunda also acknowledged that "It should therefore come as no surprise that managerial ideologies traffic in notions of both normative and rational control" (p. 386).

However, as they also noted, the period from 1980 to the present is characterized by the normative rhetoric of organizational culture. Since we are interested in new organizational forms and processes, the factors that have brought organizational culture and normative emphases to the fore must be considered. Recall from the discussion of human relations and the rational bureaucratic model that normative strategies have often been employed as a means to address the negative subjective reaction of labor to scientific management and bureaucratized forms of organization. In this sense, too much structural rationalization may necessitate normative-style appeals as a means to sustain motivation and commitment—the normative can compensate for the excessively rational.

In the current era, a much different dynamic is taking place which goes beyond Barley and Kunda's argument that there is a greater dependence on the management of labor. Rather, given what has been said about current trends in organization, there has been a clear shift away from both rational discourse and practice, and a move toward nonbureaucratic forms. Thus, the normative thrust is less a means to *compensate* for the effects of rational social control than a means to *replace* rational structures of control. It is in this context that the issue of organizational culture must be considered. In addition, the normative cultural component has been strongly associated with Japanese management systems, such as Toyotaism, and has therefore represented part of a larger managerial package to be emulated and implemented (Boswell 1987). Together, these factors help explain the growing number of articles on organizational culture since the early 1980s (Barley, Meyer, and Gash 1988).

Engineering Strong Culture: The Work of Gideon Kunda

Gideon Kunda's *Engineering Culture* (1992) is a prime illustration of the rise of organizational culture. Kunda's observational ethnographic study of a high-tech corporation captures the expanding role of culture in a nonbureaucratic workplace setting. He offered a very general and inclusive definition of organizational culture.

> The shared rules governing cognitive and affective aspects of membership in an organization, and the means whereby they are shaped and expressed . . . the shared meanings, assumptions, norms and values that govern work-related behavior; the symbolic, textual, and narrative structures in which they are encoded; and—in the functionalist tradition—the structural causes and consequences of cultural forms and their relationship to various measures of organizational effectiveness (Kunda 1992:8).

Again, this kind of definition is applicable to a wide range of normative systems extending to the earliest forms of organization. More specifically, the "cognitive and affective" refer to how organizational members understand, make sense of, and feel about their work and the organization. Organizational tasks, practices, and routines are the "means" that shape and express these cognitive and affective sentiments. In this sense, the culture is reinforced and reflected in the actual actions and behaviors of organizational members. The shared meanings, assumptions, norms, and values refer to a common way of thinking that can shape organizational behavior independent of external sanctions. These meanings, norms, and values are expressed symbolically through actions and are also embodied in the language used to describe the organization and its work. Finally, in the functionalist context, the culture should conform and be consistent with the formal structures and promote the larger objectives of the organization.

A cultural analysis of any organization might apply any or all of these concepts. However, beyond the generic description of organizational culture is the more significant claim that contemporary organizations are attempting to establish a more intensive, explicit, and systematic normative system that Kunda and others have described as strong culture.

> *Strong cultures* are based on intense emotional attachment and the internalization of 'clearly enunciated company values' that often replace formal structures and therefore no longer require strict and rigid external control. Instead, productive work is the result of a combination of self-direction, initiative, and emotional attachment, and ultimately combines the organizational interest in productivity with the employee's personal interest in growth and maturity" (Kunda 1992:10).

Though there is growing theoretical and managerial interest in strong culture arrangements, Kunda (1992:11) correctly emphasized that it represents the ongoing attempt to fashion an innovative solution to the foremost problem and age-old managerial dilemma—how to gain the compliance and control over organizational members who possess their own interests and the capacity to resist and oppose managerial prerogatives. Another reason the organizational culture may have to be stronger is to carry the growing burden placed on it in organizations like the one studied by Kunda. He described the workplace of this particular high-tech firm, referred to by the pseudonym "Tech," as vague, decentralized, chaotic, ambiguous, and controlled anarchy. More to the point, "formal and informal organizations are not readily distinguishable: informal organizing is formally prescribed, and 'culture' replaces 'structure' as an organizing principle to explain reality and guide action" (Kunda 1992:30).

Kunda emphasized the *ideological role* of the organizational culture, which suggests that it is a creation of those in positions of power and authority and is designed to legitimize the existing arrangements. The ideology at Tech is conveyed through verbal statements and written documents disseminated by management personnel, experts hired to study and report on the workings of the organization, and outside observers from the business press who report on the technology industry. The internal message emphasizes self-management, trust, and doing the right thing. There is also a concerted effort to convince employees that fulfilling their role obligation within the organization, what Kunda called the "member role," will produce a convergence of individual goals and collective interests. This represents a classic and recurring theme of managerial ideology.

In addition to the standard documents and pronouncements, Tech also hired a "culture expert" who was assigned to study the organizational culture at Tech and determine its role in promoting corporate success. Her analysis unearthed a number of themes such as a tradition of full employment, employee involvement, "ownership," rewards for success, minimal formal processes, encouragement of subcultural differences, learning from experience, tolerance for multiple viewpoints, and the organization as a free enterprise system. Finally, organizational members received materials published by external management consultants and industry observers. One such document, titled "Overview of Corporate Cultures," echoes a central theme in claiming that "if integrated into the workings of the corporate staff, the development of organizational cultures can, in part, replace the workings of outmoded cumbersome bureaucratic methods" (Kunda 1992:80).

In "decoding" these various sources of ideology, Kunda's analysis highlighted two central themes: the company's social attributes and the specifics of the member role. Metaphors conjure up images of the family, a mission, moral purpose, and progress. Kunda emphasized the cultural rather than the structural principles of organization.

> "[C]ontrol is thought of as the internalization of discipline . . . members are not constrained by enforced or traditional structures . . . decisions emerge through a political process of negotiation between innovative members. Discipline is not based on explicit supervision and reward, but rather on peer pressure and, more crucially, internalized standards of performance" (Kunda 1992:90).

Kunda also found the ideology embedded within the frequent "presentation rituals" of speeches, presentations, meetings, lectures, parties, and training workshops. Rituals are a fundamental activity of organizational life that allow the cognitive and affective principles to be presented and acted out. In this way, the culture can be demonstrated, created, and reinforced through social action. Participation in these rituals is a means for "becoming by doing" (Bowles and Gintis 1989); identities and attachments are shaped and reinforced by active involvement in ritualistic activities. At Tech, rituals are either directed toward organizational members through presentations, or experienced through day-to-day workplace activities. Kunda reported a number of presentations by upper-level management designed to both inform and motivate. These presentations generate a "sense of togetherness, common purpose, and shared excitement" but there are also those who do not attend the presentations, find the pitch monotonous, or engage in various distancing behaviors (e.g., whispering to and joking with colleagues).

Kunda applied some of the insights of symbolic interactionism (Goffman 1961) to analyze the level of attachment and engagement of organizational members. When the members of the audience are engaged and attentive, they exhibit *role embracement* which means they play along and behave in ways that suggest an identification with the speaker and the message. The ritual could not be sustained without this level of member role embracement. "Thus, the ritual frame consists of articulations and enactments of role-prescribed beliefs (the centrality of profit, the importance of technological accomplishment) and feelings (loyalty, commitment, excitement, fun, togetherness)" (Kunda 1992:106).

Equally important is the *role distancing* behavior in which members attempt to communicate some separation from the role through sarcasm, humor, and playfulness toward the ritual and the ideology. While role embracement is the model behavior, the periodic episodes of distancing are indicative of a desire by organizational members to disassociate themselves from the role of a "true believer," or one who has been totally duped by the organizational culture. On the other hand, Kunda also believed that the organizational culture can penetrate the self through the process of cognitive dissonance:

> Public expressions of support for an ideological point of view may cause cognitive dissonance: members who, under pressure, publicly espouse beliefs and opinions they might otherwise reject tend to adopt them as an authentic expression of their point of view . . . Over time, cognitive and emotive dissonance may blur the boundary between the performers' perception of an acted role and the experience of an "authentic self" (Kunda 1992:156).

The questions raised by Kunda about the impact of organization culture on the self point to the way normative control demands much more of the individual than structural control. Under more traditional bureaucratic structures, workers carried out specific job assignments because they were required. As long as they did the work, management made no heavy demand for attachment, engagement, or embracement. Workers could easily distance the self from mandated work activities. External supervision and penalties for noncompliance mean that workers have less choice or discretion: They do the work for the financial reward or they will be fired or penalized for shirking. In contrast, organizational culture, and the normative forms of control with which it is associated, bases control and conformity on the internalization of a value system. As Kunda put it, "they have entered into a contract that is more than economic, one that must contend with overt external claims on self-definition. . . In this sense, members have internalized the 'problem of control' that lies at the heart of the organization, and the private selves of members have become part of the 'contested terrain' " (p. 214–21).

Thus, Kunda believed that the reach of normative control represented by strong cultures has been extended in contemporary organizations like Tech. It is more tightly integrated into organizational practices and it demands a greater piece of the self. Normative control is also, like most managerial strategies, permeated with contradictions that stem from the tensions between the ideological and rhetorical message and the fundamental reality of the bottom-line purpose and asymmetrical employment relationship. And, in spite of the presumed efforts to penetrate and control the worker's level of consciousness, the human capacity to engage in "reflective discourse," represented by irony, sarcasm, cynicism, and humor, signals the incomplete colonization of the human factor.

Culture as Paradigm and Managerial Strategy

The rise of normative and culture theories and methods of organization can also be placed in the context of the theoretical shift from utilitarian to moral-based conceptions of human behavior. Amitai Etzioni's (1961) classic work on organizational control distinguished between utilitarian and normative forms of compliance. Utilitarian modes are based on economic reward while normative forms are based on emotional commitment and moral attachment. Etzioni argued that utilitarian methods were more appropriate for private sector profit-seeking firms ("economic organizations") and normative methods were better for "cultural" organizations that are driven by some mission or service. This distinction has become increasingly blurred as economic organizations devote as much, or more, attention to the normative as the utilitarian approach. This shift can be linked to larger theoretical developments in economics and organization theory that argue for the relevance of noneconomic, or noncontractual, bases of behavior and the more practical point that normative modes of control may be more effective for organizational success (Barley, Meyer, and Gash 1988).

The neoclassical economic position that assumes human behavior is driven by rational self-interest and material reward has been widely criticized for failing to account for the wide range of behaviors that apparently have no purely rational foundation (Etzioni 1988). The observations of trust, obligation, altruism, loyalty, and unrewarded commitment in economic exchanges and organizational behavior, and their contribution to the operation of economic institutions, have produced a paradigm shift toward the normative dimension. It is now the accepted wisdom that humans are motivated and energized by normative forces and that these may play an even greater role than economic factors.

Among behavioral economists, this shift is seen in John Tomer's (1987) "organizational capital," which he defined as "human capital in which the attribute is embodied in either the organizational relationship, particular organizational members, the organization's repositories of information, or some combination of the above in order to improve the functioning of the organization" (1987:2). Accordingly, investment in and the formation of organizational capital involves organizational redesign of formal and informal relationships, training and socialization of organizational members, and the appropriate matching of employees with work situations. Tomer argued that investments in organizational capital will address the managerial dilemma of labor control by engendering worker commitment and attachment to the firm. Worker compliance in this model is noninstrumental. Conformity and effort are unconditionally forthcoming by virtue of the normative climate created through the investments in organizational capital.

Daniel Denison (1991) addressed the cultural component of normative control more directly as an effective strategy for organizational success. Four dimensions of organizational culture enhance the effectiveness of the enterprise: (1) high levels of involvement and participation that create commitment, (2) a shared system of beliefs, values, and symbols that serves as an internalized control system, (3) the ability to interpret environmental signals and translate them into adaptable forms of behavior, and (4) a mission that provides a noneconomic basis for motivation and a general guide to appropriate behavior. Denison cited the positive association between these aspects of organizational culture and the overall economic performance of the firm. The broader implication for management is that normative regulation through organizational culture is the most cost-effective means of controlling human behavior.

William Ouchi's (1980) comparative analysis of organizational forms and his concept of the *clan* provide further arguments for the efficiency of the normative approach. The clan is a group engaged in economic exchange, or organizational activities, based on shared values and an established culture generating trust, loyalty, commitment, and dedication to the collective good. The advantage of the clan is based on the way it handles two organizational problems. The first problem is the cost associated with making sure organizational members are doing what they are supposed to do. What we have previously called the agency problem is based on the "performance ambiguity" and uncertainty that exists when people are hired and responsibility is delegated, but there is no automatic guarantee they will faithfully fulfill their contractual obligations. The clan, which is characterized by a strong culture, would presumably direct organizational action in appropriate directions without constant monitoring, supervision, and assessment. Thus, costs associated with these activities are reduced.

Ouchi called the second problem "goal incongruity." Under goal incongruity, members have different interests and therefore act in ways that might advance self-interest at the expense of larger organizational goals. Again, the common culture of the clan should minimize this problem. Ouchi recognized that the cost of creating a strong normative system can be high but believed that these costs are more than compensated by the reduction in performance ambiguity and goal incongruity. This is a further rationale for the establishment of organizational culture.

Each of these insights converge with the emerging field of socioeconomics which highlights the normative, ethical, and moral foundations of human behavior (Etzioni and Lawrence 1991). This position is advanced most forcefully by Etzioni (1988), who used the term "contextual relations" to refer to an organizational climate that generates commitment, "Many people work best, and feel less exploited, in contextual relations, in which they work, in part out of moral commitment and are treated as human beings, and not merely as commodities" (1988:75).

Etzioni distinguished between "expedient conformity"—the feeling that it pays to work hard—and "moral commitment"—the feeling that one ought to work hard. Etzioni preferred moral commitment over calculated self-interest because it will result in conformity without external constraints. Instrumental ("it pays") motives are less reliable and dependable than normative ("ought to") motives because the former are contingent on the flow of external reward. Etzioni also argued for moral commitment on efficiency grounds " to the extent that moral commitments enhance the resources that can be dedicated to economic activity rather than to supervision and verification, a higher level of morality increases productivity and the GNP" (1988:69). There is a revealing inconsistency in this argument: A system that is praised for resting on moral commitment rather than economic self-interest is justified in terms of its economic payoff.

This inconsistency betrays a larger contradiction in the normative emphases of organizational culture and socioeconomic theory. In focusing on the mechanisms generating commitment and obligation, these approaches tend to ignore the counterforces that encourage and reinforce instrumental self-interested behavior. Can moral normative sentiments be galvanized in a market system founded on self-interest, in a bureaucratic context aimed at instrumental regulation and behavior, in economic organizations whose primary goal is to maximize profit?

Clearly, management would prefer that employees be driven by moral commitment. As Etzioni noted, there will be payoffs in productivity and efficiency. But suppose organizational members decide not to cooperate. Suppose they feel no moral duty or obligation to the firm. Are they acting immorally? Can there be a moral basis for a group to advance its own "self-interest"? These questions must be considered when organizational owners begin to employ cultural, normative, and moral strategies. They recall Chester Barnard's work on "common moral purpose" and his theoretical and practical struggle to reconcile individual and organizational personalities (Barnard 1938).

Normative control and organizational culture can be viewed as a replacement for bureaucratic forms of control or a way to minimize the likelihood of shirking, lollygagging, self-interest, and opportunism. The whole question of control is itself based on the assumption that employees have different interests or goals and the organization must devise techniques to channel behavior toward the goals of one particular group. The most effective means to solve the problem would be to eliminate the fundamental antagonism of interest between bosses and workers, or principals and agents. Profit sharing is one way to reduce the antagonism. A more radical means is worker ownership which places agents in the position (in terms of material interest) of principals. As Samuel Bowles and Herbert Gintis (1990) argued, worker ownership and control would give workers a direct interest in efficiency and productivity. They would not only internalize the monitoring function but also have an interest in monitoring the effort of co-workers. Under this arrangement, self-interested behavior becomes the desirable motive as one must and will have a material interest in maximum effort.

Cultural Integration, Differentiation, and Fragmentation

This discussion of culture has been based on the assumption that it is a normative strategy used to integrate people and processes in an organization—that is, it counters the tendency toward differentiation and fragmentation by serving as a kind of social cement. It is important to recognize alternative conceptions of organizational culture. Some of these are presented by Joanne Martin (1992) who made a distinction between integration, differentiation, and fragmentation perspectives on culture.

The *integration perspective* —the approach that has been taken here—assumes that organizational culture is something that is consistently reinforced across the organization and that produces agreement and consensus on the organization's values and assumptions. The culture is described as "common" and "shared" to denote how it enhances unity and harmony.

The *differentiation perspective* in contrast, recognizes the inconsistencies and lack of consensus across the organization. For example, there may be little relationship between the espoused culture and the actual forms of behavior within the organization. There may also be little agreement across different units, departments, and work groups over the basic operating assumptions and mission of the organization. Rather than viewing this as an absence of organizational culture, Martin has reminded us that it is simply one cultural form among several. The inconsistency and lack of consensus can be the product of powerful but competing cultural forces within a single organization.

In many ways, our analysis of unintended consequences of differentiation and divisions of labor has rested on the assumption that these will generate competing visions, loyalties, or subcultures. The notion of a larger organizational culture is then seen as the antidote to the emerging divisions and tensions. However, it is also critical to note that the organizational subcultures do not necessarily undermine organizational effectiveness. Tightly knit work groups or teams that share a common set of values and assumptions may be particularly effective and productive.

The third perspective on organizational culture—*fragmentation*—identifies what is probably one of the most common scenarios in the real world. Here there is simply confusion and ambiguity over the organization's core values and essential premises. The inability to articulate a coherent vision and consensus over values and goals may be due to the contradictions and paradoxes of organizational life that permit a variety of legitimate visions and courses of action. This represents a kind of normlessness or anomie that can potentially paralyze organizational actors. There is no overarching culture nor any local or subcultural value system. If there is confusion or no sense about what an organization values, or how one goes about affirming the core principles, organizational effectiveness is likely to suffer.

The Learning Organization

The final continuing organizational trend to be considered is the learning organization—"continuing" because, even though the concept of a learning organization has been around for at least 10 years, it continues to fuel models of organization based on the processing of knowledge and information (Huseman and Goodman 1999).

However, before the main points of this approach are presented, it would be remiss in a text devoted to organizational tensions, contradictions, and paradox if it did not draw attention to the important argument of Karl Weick and Frances Westley (1996:440):

> Organizing and learning are essentially antithetical processes, which means that the phrase "organizational learning" is an oxymoron. To learn is to disorganize and increase variety. To organize is to forget and reduce variety. In the rush to embrace learning, organizational theorists often overlook this tension.

It is true that the formal organization of a process or activity can result in an end to learning and a blind reliance on standardized operating procedures and institutionalized practices. This was one of the major problems associated with the mass production/scale economy model of Fordism. The perfection of the model, its ultimate organization, rendered the system incapable of adjustments and adaptations to new conditions and information. Therefore, the concept of a learning organization invites disorganization and a constant assessment and analysis, rather than the acceptance, of standardized procedures.

Paul Senge's Five Disciplines

The notion that an organization is an information processing entity, capable of learning, conforms with the *brain metaphor* of organization (Morgan 1997). The human brain's ability to collect and process information and stimuli, reflect and respond quickly, flexibly, and adaptively are understandably desirable organizational traits. This learning approach to organizing and managing is most widely associated with the work of Paul Senge in *The Fifth Discipline* (1990).

Senge's suggestions for those who manage organizations will resonate with sociologists because his framework emphasizes systemic and structural analysis. Given the importance of this work and its enormous influence on management and organizational theory, Senge's work will be considered in some detail.

Senge advanced five "disciplines" that are the essence of his approach to and prescriptions for the learning organization: personal mastery, mental models, team learning, shared vision, and systems thinking. "Systems thinking," the fifth discipline, ties the other four together.

Personal mastery, the first discipline, is an individual-level process that involves developing a vision or goal and the means to determine whether the vision has been realized. Here, Senge had in mind the ultimate goals that one may devote an entire lifetime to achieving. To realize the vision, one must constantly assess where one stands and what must be changed to move toward the grand objective. This is an individual-level version of the continuous improvement process. The gap between one's current location and ultimate destination—a kind of performance gap—produces "creative tension" that motivates further action and effort. Again, these ideas are directly related to the Japanese approach discussed earlier under the concepts of Kaizen and the paradox of ultimate goals in the lean production model.

In this scheme, it is not enough to simply react to changing demands and conditions. One must constantly evaluate the underlying causes of performance gaps and implement meaningful strategies. This is what Senge referred to as *generative learning* which is proactive, rather than *adaptive learning,* which is reactive. The latter form of learning is a coping strategy, while the former is a creative strategy.

The second discipline is *mental models.* This notion is now widely discussed in organization and management theory and refers to the cognitive sense-making schemes that organizational members employ. Mental models are akin to the organizational metaphors used to conceptualize how an organization works and achieves its objectives (Morgan 1997). For example, if one's mental model conceptualizes the organization as an assemblage of interrelated and interchangeable parts that mechanically operate to produce some output, this will shape how one thinks, acts, and manages in an organization. An enormous amount of management literature today is aimed at changing and shaping these mental models in the hope of altering organizational behavior; this is also a central objective of the learning organization literature.

Team learning is the third discipline. This refers to the process of aligning and developing the capacity for teams to generate knowledge, learn, and act. While Senge emphasized the individual-level processes of personal mastery, he viewed teams as the fundamental unit of modern organization. The most important process at this level is "dialogue," a process that requires participants to suspend their assumptions, treat one another as colleagues, have a facilitator direct and mediate the dialogue, and entertain and experiment with new and different ideas. In this context, dialogue is itself developmental and process oriented, designed to reshape the way people interact, think, and learn. Creative and innovative ideas require this open-ended approach to team interaction. This conforms with a central feature of the postbureaucratic organization discussed earlier.

The fourth discipline is *shared vision*. This relates to the long-term goals and objectives that individuals set for themselves, but it can also apply to the larger organizational collective. The normative and cultural modes of organizational socialization and control, outlined above, typically seek to shape some long-term vision for organizational members. To generate the creative tension for teams and the larger organization, a shared vision must be established. This can be used as a continual criterion for evaluating progress and generating further action.

The fifth and final discipline is *systems thinking*. This mode of thinking works in an ensemble with the other four disciplines. Systems thinking provides the most effective mental model for personal mastery, team learning, and the realization of shared vision. Senge's elaboration of systems thinking has significant affinities with the sociological perspective. He argued that "structure produces behavior, and changing underlying structures can produce different patterns of behavior. In this sense, structural explanations are inherently generative" (1990:53).

In the context of an organization, this means that the organizational structure shapes patterns of relationships between positions and people. These relationships produce patterns of behavior and organizational action. However, this behavior is typically experienced as short-term events or "snapshots." If we do not use systems thinking, and restrict ourselves to analyzing and dealing with or predicting "events," we are engaged in adaptive rather than generative thinking. In this scenario, organizations will simply develop strategies and methods to manage events. But these events are the product of larger structural or systemic forces. Therefore, adaptive methods are palliatives, or coping strategies, that do not get at the source of the behavior. Systems thinking, in contrast, allows people in organizations to connect events with structures and, in the process, learn how to develop effective techniques for altering organizational behavior and events. Systems thinking forces people to recognize the interrelationship between structures, behaviors, and events and the associated contradictions that plague organizations. Senge provided a wide variety of examples and applications of his model.

Analyzing Organizations as Systems

Senge's model for systems thinking is closely related to the notions of paradox and unintended consequences highlighted throughout this text. More specifically, a systems thinking analysis of organizational dynamics can show

how managerial actions designed to solve a problem or advance a goal have consequences that exacerbate the problem or undermine the goal.

Take the problem of a low level of work effort on the part of employees. Let's assume that the actual systemic cause of the problem is the bureaucratic organization of work which severely limits the level of discretion and autonomy exercised by the workers. Because they are unable to exercise mental skills, employees become bored and withdraw their maximum effort. A "symptomatic solution" is to increase the level of supervision and monitoring to ensure that workers expend sufficient effort. However, the unintended side effect is to further increase levels of management/supervisory hierarchy. While the ultimate "structural solution" would be a reduction in the hierarchy and supervisory management structure—and to allow workers greater latitude and discretion—the symptomatic solution renders this fundamental solution increasingly difficult. In short, the symptomatic solution further contributes to the fundamental cause of the problematic behavior.

This part of Senge's analytical model is closely related to the work of Gregory Bateson (1979) and Chris Argyris (1982). Bateson distinguished between first-order and second-order changes in systems. A *first-order change* is a response that involves increasing or decreasing some existing process. It is an adjustment. In our example, the symptomatic solution is a first-order change, an adjustment which in this case brought about an increase in the level of supervision. A *second-order change* involves doing things or structuring the organization in a qualitatively different fashion. Eliminating the supervisory hierarchy and creating autonomous teams would be a second-order change.

Similarly, Argyris (1982) distinguished between single-loop and double-loop learning. *Single-loop learning* is a response to a problem that is carried out in the context of the existing assumptions and structures. In our example, the existing assumption is that work effort requires hierarchical controls. Thus, a reduction in effort produces more controls. This is the "symptomatic solution" or "first-order change". *Double-loop learning* connects the problem to the very structures and assumptions that guide the organization. It involves an evaluation of the assumption and a greater likelihood for a structural solution or second-order change. If effort is low under the existing system, maybe the assumptions underlying the organizational structure are invalid. This is a transformative mode of learning.

Organizational analysis using systems thinking provides one way to identify leverage points in the organization. One of the laws of the fifth discipline—systems thinking—is the adage that "small changes can produce big results." If one can locate the structural systemic source of organizational action and behavior, and direct interventions toward these strategic locations in the organization, the results are potentially enormous. Gareth Morgan (1993) and Morgan and Asaf Zohar (1996) applied this principle to the notion of the *15 percent solution.* They argued that most efforts of organizational change are frustrated by a desire to address each and every problem when, in reality, it is difficult to influence more than 15 percent of one's environment. Therefore, they suggested avoiding the tendency toward an overload in organizational change by implementing high-leverage decisions that can have "quantum" consequences over time.

The concept of a learning organization and organizational learning has captured the imagination of administrators and managers in both public- and private-sector organizations (Chawla and Renesch 1995). Many of the ideas in Senge's work are derived from earlier work on systems thinking (Weinberg 1975), personal development (Fritz 1989), mental models (Argyris 1990, 1993; Schon 1983), and teams (Bohm 1990). The synthesis of this diverse literature, in service to organizational change and transformation, contributes to the appeal of the learning model. Most of the models of emerging organizations reviewed in this chapter seek to develop methods for collecting, distributing, and creating information and knowledge. This is accomplished through teams, continuous improvement schemes, the translation of implicit into explicit knowledge, the sharing of information, collaboration, and the exploitation of information technology. Many organizations also seek to transform the organizational culture to support new mental models that encourage questions, ideas, experiments, and the critical reflection required for genuine learning (e.g., Handy 1995b; Huseman and Goodman 1999).

As with the other organizational models discussed in this text, the learning organization faces the same kinds of contradictions and dilemmas. Organizations continue to seek to control and regulate human behavior. Authority, hierarchy, and bureaucratic routines are the standard mechanisms to address this objective. These elements operate to discourage and limit human learning. An advocate of the learning organization, Charles Handy (1995b:48) directly confronted the issue: "It is an upside-down sort of place, with much of the power residing at the organization's edge. In this culture, imposed authority no longer works . . . This organization is held together by shared beliefs and values, by people who are committed to each other and to common goals—*a rather tenuous method of control* [emphasis added]." Thus, the long-term durability and success of the learning model of organizations will depend less on the appealing rhetoric that tends to dominate the literature (e.g., curiosity, forgiveness, trust, togetherness, community, wisdom, dialogue) and more on the organizational structures within which people work.

What's Happening on the Ground?

This chapter concludes with a brief consideration of whether any solid relationship exists between the vast and seemingly continuous transformation of organizational forms and the expressed experiences and attitudes of workers and managers. A major study of 2,500 U.S. employees by the consulting firm of Towers Perrin reveals some interesting patterns (Towers Perrin 1997). First, it reported that employees are now well aware of the need to continually learn new job skills as a condition for job security. The rhetoric emphasizing learning, training, participation, and responsibility, has had a significant impact on employees' orientation toward work. However, the study's primary investigator found that the success and internalization of the message has created a

> paradox that is beginning to emerge in employee attitudes. As employees take more responsibility and control in their jobs, their sense of satisfaction and motivation is increasing. At the same time, their acceptance of more responsibility heightens their expectations that they will have the opportunity to demonstrate their capabilities and be rewarded for their contributions. . . But because their expectation is not being fully met, doubts about workplace fairness are starting to grow (Towers Perrin 1997).

More specifically, the study found considerable employee skepticism regarding reciprocity. While the survey was conducted during a period of unprecedented economic expansion and high corporate profits, there was either no improvement or a decline in employee attitudes (compared with 1995) regarding a sense of shared destiny with the firm, the extent to which employees feel connected to the company's mission, and views about how well the company is managed.

Furthermore, there were significant declines in employee beliefs that "the company fills jobs with the most qualified candidates" (down from 55 percent to 49 percent), top performers receive more pay (48 percent to 44 percent), promotions are fair (51 percent to 45 percent), the company considers employee interests in making decisions affecting them (50 percent to 41 percent), or that workplace polices are administered fairly (59 percent to 56 percent). The perceived inequity or absence of a quid pro quo appears to be fueling the discontent of employees or, as the report indicates, the employee "attitudes suggest there is a significant component missing in today's workplace: consistent evidence of the partnership employers say they want to create with their employees" (Tower Perrin 1997).

In a separate survey, the American Management Association found that managers too reported severe obstacles to organizational effectiveness that continue to plague their firms in spite of restructuring and reorganization (American Management Association 1999). Managers were asked about the prevalence of bureaucracy, miscommunication, skepticism, misconceptions, procrastination, traditions, and avoidance. These are factors widely viewed as the most common obstacles to effective organizational action. The largest percentage of managers cited miscommunication (misunderstanding or lack of adequate communication, 49 percent) and traditions (long-standing practices that have no current relevance or benefits, 43 percent) as the most highly prevalent factors. These two factors were linked, respectively, to turnover and an inability to compete successfully.

While longitudinal data extending over a 20- to 25-year period would be the optimal means to gauge the impact of organizational changes, these snapshots indicate the tensions that emerge as employee expectations are changed and common organizational problems persist. In terms of the persistance of organizational problems, miscommunication may become a larger problem as hierarchical and bureaucratic communication mechanisms are replaced by less direct or explicit commands. The reliance on "traditions" may be related to the miscommunication problem as the organization manages uncertainty by falling back on familiar routines and practices as guides to action.

Another set of developments also could be interpreted as a less than positive endorsement of organizational changes. This is reflected in the rising proportion of employees who would opt for union representation in the workplace. According to polling data collected by Peter D. Hart Research Associates, reported in *Business Week,* the percent of workers who would vote for a union has increased from 30 percent in 1984 to 43 percent in 1999 ("Commentary: All's Not Fair in Labor Wars," *Business Week,* July 19, 1999, p. 42). The rapid changes and increasing flexibility that affect job security and benefits may be responsible for this trend. However, unions only win half their elections in the private sector. This seemingly paradoxical situation—relatively high levels of expressed support for union representation coupled with relatively low levels of organizing success—has been attributed to the antiunion tactics of private employers. Research based on data from the National Labor Relations Board (NLRB) indicates that companies are increasingly likely to use aggressive tactics—some illegal—to prevent union organization of their workforce. Again, this reflects the two faces of flexibility and restructuring. On the one hand, they might produce a less rigidly bureaucratic and potentially more participatory workplace; on the other hand, private employers who desire greater flexibility may view union-based collective bargaining agreements as obstacles to this objective.

Finally, there are the findings from the Worker Representation and Participation Survey of 2,400 American workers reported in Richard Freeman and Joel Rogers's *What Workers Want* (1999). The central focus of the research is the issue of organizational governance and, more specifically, the division of authority and influence between workers and managers. One of the primary findings of the study is captured in what Freeman and Rogers labeled the *representation/participation gap.* "American workers want more of a say/influence/representation/ participation/voice (call it what you will) at the workplace than they now have" (1999:4). This refers to a greater desire for individual and group participation, and joint decision making, on workplace issues.

In this context, it is important to note that management initiates and directs most of the emerging and new organizational forms reviewed above. While these forms may be designed to increase commitment and involvement, they may not necessarily be devoted to expanding participation and decision-making power among workers. Further, while there seems to be an increasing number of employee-involvement and human resource programs, "most think these programs do not go far enough in devolving authority to employees . . . most participants in such programs believe that the programs would work much better if management gave greater decision-making power to workers" (Freeman and Rogers 1999:6).

When workers were asked about the primary reason for the lack of desired workplace influence, they indicated "management resistance." Workers believe that most managements do not want to share power or permit workers much independence in decision making (1999:5). This is an interesting finding. Much of the discussion in previous chapters has centered on worker resistance to managerial initiatives and the way this shapes organizational outcomes. The term *management resistance* indicates the other side of this dynamic process. Worker requests and pressures for greater decision-making power and control are assessed and evaluated by management in light of its interests, and either resisted or opposed. The workplace attitudes of the managers surveyed in the study confirm the perceived intransigence. "Many are antiunion. Many oppose programs that would keep them from making the final decisions about workplace governance." On the other hand, "much of management favors a more substantial employee voice in joint committees" (1999:7).

The results of this survey and the one on union representation remind us that the organization remains a contested terrain and that labor-management divisions continue to shape organizational conflict and struggle. Also, many of the new organizational developments highlighted here represent the more forward-looking managerial initiatives that are not necessarily widespread across the organizational landscape. It is probably safe to say that most workers are employed in organizations that continue to employ highly bureaucratic organizational techniques with only minor variations in human-resource style initiatives.

More generally, these and other findings point to the considerable gap and slippage between the rhetorical and structural changes associated with new organizational forms and the actual impact on the work experiences of the human resource.

Summary

1. Much of the literature on emerging organizations is also couched in the language of postbureaucracy. Bureaucratic principles, once the foundation for administrative structure, are being deliberately demolished by many organizations. This amounts to a kind of dis-organization represented by firms that emphasize interaction, collaboration, and informal structure. A fundamental feature of these new organizations is the restructuring of physical space to realize the alternative social organization of work.

2. Organizational culture, also a long-standing element of organization theory, has taken on greater importance in the current era. As traditional bureaucratic and structural systems of control are challenged or eroded, normative cultural systems are employed as a means to pick up the potential slack in social control.

3. The metaphor of the organization as a brain has stimulated an interest in the learning organization. Using systems thinking, this prescriptive organizational approach encourages systematic means to reflect on organizational practice in an effort to generate continuous learning and transformation.

4. The wide-ranging organizational developments highlighted in this chapter have been analyzed in the context of unintended consequences and unresolved tensions. The available data on employee attitudes indicate a great deal of ambivalence concerning the inconsistencies between the rhetoric of change and the reality of the workplace. This confirms the difficulty in making sweeping assumptions about wholesale change from one organizational form to another.

8

TECHNOLOGY AND ORGANIZATIONAL TRANSFORMATION

The last two chapters have referred to various technologies used in old and emerging organizational forms. This chapter will explicitly examine the role of technology, both in theories of organization and as a harbinger of organizational transformation. With the digital revolution and the proliferation of new information technologies, one must ask whether these new technologies are playing a qualitatively different role in shaping organizational structure and process.

In the organizational literature, technology has been defined as the means, activities, and knowledge used to transform materials and inputs into organizational outputs (Scott 1987:18). This definition is deliberately wordy because so many different technologies might be employed by any organization.

As a simple example of organizational technology, take the case of a raw material, say a piece of wood, entering an organization in the form of a log (the input) and leaving the organization as two-by-fours (the output). The technology includes the machinery and knowledge applied to the task of transforming the log into pieces of smooth lumber. This is the *core technology* of a lumber mill. Other forms of technology are likely to be employed by the organization that would be *peripheral* to the central core transformation process. For example, those working in the accounting, billing, and shipping offices of the organization might use computers and spreadsheet software to process information about inventory, sales, and suppliers. Technology is applied to these activities but they do not represent the core activity of the organization.

Technology and Organization Theory

The classic works on technology and organization have attempted to correlate the form of core technology with other organizational characteristics. Thus, an initial task was to delineate the significant variations in technologies across organizations (see Table 8–1). Some of the most influential contributions were made by Joan Woodward, Robert Blauner, James Thompson, Charles Perrow, and members of the Tavistock Institute.

Joan Woodward

Joan Woodward (1958) distinguished three types of core technology and associated labor processes. *Small batch and unit production* technologies produce items one unit at a time, in small numbers, in response to a restricted number of orders for the product. This kind of technology is associated with a labor process in which a worker is involved at every stage from start to finish. This technology is also regarded as the least technologically complex.

Large batch and mass production technologies produce a large number of the same items at the same time for an undifferentiated mass market. The labor process under this technology typically involves a more rigid division of labor along the lines of the Fordist assembly line. The level of complexity in this case is moderate.

Continuous process production is a technology that takes a raw material and subjects it to a continuous transformation process that cannot be divided into distinct and separate operations. A chemical plant, for example, will feed various chemical ingredients into a flowing liquid and apply different physical conditions (e.g., mixing, heating, cooling) as the ingredients move from the beginning to the end of the manufacturing process. Labor activity involves oversight of the technology, which automatically regulates and monitors the production process. There is no direct physical human contact with the manufactured materials. This form of technology represents the highest form of technical complexity.

Woodward correlated these organizational technologies with different management structures. She concluded that mass production technologies tend to be associated with centralized and bureaucratic forms of management while small batch and continuous processing technologies are most successful when coupled with decentralized management structures (Table 8–1A).

In linking technology with management systems, Woodward's analysis suggests that the technology employed determines the degree of latitude and autonomy exercised by workers. Of the technological types identified by Woodward, those with the greatest levels of autonomy would coexist with batch and continuous processing technologies. Mass production, on the other hand, would tend to exist with a labor process that restricts the exercise of worker autonomy.

TABLE 8–1 Perspectives on Types of Technology and Organizational Characteristics

---

A. Woodward's Model

Technology Type	*Associated Organizational Characteristics*
Unit and batch production	Decentralized decision-making structure
Large batch and mass production	Centralized bureaucratic decision-making structure
Continuous processing	Decentralized decision-making structure

---

B. Blauner's Model

Technology:	craft	machine	assembly-line	process
Industry:	printing	textiles	automobiles	chemical

C. Thompson's Model

Technology Type	*Associated Organizational Characteristics*
Long-linked technology	Standardized sequentially interdependent linear process
Mediating technology	Standardized procedures mediating transactions
Intensive technology	Unstandardized applications of machines and knowledge

---

D. Perrow's Model

Technology Type	*Associated Organizational Characteristics*
Routine technologies	Low task variability–high task analyzability
Craft technologies	Low task variability–low task analyzability
Engineering technologies	High task variability–high task analyzability
Nonroutine technologies	High task variability–low task analyzability

---

Robert Blauner

Robert Blauner's well-known study, *Alienation and Freedom (1964),* advanced a hypothesis based on the logic derived from Woodward's analysis. In examining the relationship between types of technology and the degree of worker alienation (defined as a combination of powerlessness, meaninglessness, isolation and estrangement), Blauner advanced the inverted U-curve pattern shown in Table 8–1B. His research of different industries indicated low levels of alienation under the simple craft technology employed in the printing industry, higher levels of alienation in the textile industry where workers tend the machines, the highest level of alienation in the auto industry using the assembly line technology, and low levels of alienation in the continuous process chemical industry. Together, Woodward and Blauner suggested that the core technology used by an organization determines and shapes the management and authority structure.

James Thompson

James Thompson (1967) also proposed a method for classifying the types of technology used by both manufacturing and service organizations (Table 8–1C). *Long-linked technologies* are most common in manufacturing and involve a linear process that begins with raw materials and proceeds toward a finished product. Both mass production and continuous process qualify as long-linked technologies.

Mediating technologies are those used by organizations that link clients or customers interested in engaging in a transaction. For example, employment agencies bring together employers and job seekers; banks join investors and borrowers. These organizations develop procedures and services for, and process information about, producer and consumer needs. The Internet has greatly expanded the role of this technology as the global computer network generates entry points, or "portals," that link Internet users and consumers with every conceivable kind of supplier and service (see Hagel and Singer 1999).

Thompson's third type, *intensive technologies,* are those forms of hardware and knowledge used to change some specific object. For example, medical technology is used to diagnose and treat a patient's disease; laboratory technology is used in university research to conduct experiments; software is used in computer-mediated instruction to train and educate people.

Charles Perrow

Another widely used framework for the analysis of organizational technology was proposed by Charles Perrow (1967). His model has the advantage of being applicable to a wide variety of tasks and activities beyond the core technologies. Perrow used two dimensions—task variability and task analyzability—to classify organizational technologies. *Task variability* refers to the degree to which the labor process involves routinized standardized procedures (nonvariable) or whether it includes a wide range of exceptions (variability) that must be managed. *Task analyzability* refers to the degree to which formal procedures are required for handling the nonstandardized exceptional cases (analyzability) or whether exceptions require workers to improvise (non-analyzability). In typology form, these two dimensions yield four kinds of organizational technology (see Table 8–1D).

Routine technologies involve standard operating procedures coupled with systematic procedures for dealing with exceptions; thus low variability and high analyzability. Assembly line production fits this pattern.

Nonroutine technologies possess the opposite characteristics. There are no standardized routines used to approach the work (high variability) and no formal procedures to deal with uncertainty (low analyzability). Research and development work fits this pattern.

Craft technologies entail standard procedures for most tasks, but when exceptions and problems occur workers must innovate and invent solutions due to the inability to formalize all possible contingencies. Carpentry fits this pattern.

Last, *engineering technology* is characterized by high variability because the work cannot be reduced to a standardized protocol, yet the range of problems have predetermined and formalized solutions (high analyzability). Financial accounting work fits this pattern. The variety of cases confronted are managed with a set of specific rules, procedures, and forms.

Perrow's model conceptualizes task-related technologies in the context of rational bureaucratic (or what he calls neo-Weberian) principles. A highly bureaucratized organization seeks to standardize task activities (low variability) so that they can be managed with formalized procedures; even the small number of exceptions should have a formal protocol. This kind of organizational technology is designed to reduce or eliminate human discretion. It represents a high level of formal control.

While organizations would prefer to have predictable standardized inputs and demands, most face some degree of uncertainty. Therefore, at the other end of the spectrum where tasks involve a wide variety of tasks and, consequently, many exceptions, it is unlikely that formal bureaucratic controls will suffice. Task-related technologies may therefore involve low variability and high analyzability. Action in this situation must be based on informal emergent decision making and inventiveness. Such tasks are carried out by those who are socialized to select the appropriate strategies independent of formal constraint. Perrow (1986:22) has described the role of professionals as "personnel who have complex rules built into them." The strength of Perrow's technology framework lies in its inherent connection to broader organizational principles—formalization, decision making, social control, environmental pressures—and its application to a range of different tasks within a single organization.

Tavistock Institute

A final tradition in the literature of organization theory comes under the heading of sociotechnical systems and is based on the work of Eric Trist and his associates at the Tavistock Institute. In describing organizations as both technical and social systems, Trist (1981) recognized the associated tension that resulted from the "core interface . . . between a nonhuman and human system." The technical side of the organization involves the application of instrumentally logical methods for the completion of tasks. The social side of the organization involves the needs of and relationships among humans.

The sociotechnical approach stemmed from a study by Trist and Kenneth Bamforth (1951) of technological innovations in British coal mines. In an effort to rationalize the mining process, mine owners introduced mechanization to enhance the extraction of coal from the mines. The increased technical complexity resulted in a reorganization of social relations and job tasks (through what was known as the longwall method). Prior to mechanization, the organizational structure involved small groups working as teams (using the shortwall method). After the introduction of the new technology, the organization of production resembled the factory model with greater specialization and segregation of work tasks and reduced autonomy. Instead of enhancing the productivity of the enterprise, the new system created an assortment of problems.

> The social integration of the previous small groups having been disrupted, and little attempt made to achieve any new integration, many symptoms of social stress occur. Informal cliques which develop to help each other can only occur over small parts of the face, inevitably leaving some isolated; individuals react defensively . . . they compete for allocation to the best workplaces, there is mutual scapegoating across shifts . . . Absenteeism becomes a way of the miner compensating himself for the difficulties of the job (Pugh, Hickson, and Hinings. 1985:85).

Theoretically, Trist and his colleagues argued that the technical and social (or nonhuman and human) features of organization require an optimization of the relationship between technical imperatives and the social and psychological needs of workers. Practically, this insight was reflected in the implementation of a "composite longwall method" that reintroduced the autonomous work groups while still utilizing the new technologies for the extraction of coal. Thus, the tension created by the introduction of technology and the associated reorganization of production prompted human-generated consequences that challenged both technologically deterministic organization theory and the managerial efforts to institute technical forms of social control.

Taken together, the classic technology typologies of Woodward, Thompson, Blauner, and Perrow, and the work of the Tavistock Institute, provide a means to classify and differentiate organizational technologies. However, they all predate the implementation of qualitatively unique forms of information technology that have infiltrated in varying degrees almost every organization. These technologies have forced theorists to rethink the old typologies and to develop new ways to conceptualize the transformative impact of technology (DeSanctis and Fulk 1999).

Entering the Age of the Smart Machine

In her book *In the Age of the Smart Machine* (1984), Shoshana Zuboff posed profound and defining questions about the relationship between information technology, work, and organization. Most generally, she asked how and in whose interest would technologies be used and how would they affect the human factor of production? She outlined several alternative visions which continue to frame the debate over the consequences and appropriate application of organizational technology (see Table 8–2).

TABLE 8–2   Alternative Visions of the Impact of Technology on the Organization

Organizational Dimension	Positive Vision	Negative Vision
Conception and distribution of knowledge	New forms of skill and knowledge are generated to exploit the new technology; workers exercise greater critical judgment in applying technology to tasks; new forms of mastery, meaning, and opportunity pervade organizations	Intelligence lodged in the machine; humans exercise no critical judgment and are dependent and passive; human senses no longer generate knowledge; results in disorientation, meaninglessness, apathy, and alienation
Relations of authority	Organizational behavior is transformed in the direction of greater collaboration and mutual responsibility; managers and workers break out of their functional and vertical relationships and create new roles which blur the lines of authority and decision making	Managers use the technology to reinforce, reestablish, and reproduce their legitimacy; hierarchical distinctions are erected between those who can use and understand the abstract scientific principles of the smart machines and those who cannot
Methods of coordination	The technology becomes a rich resource that permits innovative methods of information sharing, exchange, and collaboration; the wide and open access to information allows a climate of collective responsibility, mutual ownership, and team problem solving	The new technology is used as a potent method for controlling and monitoring workers; management becomes a form of remote and automated surveillance and administration; a climate of distrust pervades the organization as workers seek new forms of resistance

Source: Shoshana Zuboff, *In the Age of the Smart Machine* (New York: Basic Books, 1984), pp. 5–7.

Among the central questions: Will technology prevent workers from translating their experiences into skill and knowledge and shift all intelligence to the machine, or will technology reduce physical labor while expanding mental and conceptual job skills? Will technology create greater divisions between conception and execution, or will technology break down the vertical divisions and generate new multiskilled roles for managers and workers that reduce the need for authoritative control? Will smart machines be used as a more advanced and sophisticated form of technical control to monitor work effort and compliance, or will they become a resource permitting all workers to share and exchange information, collaborate, and solve problems collectively?

Zuboff argued that the smart machines used in today's organizations are qualitatively distinct from earlier forms of machine technology, as is their impact on the organization and its workforce. Information technologies do not just *automate;* they also *informate.*

Automating machines are designed to replace the physical motions and actions of human labor with an automated process subject to greater continuity and control. For example, an assembly line automates the movement of a product from one workstation to another. *Informating machines,* in contrast, "generate information about the underlying productive and administrative processes through which an organization accomplishes its work" (Zuboff 1984:9). Information technology machines can be programmed to carry out not only physical tasks (automate) but also to record and store information and data (informate) on the production process. This represents a major advance over earlier forms of organizational technology. Any analysis of the organizational impact of technology must consider this qualitatively new dimension. Together, automated and informated tasks weaken or eliminate a physical hands-on labor process and shift work activities toward the comprehension and interpretation of information. An example from the furniture industry:

> Plant 12, Pulaski Furniture Corp.'s new $20 million factory in Pulaski, VA, is a gleaming testament to technology's capacity for reordering work. Computerized equipment shapes wood with spurts of laser beams; an automated machine instantaneously cuts eight pieces. Each would take a craftsman 30 minutes by hand.
>
> This is labor-eliminating automation at its most severe: Plant 12's 125 workers manufacture more furniture than five times as many people at Pulaski's much larger Dublin (VA) operation . . . It also leaves 60-year-old Howard Frazier strangely out of place. Having fashioned furniture by hand for 40 years, he now advises a new breed of machine operators, 90 percent of them computer-literate. "They have good educations and they know about computers, but they don't know a lot about building furniture," Frazier says. ("Rethinking Work: Special Report," *Business Week,* October 17, 1994, p. 80.)

One of Zuboff's major insights is her subtle analysis of the de-skilling and re-skilling process in organizations. For most production workers, skill is developed out of hands-on, sensory-involvement with the labor process. Knowledge is based on a sentient relationship with materials and machines. The furniture maker who claims that the machine operators don't know much about building furniture does so because their computer knowledge is divorced from the physical process of holding, measuring, and directly cutting wood. These are what Zuboff calls the *action-centered skills* which are forms of competence based on physical activities and performed in response to sensory cues (Zuboff 1984:61).

In the pulp and paper mills she studied, Zuboff found that the introduction of new technology eliminated the workers' direct connection with the production process. Mediated by computers, the action-centered skills were no longer relevant. Judgments and decisions once based on a worker's experience, feel, and intuition were programmed into the machines. Action-centered skill was replaced with *intellective skill* involving the interpretation of abstract symbols that are remote from but still representative of a physical production process. This entails, for example, reading dials and interpreting messages on a computer screen. For many workers this transition created "epistemological distress." "Computer mediation seems to bathe action in a more conditional light: perhaps it happened; perhaps it didn't. Without the layered richness of direct sensory engagement, the symbolic medium seems thin, flat, and fragile" (Zuboff 1984:81). The concepts of de-skilling and re-skilling take on a deeper meaning in this context.

The introduction of computer technology translates the action-centered skills into explicit data. For this translation to produce a parallel shift toward worker empowerment will depend, according to Zuboff, on the training and nurturing of intellective skills in the workforce and the requisite opportunity to exercise and perform these skills in a nonhierarchical environment. Traditional authority structures must be transformed if the workers are to apply the new technology to the labor process effectively. As Zuboff explained, "The informating process sets knowledge and authority on a collision course. In the absence of a strategy to synthesize this force, neither can emerge a clear victor, but neither can emerge unscathed" (1984:310).

A third question about the application of informative technology concerns its use as a means to control and monitor the labor process. Zuboff used the term *information panopticon* to raise the specter of a form of surveillance capable of automatically and continuously recording, as hard objective data, all organizational activities. From a managerial perspective, this capacity might provide a final solution to the "agency problem"; that is, the accountability and responsibility of employees can be empirically validated; inefficiency and shirking can be detected and sanctioned. In practice, Zuboff observed that many managers used the electronic recording system as a substitute for the more direct and personal modes of interaction and evaluation formerly used. Instead of impressionistic, subjective, qualitative data, managers could base their evaluations on systematic, objective, and quantitative data. "There was a distinctive shift toward less interaction, less engagement, and more impersonally administered relationships" (1984:334). Paradoxically, this objective and systematic accounting system replaced the interactive modes of supervision and assessment on which productivity-enhancing human relations principles are based. Again, the action-centered skills that might be associated with human relations management techniques are supplanted by intellective skills directed toward managing through the interpretation of hard data.

Alternatively, the electronic workplace accounting system has the potential to be used as an information gathering mechanism devoted to worker instruction, training, and quality improvement. Workers could also use objective data to evaluate and validate their own performance independent of the potentially subjective and arbitrary managers. In this way, the information provides workers with both a language and an objective record to confront their managers (1984:356). Under this form of empowerment, rationality triumphs over authority, but this can only be realized in an organization that allows free and equal access to the empirical record. As Zuboff put it, "Because rationality has no guile, it can also work to limit authority."

Information Technology and Organizational Change

Let's now turn to an examination of the relationship between the developing information technologies and the emergence of new organizational forms. The question of cause and effect should be considered here; that is, have new information technologies determined the trajectory and shape of organizational structures and change? Or has the effort to restructure and develop a more flexible organizational form stimulated innovations in information technology? Another possibility is that the two processes of organizational transformation and information technology have progressed independently but are now tightly connected and interdependent.

In a chronological sense, the crisis of Fordist-style organizational forms preceded what is now thought of as the information technology revolution. Microelectronics, digital computing, telecommunications, and virtual networks emerged in a comprehensive fashion in the mid-1980s and the pace of development has increased exponentially since that time. Thus, the search for flexibility and the existence of flexible organizational forms (e.g., the Japanese models) preceded the technology revolution. Today, however, they are closely linked and seem to be mutually stimulative. Information technologies now seem to enhance the prospect of flexibility

> The information technology paradigm is based on *flexibility.* Not only processes are reversible, but organizations and institutions can be modified, and even fundamentally altered, by rearranging their components . . . Turning the rules upside down without destroying the organization has become a possibility, because the material basis of the organization can be reprogrammed and retooled (Castells 1996:62).

The Organizational Impact of Information Technology

Emerging information technologies give rise to production processes characterized by several critical features. First, value added is generated by innovations in both production process and product development activities. The application of information can improve the production *process* and enhance the versatility of the actual product or service delivered. This is a defining element of the new organizational paradigm (Castells 1996).

Second, efficiency rests on the ability to automate standard procedures and routines while at the same time devoting human energy to analysis, decision making, reprogramming, and system feedback activities "that only the human brain can master." Manuel Castells believed that the application of information technology "increases dramatically the importance of human brain input into the work process" and also stimulates a "greater need for an autonomous educated worker able and willing to program and decide entire sequences of work" (1996: 241).

Third, the potential for the greater application of human brain power is represented by the employment of "open processes" that "manage rather than reduce complexity" (Kolodny et al. 1996). The greater use of open processes represents a shift from the bureaucratic effort to create formal rules and procedures that limit worker discretion, to those that emphasize innovation, brainstorming, creative problem solving, and responsible engagement. These become an increasing part of the labor process as routine and standardizable procedures are automated.

This need to manage uncertainty, rather than reduce or eliminate it (Kolodny et al. 1996), is due to the ineffectiveness in a rapidly changing environment of the rigid formal procedures once used to eliminate uncertainty. Information technologies provide a means to better manage the inevitable uncertainties by providing workers with the necessary information to construct knowledge-based methods for handling a variety of contingencies.

Fourth, information technologies, such as groupware, allow information and databases to be shared and accessed by functionally differentiated departments and units. This advances the objective of integrating functionally distinct but highly interdependent organizational activities in a nonlinear, rugby-style, interaction pattern. The study of a variety of firms by Harvey Kolodny and his associates found that "new integrative approaches include: shared use of common databases; computer integrated manufacturing practices; simultaneous or concurrent engineering to expedite the design-to-manufacture transition; flatter organizational structures with more horizontal communication; self-regulating work teams; and some not-so-new coordinating mechanisms such as project management teams" (Kolodny et al. 1996:1472).

A final observation of the research by Kolodny's associates concerns the notion of *enlarged rationalities*—"that organizations may be able to entertain different and even conflicting outcomes simultaneously." The dilemma of trade-offs (Aram 1976) that faces most organizational choices—such as high quality or lower costs, differentiation or integration—can be better managed, balanced, and anticipated with the application of information technologies that allow simulations, feedback, and advanced forecasting. The ability to consider and pursue several potentially contradictory objectives simultaneously may prove to be a significant asset in the "age of paradox" (Handy 1994).

Information Technology and Social Organization

Each of these emerging organizational principles and practices have been associated with the application of information technologies. More accurately however, these technologies *enhance and facilitate* the shift toward alternative, flexible, nonbureaucratic, organizational forms. They do not *determine* these changes. Kolodny's analysis indicated that the realization of an "emerging organizational paradigm" employing these practices is contingent on the beliefs and ideas of engineers and managers (the design principles) and the implementation strategies employed (the design implementation). Team-based design principles coupled with participatory implementation strategies were found to be the necessary conditions for the efficacious application of information technologies. This confirms the importance of the social organization in shaping the impact of technology.

Further support for the importance of the social dimension is provided by several studies that have examined the organizational consequences of introducing groupware technologies such as Lotus Notes. These software technologies require a hardware network that links organizational members and allows them to communicate, collaborate, share information, asynchronously develop and complete projects, and access information databases. The purchase and application of this collaborative software does not automatically transform the organization into a flexible collaborative enterprise. This transformation depends on the prevailing *mental models* about the relationship between technology and work, and the *structural properties* (such as policies and reward systems) of the organization (Orlikowski 1992).

This study found an unsuccessful application of groupware technology owing to the use of the dominant mental model of software as a stand-alone application rather than as a collaborative communication tool. For this reason, the groupware was neither widely used nor correctly employed. The organization did little to change these conceptions or communicate the purpose and potential of the groupware. Structurally, this particular organization also allocated rewards on the basis of billable hours charged to clients. Using the groupware was not viewed as a client-related activity and was therefore deemed a "waste of time" in terms of a renumerated activity. Furthermore, the promotion system in this organization fostered an individualistic and competitive culture that served to discourage the collaborative or information-sharing objectives of groupware. Together, the prevailing mental models and the reward and promotion structure rendered the information technology ineffective.

Similar patterns of inattention to the social dimension have been reported in other industries. David Upton and Andrew McAfee (1997) conducted a quantitative analysis of the impact of computer-integrated manufacturing (CIM) technology in the fine-paper industry. They noted that strong pressure had been exerted to build plants that can switch between products quickly and reliably, and respond to growing market volatility and product proliferation. Upton and McAfee were interested in examining whether the computer-integrated methods implemented in many plants in this industry would advance these goals of quick response with little penalty. The ultimate penalty in this industry is "catastrophic failure rate." This means a "paper break" requiring the production process to be shut down, repaired, and restarted at great expense.

The two-year study of 61 paper plants concluded that "the computer automation of the production process increased the rate of catastrophic failure in the paper plants." The explanation for this finding is revealing:

> The use of computer integration to provide this flexibility is an example of a *structural* solution to the development of the capability. Such solutions are attractive, since the costs are definable and "once-off" (even if the benefits must be justified partly on faith). However, there is growing evidence . . . that flexibility is best facilitated through *infrastructural* solutions—that is through solutions which rely on dismantling inappropriate measurement systems, nurturing the right skills in the workforce, and focusing managerial attention on the development of flexible capabilities. This is unfortunate, since it implies that flexibility cannot simply be bought, but must be built through a painstaking process of skill-building and organizational development (Upton and McAfee 1997:31).

The researchers do not argue that flexible technology is ineffective, only that it cannot be inserted into an organization as a "structure" in isolation from the broader social processes or "infrastructure" of the enterprise.

Another study in the same industry by Steven Vallas and John Beck (1996) examined how the shift toward greater flexibility—particularly the application of computerized Distributed Control Systems, quality standards assessment, and advanced information systems—affected the transformation of work. The new technology was designed to gain greater control over all aspects of the production process and monitor the flow and quality of each production stage. This required worker training and the upgrading of skills. It also resulted in the "disproportionate growth in the number of process engineers involved in each mill's production process" (1996:349). The introduction of the technology and the growing presence of process engineers had the net effect, according to Vallas and Beck, of *devaluing the traditional craft knowledge* previously employed by the workers and increasing the constraints on the workplace discretion of manual workers.

These are not the kinds of changes normally associated with the transition toward a more flexible organizational form, yet they represent one example of the kinds of contradictions, or limits, that emerge in the effort to transform different but related aspects of the production process. In this case, the technology brought expert personnel, a new production vocabulary and knowledge, and a shift from human discretion to distributed control. This may enhance the flexibility of the production process without expanding worker discretion and autonomy. In this environment, the familiar contradictions emerge:

> On the one hand, mill managers want operators to maintain high levels of commitment to the quality of output, and thus to scan their process controls with the utmost patience. On the other hand, mill managers have embraced a conception of work that places growing limits on craft workers' traditional discretion and demands that production settings be defined in accordance with the logic of technical expertise. Thus, even as they take some halting steps in the direction of greater flexibility, these mills are pulled even more decisively in the direction of a technocratic operational regime (Vallas and Beck 1996:356).

Vallas and Beck's observation provides a nice complement to the findings reported by Upton and McAfee. The performance results of the new integrated technology were less than satisfactory because of a disregard for the larger "infrastructural" or, more accurately, human social processes related to skill building and organizational development. The shop floor relations examined by Vallas and Beck point to one obvious area for further managerial attention.

More generally, these cases reinforce the central organizational theme regarding unintended consequences and paradoxical effects (see also Victor and Stephens 1999; Poole 1999). As it applies to technology, this point is well illustrated in Edward Tenner's book, *Why Things Bite Back* (1976), which provides an answer to the question posed by the title:

> Revenge effects happen because new structures, devices, and organisms react with real people in real situations in ways we could not foresee. There are occasional reverse revenge effects: unexpected benefits of technology adopted for another reason. Like revenge effects themselves, reverse revenge effects are a rough but useful guide metaphor: in one case, for the way reality seems to strike back at our efforts, and in the other, for the equally unexpected ways in which we benefit from the complexity of the world's mechanisms (1976:9–10).

Additional Consequences

Some further examples show how the application of the information technologies, alongside the reorganization of tasks and positions, can produce qualitatively new forms of organization. These trends suggest a horizontal or network-based organizational structure (Castells 1996; Powell).

> The corporation has changed its organizational model . . . *The main shift can be characterized as the shift from vertical bureaucracies to the horizontal corporation.* The horizontal corporation seems to be characterized by seven main trends: organization around process, not task; a flat hierarchy; team management; measuring performance by customer satisfaction; rewards based on team performance; maximization of contacts with suppliers and customers; information, training, and retraining of employees at all levels (Castells 1996:164).

Some of these patterns of organizing have already been suggested in our discussion of flexible, lean, and postbureaucratic forms. Other aspects, particularly those concerned with the interorganizational relations between firms, will be considered in Chapter 10. What is worth elaborating here are other internal organizational transformations associated with what is variously called the network enterprise, network capitalism, the horizontal corporation, or the horizontal firm. The widespread use of network and horizontal conceptions indicate the perceived importance of and trend toward greater interactive, collaborative, and nonbureaucratic work arrangements. One of the central features of this transformation within the firm can be seen in the shift from the job to the project.

> [W]ork today is evolving in terms of how it is conducted, and it is changing into short-term projects often performed by teams. Consequently, the organization of work is likely to be much less frequently honeycombed into a pattern of highly specified jobs . . . This form of production integrates conception and execution, with design and production running on parallel tracks . . . These new arrangements are deeply corrosive of the old system of sequential steps, linear design, and vertical integration that provided worker and manager alike with security (Powell).

The demise of jobs, in this scenario, represents a monumental transformation. Jobs, job titles, and job descriptions have been central principles shaping human identity and the definition of formal organizational activities. When individuals no longer have a job linked to a career, but are instead members of a team working on a project, individual security and performance are replaced by rapidly shifting demands and collective accomplishments. When work is organized in this fashion, centralized hierarchy and strict functional differentiation must also be abandoned. Further, forms of information technology, such as groupware, can then play a role in facilitating communication and the exchange of information among project team members. Again, the information must be joined with structural reorganization in order to avoid what Walter Powell described as the "mismatch" between the technologies designed to level hierarchy and the centralized structures that reinforce status orders.

Lynda Applegate's (1995) extensive analysis of information technology and organizational change suggests that current and increasingly available information and communication systems will allow a truly qualitative transformation of organizational structure and process. Earlier efforts at organizational reform attempted to reduce decentralized control and provide managers with greater decision-making power. However, this created problems because the information processing infrastructure revolved around mainframe computer systems based on centralization and hierarchy. This thwarted efforts to truly reorganize the decision-making and communication structure. According to Applegate (1995:36), a gap remained between the "information process and communication demands of the matrix" and the "technology to support both lateral and vertical information sharing and communication." She believed this extended challenge combining centralization and autonomy could be resolved with the introduction of state-of-the-art systems of information technology. She wrote:

> The "networked IT revolution" of the 1990s—reflected in the emergence of distributed, client-server systems, electronic data interchange with customers, suppliers, and business partners, and the growing interest in electronic commerce—provides an information processing and communication infrastructure that matches the information and communication requirements of a firm wishing to operate as if it were both big and small (1995:36).

In this rendition of the informational technology-organizational structure interface, technology does not determine the outcome but enhances the realization of intended objectives.

Public-sector organizations are also employing information technologies as a means to enhance and extend their operations (Ghere and Young 1998; Percy-Smith 1996; Alexander and Grubbs 1998). Richard Ghere and Brian Young (1998) pointed to the five critical organizational functions advanced by the new technologies: access engineering, substantive policy communication, record keeping, decision-making support, and vehicles of informal communication. *Access engineering* refers to the infrastructure designed to "extend network access between government and citizens." Citizens now have easier access to government documents and services, and the technology in turn has facilitated a greater consumer orientation in government. *Substantive policy communication* is also presumably expanded as a wide range of constituents can access policy proposals and communicate reactions and opinions. *Record keeping* has been brought up-to-date as well. Records can now be stored more efficiently, disseminated electronically, and accessed remotely. *Decision-making support* is enhanced to the degree that decision makers are able to access all the necessary information on which to base policy decisions. Again, electronic storage and retrieval can contribute to this function. Finally, a greater proportion of the *informal communication* within public organizations is conducted electronically. While this may increase organizational interaction, Ghere and Young pointed to the emerging issue of whether electronic forms of communication are subject to the same "open records" provision as conventional intra-agency mail. In short, what is private and what is public?

Related to the last point, Ghere and Young raised the important and persistent question about the unintended organizational consequences of these technologies. With the advent of electronic record keeping and access, long-standing operating procedures will have to be reassessed or replaced. This has a destabilizing effect on the entire organization. Further, the greater access to public policies and actions can increase the challenges and criticisms by antigovernment and taxpayer forces. Lastly, managing and dealing with the array of technological applications, consequences, and safeguards may result in the proverbial "displacement of goals" as public administrators become obsessed with the technological means rather than the public service ends of government operations.

The Virtual Organization

Any discussion combining the topics of information technology and new organizational forms will inevitably raise the issue of the virtual organization. The literature on the virtual organization has proliferated over the past 10 years along with the number of definitions and applications of the concept.

Definitions and Characteristics

One of the earliest forays into the topic was undertaken by William Davidow and Michael Malone in *The Virtual Corporation* (1993) which, as is common in much of the popular management literature, defined the *virtual corporation* as an organization that has adopted any and every trendy management idea and buzzword. Thus, the virtual corporation employs computer design in the product development process; collects and analyzes information on and shares information with customers, suppliers, and distributors; utilizes flexible, team-oriented, quality-conscious, lean production processes; and allows employees to exercise autonomy, responsibility, and continuous learning.

More recent works have identified some of the key and distinctive features of the virtual organization that are related to the interaction of information technology with alternative structural arrangements. Although the term *virtual* is often applied to any application of digital technology, it was originally used to describe the way a computer can generate *virtual memory*. This referred to the ability of the hard disk to simulate additional memory or random access memory (RAM) that exceeded the physical technical specifications and capacity of the machine. As applied to the organization, virtual memory suggests that a virtual organization possesses abilities and capacities beyond what would be expected from mere appearances (Goldman, Preiss, and Nagel 1997).

For example, we often confine our image of an organization to the physical location of a building, office, or factory made up of departments and units in which people work. A virtual organization would possess an operating capacity that could not be represented by, and that would extend beyond, these familiar organizational traits. More specifically, there might be no physical location for the organization; the units, departments, and offices might not exist under or within a single, clearly defined, organization; there may be no physically copresent human labor process in the virtual organization requiring people to assemble in a single location. In this sense, the structure and capacity of the organization defies the conventional notion of a bounded and physically situated organizational entity.

The question then arises: How is the virtual organization able to expand its capacity? Here the interaction of the technological and structural features of the virtual organization must be considered. Technologically, virtual organizations are enabled by information technologies that allow interaction, communication, and collaboration to take place without face-to-face contact in a common physical location. A computer network that links teams and employees, and distributes information anytime and anyplace, facilitates the realization of the virtual form (Lipnack and Stamps 1997). For these reasons, information technologies are closely associated with the rise of the virtual organization. People can work without physically locating themselves in an organized workplace. It can be accomplished through "homeworking" or telecommuting; "hot desking," which involves the use of shared work space just when needed; and "hoteling" which allows workers to set up a temporary work space in the facility of another firm (Barnatt 1995; Snizek 1995).

While these virtual office practices are associated with the larger objective of flexibility and customer support, they are also driven by an effort to reduce costs. Siemens Communications Ltd., a subsidiary of the transnational information technology company, encourages these new work practices in its online "Flexible Working Guide" (Siemens Communications Ltd. 1998) and emphasizes that "office space is one of the most significant fixed costs. For a business to work effectively, building management must be controlled . . . By introducing hot-desking you can reduce the total number of desks required in your company whilst providing users with all the services associated with a permanent office desk." These forms of consulting advice are a useful reminder that a significant portion of what falls under the glamorous title of the virtual organization or "alternative officing" is driven by some very basic bottom-line considerations.

However, a major component of the virtual organization is the communication and information networks that preclude the need for the centralized or agglomerated location of employees. If this trend continues, it will be increasingly the case that, as Charles Handy expressed it, "work is what you do, not where you go" (Handy 1995a:42). As with other technological applications, the virtual office will likely yield some unintended human consequences. Interaction dynamics, sense of community, and organizational connectedness through "ownership" of physical office space may be negatively impacted under the virtual organizational arrangement (Snizek 1995).

As the association of work with a physical workplace location and environment slowly erodes under the virtual organization system, the notion of organizational borders begins to be challenged. The new system has promoted the related phenomenon of the borderless organization (Jarillo 1995; Ashkenas et al. 1996).

The borderlessness of the virtual organization refers to a key structural element of this organizational form: temporary collaboration, networking, and alliances between firms. These interorganizational arrangements (discussed further in Chapter 10) again give the virtual organization a reach that extends beyond its apparent capacity. What we have previously described as the "network enterprise" or the "horizontal corporation" is a fundamental element of the virtual corporation. Just as there is a greater emphasis on teams and projects *within* the organization, there is now a growing trend toward partnerships and joint ventures *across* organizational borders. A major consequence of this trend for intraorganizational structure is the elimination of departments and units that do not represent a core competency, or value-added link in the production chain. If other firms that are more adept or experienced with these peripheral activities can provide these resources when needed, the organization itself is more flexible and lean. It also means that those workers who are retained will increasingly be interacting with a wider range of unfamiliar personnel from other firms.

A particularly powerful example of a virtual organization is Verifone, Inc. Verifone designs, manufactures, markets, and services electronic credit card payment systems. It is the global leader in credit card "swiping" machines used to authorize Visa and MasterCard payments. It also represents a virtual organizational model (Taylor 1995). Verifone has no corporate headquarters or recognized national origin. The company employs 3,300 people worldwide and operates continuously without regard to the limitations of time and place. This is made possible by a worldwide computer network that provides immediate online access to all company information and data. Driven by a "culture of urgency," software projects involve the input of programmers and engineers in Bangalore, Dallas, and Hawaii who write a computer code, test it, and eventually integrate it into the products and software. The activities proceed in a parallel rather than serial fashion. There is no "downtime." As Verifone's CEO emphasizes, the competitive edge rests on the fact that "people are distributed around the world" and the company is "insensitive to distance and time" (Taylor 1995).

Further Consequences

The various characteristics of the virtual organization—physical decentralization, telecommuting, teams and projects, partnerships and alliances—are likely to produce some significant unintended consequences for organizations. Several can be considered here.

First, the emergence of these horizontal, network, and virtual organizations raises the fundamental issue of social control. As hierarchial control systems are dismantled, as employees are able to exercise greater discretion, as a greater proportion of work is performed away from the physical workplace, and as the ability to physically supervise and monitor employees is diminished, alternative modes of social control must be devised and implemented. The "agency problem" in the virtual organization is increasingly addressed through normative strategies of labor control, or what some have called "infor-normative" control (Frenkel et al. 1995). The CEO of a virtual organization explained it this way:

> Given that the key objective of virtual corporation is to provide for ultimate adaptability and flexibility, monitoring may not be of much use. The key emphasis is on empowerment and self-control of the employees . . . This issue is related to the company's broad vision and strategic goals which are communicated through the shared culture and common corporate values.
>
> I am not suggesting that the virtual corporation cannot use technology for "monitoring" employees' work . . . The traditional "monitoring" by means of "observing" every move of the employee may not be necessarily conducive to the agility that is the key objective of the virtual corporation. ("Virtual Corporations, Human Issues and Information Technology," *Training and Development,* May 1997, p. 30.)

The transition toward virtual-style organizational forms also raises a second issue: How will organizational members make sense of and interpret their work-related activities. Karl Weick's (1995) notion of organizational *sensemaking* refers to the frame of reference people use to make sense of organizational stimuli and how this process influences action. The most common frame of reference, labeled the *generic subjective,* entails the elements of formal social structure, such as roles and rules, that shape organizational understanding and behavior. The "generic subjects" are the interchangeable people that can be slotted into the formal positions in an organizational structure. As these formal controls associated with rational bureaucratic organization subside, the sensemaking process is also transformed. Weick (1995:174) addressed this change:

> Consider, for example, the current movement away from hierarchy and vertical organization toward projects, horizontal structuring, and self-managed teams . . . The routines, roles, and expectations that allow for generic subjectivity and interchangeability seem to be giving way to intimacy, discretion, close proximity, and smaller sized collectivities where people work primarily as collaborators rather than as experts. If units keep changing their mission, size, and composition, then generic descriptions become meaningless. This suggests that intersubjective sensemaking—or perhaps some new social form—may be a new defining property of organizations . . .

The greater prevalence of multifunctional teams that form and re-form around different projects may produce this new organizational mode of intersubjective sensemaking. It seems less structural and more emergent. It develops out of the close interaction among team members. However, if the number of team projects increases while the duration decreases, and there is an increasingly likelihood that teams will be composed of unknown personnel from one's own firm as well as other firms, there will be far less time to develop the intersubjective sense and trust usually required for effective group process.

This raises a third potential problem for the virtual and network organizations. One of the most familiar forms of trust is "knowledge-based trust" (Shapiro, Sheppard, and Cheraskin 1992; Lewicki and Bunker 1996). This is founded on knowledge about other people that is accumulated over extended periods of interaction, communication, and "courtship." In the emerging work organization, this form of trust will be more difficult to establish.

Different forms of trust, such as what Debra Meyerson, Karl Weick, and Roderick Kramer (1996) described as "swift trust," might be discovered. *Swift trust* is established in the "temporary groups" that (1) work on tasks with a high degree of complexity; (2) depend on the diverse skills of relative strangers; (3) are involved in high-risk, high-stakes outcomes; but (4) lack a formal or normative structure to coordinate behavior and interaction. "In many respects, such groups constitute an interesting organizational analog of a 'one night stand':

they have a finite life span, form around a shared and relatively clear goal or purpose, and their success depends on a tight and coordinated coupling or activity" (Meyerson, Weick, and Kramer 1996:167). Under such conditions, trust must be established rapidly, using the available sense-making information. "Category-driven information" is used in such situations. This involves a set of role expectations based on the type of organization one represents, the specific occupational specialty one practices, or the stereotypes associated with people who practice a particular craft. Swift trust is reinforced when team members live up to these expectations and behave in a manner consistent with the stereotypification. Thus, people interact with roles rather than personalities.

Trust is also established more easily if members of a group possess resources that will be required for future projects. Members will then be driven to act responsibly in order to maintain a good reputation. The assumed desire of all team members to be included in future projects serves to encourage competence and conscientious dedication to the task at hand. The mutual knowledge of the importance of reputation for inclusion in partnerships and projects is both a controlling and reassuring force in temporary groups. The increasing use of temporary teams "suggests a rather rich and complex phenomenology—what may be most distinctive about swift trust in temporary systems is that it is not so much an interpersonal form as it is a cognitive and action form . . . swift trust is less about relating than *doing*" (Meyerson, Weick, and Kramer 1996:191).

The discussion of the dynamics surrounding social control, sensemaking, and swift trust is just one reminder of how the radical transformation of organizations can have large consequences for fundamental human organizational processes (see also Victor and Stephens 1999).

Summary

1. Much of the study of technology in organization theory has been devoted to determining the relationship between technological applications and organizational structures and processes. Some accounts assume that particular production processes require a particular technology which then determines the organization of production. Others are based on the notion that the technologies are not neutral but employed for the purpose of controlling workers or reinforcing class divisions.

2. The emergence of highly sophisticated information technologies has further complicated the analysis of the relationship between technology and organization. These technologies allow organizational processes to be both automated and informated. They

also facilitate organizational flexibility, decentralization, information sharing, collaboration, and communication. Again, these technologies can be used either to expand human involvement and brain power in the organization or to monitor and penetrate every aspect of the labor process.

3. Regardless of the intended purpose, technology can "bite back" with unintended consequences. The obsession with technological applications can produce a displacement of goals; technology can disrupt and cripple production systems; the technology can devalue traditional skills and create alienation and disaffection; it can decentralize and enhance autonomy while at the same time undermining a sense of community and organizational attachment.

4. Technology is a major force fueling and reinforcing the new organizational forms. While technology has always been a central focus of organizational theory, the explosive proliferation of information technology and computer networks has had a profound influence on the organization of the labor process. Notions of virtual organization challenge traditional conceptions of the organization as a tangible and bounded entity.

THE ENVIRONMENT AND THE ORGANIZATION

How an organization learns about its environment, how it attends to the environment, and how it selects and processes information to give meaning to its environment are all important aspects of how the context of an organization affects its actions.

Jeffrey Pfeffer and Gerald Salancik, *The External Control of Organizations.*

One of the fundamental insights of sociology is that individuals operate in a social environment and context that has a powerful influence on their behavior. If this idea is applied to organizations, it leads us to acknowledge and incorporate the role of external forces and interorganizational relations into our model of organizational structure and action. Thus far, the greatest attention has been devoted to *intraorganizational* level theories that focus primarily upon the internal structures, processes, and dynamics of organizations. However, all of these internal elements can be influenced and shaped by forces operating outside the organization. The role of these factors will be made much more explicit in this chapter as the significant contributions from contingency, resource dependence, population ecology, and institutionalist theories of organization are reviewed. The chapter concludes with a discussion of the political-economic environment.

If there is a general heading under which environmental theories can be placed, it is the "open systems model." In this view, organizational systems and structures are penetrated by and subject to a wide variety of external influences. The particular way in which these external influences shape an organization is what distinguishes the various theories that fall under the rubric of the open systems model. The area or space that contains these influences, lying outside the organization, is the *environment.*

FIGURE 9–1

The organization and the environment

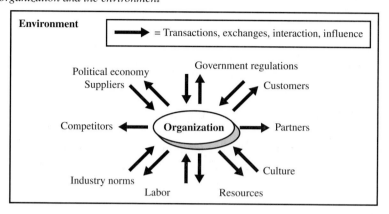

Figure 9–1 presents an environmental conception of organization that includes some of the different environmental forces that can influence an organization: customers, suppliers, competitors, partners, industry norms, government, labor, culture, and the political economy. For example, customers can make demands on a firm that result in product changes; customers can take their business to another firm which might then prompt a change in organizational strategy; component suppliers can become unreliable or raise prices which might lead the organization to manufacture its own components; labor might organize a union which then requires the organization to develop labor-management procedures or provide higher wages and benefits; cultural expectations about corporate responsibility or environmental protection might require a firm to change its production techniques; government regulations might require affirmative action procedures for recruiting and hiring workers which will affect human resources practices and the composition of the workforce; the political economy might be characterized by high interest rates which will affect the ability of the organization to borrow capital and invest in new projects; competitors might make a strategic blunder that results in an unexpected windfall in business and profits for a particular firm. In each one of these stylized cases, something outside the boundaries of the organization influences its internal operation.

An open systems/environmental model points to a crucial fact of organizational life: *The existing internal structure, strategy, and success of an organization is heavily influenced by the environmental forces in which it operates and with which it interacts and competes.* This proposition poses a challenge for many organization and management theories. It suggests that (1) organizational owners and managers are externally constrained in their ability to implement any organizational structure and strategy, and (2) any "one best way" to organize depends on the environment in which the organization operates. These two points will be further elaborated in a review of the major environmental theories and related organizational studies.

Contingency Theory

When something is said to be "contingent" it means that *it depends* upon events or circumstances. As it applies to organizations, *contingency* means that the effectiveness of a particular organizational structure or strategy depends upon the presence or absence of other factors. In this sense, there are no *absolutely* right or wrong structures or strategies. Instead, rightness or wrongness must be gauged *relative* to the situation, the circumstance, or the other factors. Many of these "other factors" are external to or exist in the environment of the organization.

Paul Lawrence and Jay Lorsch

Contingency theory has its origin in a number of well-known organizational studies that examined the relationship between the internal organizational structure of firms and the environmental demands placed upon these organizations. One of the best-known studies was conducted by Paul Lawrence and Jay Lorsch (1967) who examined 10 firms in three different industries: plastics, food, and containers. The central research question was whether variations in the environments of the three industries would correspond with differences in the internal structuring of the firms.

One especially important dimension of an organization's environment is the *degree of certainty/stability,* defined by levels of competition, changes in product innovation, and the predictability of the supply of and demand for inputs and outputs. A highly stable and certain environment has low levels of competition, few changes in product design, dependable supplies of required materials, and dependable demand for the final product. Unstable, uncertain environments are characterized by high levels of competition, rapid product innovation, and unpredictable access to supplies and markets.

In comparing the environments of the three industries, Lawrence and Lorsch viewed plastics as the least stable and certain, containers as the most certain and stable, and food as falling somewhere in between. Returning to the research question: Do variations in the environments in terms of stability and certainty between the firms correspond with differences in the internal structuring of the firms? The measure of internal structure was the degree to which the organization employed a rigid formal structure or a flexible informal structure. The

TABLE 9–1 Lawrence and Lorsch's Contingency Relationships

Type of Business Organization	Environmental Characteristics	Internal Structure
Plastics	Highly unstable and uncertain	Flexible/informal
Food	Moderately unstable and uncertain	Moderately flexible/informal
Containers	Highly stable and certain	Rigid/formal
Organization Subunit		
Manufacturing	Highly stable and certain	Rigid/formal
Sales	Moderately unstable and uncertain	Moderately flexible/informal
Research and development	Highly unstable and uncertain	Flexible/informal

expected relationship can be stated in the form of a hypothesis: The greater the degree of certainty/stability, the greater the rigid-formalized structure. This relationship and the pattern of results are presented in Table 9–1.

The results support a positive relationship between environmental certainty and the formalization of organizational structure. However, the results do not speak for themselves. It is important to understand the theoretical rationale underlying the empirical pattern. Contingency theory explains this pattern in the context of an adaptation process. In a stable and certain environment, organizations can develop a fixed and highly formalized set of practices and routines. In an unstable and uncertain environment, organizations are forced to constantly adapt to new conditions which require a more flexible, less formalized structure. Given this relationship, there is no one best way to organize. Furthermore, the success of the method employed will depend upon the environmental conditions that the organization confronts in carrying out its tasks.

A second important component of Lawrence and Lorsch's research must be mentioned. Within each firm, the researchers identified three distinct subunits—manufacturing, sales, and research and development—which point to a fundamental division of labor or, more precisely, differentiation within these organizations. Just as the firms themselves face varying levels of stability and certainty, so do the subunits. Research and development units face a more uncertain environment than sales, which faces less certainty than the manufacturing units. Research and development units must keep up with the latest innovations and developments in their field and experiment with alternative products and techniques. Sales must stay tuned to changing market conditions. Manufacturing, in contrast, must establish a fixed set of production processes and routines. Thus, it is hypothesized that research and development subunits will be the least formalized and manufacturing subunits the most formalized in structure. Or, in the language of Lawrence and Lorsch's *contingency hypothesis,* the subunits within the organization must be designed to conform to the demands of the environment with which they interact. The pattern of expected relationships and the confirming empirical results are also presented in Table 9–1.

Lawrence and Lorsch's analysis of subunits within the organizations indicates the fundamental organizational tension existing between differentiation and integration. The subunits were not only segmented physically and departmentally, but also in terms of the professional socialization, cognitive orientation, and organizational interests of their members. Lawrence and Lorsch placed a great deal of emphasis on the importance of establishing integrative mechanisms to counter the centrifugal forces that differentiate and fragment employees. Thus, their model reflects the larger contradiction between a differentiated subunit structure matching environmental demands, and integration strategies designed to coordinate and establish solidarity among subunits. Organizational solidarity is tested when research and development is focused on long-term projects, sales is fixated on short-term sales, and manufacturing is concerned with containing costs.

According to Lawrence and Lorsch, the most effective firms are those that can effectively balance the conflicting demands for subunit environmental congruency (differentiation) with cooperation and coordination across subunits (integration). This involves integrative departments, cross-functional teams, and paper systems. The summary and prescriptive message derived from the work of Lawrence and Lorsch is that the success of the organization is contingent upon appropriate differentiation—characterized by a congruency between subsystems and the environment—alongside effective integration of the subsystems within a single organization. In short, successful organization requires a delicate balance between differentiation and integration.

It is also worth noting that the convergence of the two central organizational tensions outlined in Chapter 2 appear in Lawrence and Lorsch formulations (1967:8–13). First, we have already seen how subunit differentiation necessitates the implementation of integrative mechanisms. Second, in elaborating the reasons for integrating the differentiated units, the focus is placed on the way subunit specialization impacts the human factor. The various subunits—research and development, sales, and manufacturing—shape the sentiments, motives, and interests of their personnel. This in turn creates greater social cohesion and unity *within* units but generates conflict *across* units. This conflict can undermine the larger objectives of the organization. Integrative strategies are designed to create greater unity among the human elements within the organization.

Tom Burns and G. M. Stalker

The research of Tom Burns and G. M. Stalker (1961) complements the findings of Lawrence and Lorsch and provides further support for a contingency approach to organizational structure. Burns and Stalker examined the internal structure and management style employed by four types of firms: rayon textile mills, electrical switch gear manufacturers, radio-TV manufacturers, and electronic development firms. They discovered a great deal of variation in management styles and structures that led to their distinction between mechanistic and organic organizations.

Mechanistic organizations are characterized by narrowly specialized routine tasks, formal hierarchy, organizational charts, a clearly defined authority structure, vertical communication, top-down decision making, and an emphasis on obedience and loyalty.

Organic organizations are characterized by specialized areas of knowledge, employee contributions to the larger organizational task, frequent redefinition and reformulation of task responsibilities, horizontal or lateral forms of communication and interaction, a high proportion of mental labor, the sharing of information and advice, and a focus on commitment to the larger collective interests of the organization.

The distinction between the mechanistic and organic organization is closely related to Lawrence and Lorsch's dichotomy of formal and informal. Again, the key question is whether there is any relationship between the organic and mechanistic organizational types and the particular industrial environment. Burns and Stalker distinguished variation in the environment along a stable-unstable continuum which is similar to Lawrence and Lorsch's distinction between certain and uncertain environments. They found that organic organization is more common in electronic firms that face and must adapt to an unstable environment. Textile firms, on the other hand, are much more likely to employ a mechanistic organizational system within a relatively stable environment. Thus, in spite of the widespread debate over the absolute superiority of either the organic or mechanistic organization, the lesson from Burns and Stalker is that it depends upon the industrial environment.

Formal bureaucratic and mechanistic organizations might represent a successful form under stable environmental demands while the polar opposite—organic organizational systems—appear most effective in a less stable environment. As has been noted, emerging organizational forms increasingly characterized by a nonbureaucratic structure have been linked to what is assumed to be a much less certain and more unpredictable organizational environment. This was one of the environmental challenges that led to the demise of the Fordist model.

Contingency theory laid the groundwork for an approach to organizational analysis that views organizations and their various subsystems as adaptive entities in relation to their environment. The notion of adaptation to the environment has its roots in the biological sciences and has been applied to the analysis of the evolving complexity of biological organisms. In this sense contingency theory implies that environments determine, to a large extent, what the internal structure of an organization will look like. To put it another way, the success of the organization depends upon conforming to the demands placed on it by the environment. Most generally, this model advocates the importance of *requisite variety* which refers to the need for successful systems, from organizations to whole societies, to match their internal structure with the variation and complexity that exists in the environment (Ashby 1960). This allows the system to adapt and "survive."

The idea that the environment determines the internal structure and ultimate "survival" of the organization has been most fully developed by population ecology theorists. In examining their arguments, think about the organization-as-organism metaphor (Morgan 1997) outlined in Chapter 1.

Population Ecology Theory

The Concept of Population

The first point to emphasize about population ecology theory is that the analytical focus is not on the individual organization or the relationship between a focal organization and the environment but on *organizational populations*. This refers to groups of organizations that carry out similar functions and activities, compete with one another, and utilize the same kinds of environmental resources. Therefore, the research question extends beyond identifying what kind of organizational strategies are best suited for a particular environment and attempts to explain the variation, longevity, diversity, birth rates ("foundings"), and death rates ("failures") for particular organizational populations (Aldrich 1979; Hannan and Freeman 1977, 1984; Freeman, Carroll, and Hannan 1983).

One can think of a population as a collection of organizations in a particular industry. These organizations carry out similar activities in terms of the products produced and the resources expended. Any population will have some variation in the structure and strategy of the various organizations. A central question is whether a particular environment, or ecosystem, can support a wide variation of organizational forms or whether, given relative resource scarcity, some organizations are *differentially selected* by the environment for survival. The basis for organizational selection is presumed to be some match between the organizational structure and the ability to acquire resources from the environment. Those that are best able to acquire resources survive; those that are unable to do so die.

The process of environmental selection is further reinforced by the action and resource allocations of relevant actors and organizations within the larger ecosystem (e.g., investors and consumers). Successful organizational forms in the population may be imitated by existing organizations or adopted by newly forming organizations; in the process they are retained in the organizational population.

Demographic, Ecological, and Environmental Processes

The actual empirical analysis of this process, and the determination of the factors contributing to organizational births, deaths, and life expectancies, have focused on characteristics of the population, characteristics of the environment, or specific organizational traits that might predict longevity or an early death. Joel Baum (1996) noted three distinct themes—demographic, ecological, and environmental processes—in his analysis of the research literature.

Studies of the *demographic processes* in organizations examine, for example, the liability (or asset) of newness, adolescence, obsolescence, and smallness. These terms refer to the age and size of the organization. Efforts to establish support for empirical patterns between these demographic characteristics and organizational survival have been mixed. Equally plausible arguments can be made for positive or negative relationships between each characteristic and longevity. This is a serious problem with this research literature and the theoretical model on which it is based.

A second area of empirical investigation is *ecological processes.* Ecological processes include a consideration of the distribution of resources in an environment, death rates and birth rates, and population density. In terms of resources, population ecologists have developed the concept of *niche-width* to describe the extent to which environmental resources are finely concentrated, allowing small specialized organizations to locate a resource niche for survival, or whether environmental resources are *coarsely dispersed,* favoring larger generalist organizations.

Births (foundings) and deaths (failures) are also measures of ecological conditions that might influence organizational success. A surge of foundings reflects a fertile resource environment that tends to encourage further births. Over time, however, competitive pressures in the swelling population may result in a drop-off in the founding rate. Likewise, a surge of organizational failures may initially free up resources for other organizations, but over time high failure rates signal larger deficiencies in the resource base of an organizational ecosystem.

Environmental processes refer to changes in the institutional and technological profile of organizational environments. At this level the familiar environmental concept of turbulence (or what we have called uncertainty/instability) plays a more prominent role. For example, an organizational population will be affected by changes in legal rules, government regulations, or regulatory policies that certify and establish requirements for organizations. Rapid changes in technology will also impact the competitive ability of organizations and the likelihood of a shakeout in organizational populations.

Structural Inertia

A major question and challenge for the population ecology model is to explain the extent to which organizations are capable of exercising any agency in determining their fate, or whether the environment somehow determines success and failure independent of organizational decisions and strategy. Population ecology theorists assume that organizations are structurally incapable of acting effectively to alter or determine their fate. This assumption is closely related to the concept of *structural inertia* (Hannan and Freeman 1977).

> Structural inertia theory asserts that existing organizations frequently have difficulty changing strategy and structure quickly enough to keep pace with the demands of uncertain, changing environments . . . it depicts organizations as relatively inert entities for which adaptive response is not only difficult and infrequent, but hazardous as well (Baum 1996:77–78, 99).

The concept of structural inertia points to a fundamental paradox for organizations. On the one hand, organizational success requires establishing predictable routines that produce consistent and reliable results over time. This often locks organizations into established and fixed procedures. Organizational forms that establish these patterns are also said to be favorably selected by the environment (Singh and Lumsden 1990). On the other hand, as external conditions change, organizations must be able to adapt and alter established, but obsolete, patterns of activity.

Population ecology theorists also believe that the environmental forces encouraging consistency and reliability render organizations structurally inert in the face of changing environmental demands. Thus, the characteristics that facilitate selection and longevity at one point in time may ultimately spell the demise of organizations during turbulent phases.

Herbert Kaufman (1985) provided a richer and more interesting explanation for the inability of organizations to adjust to a volatile environment. While operating in the context of a "natural selection" framework, Kaufman was willing to incorporate and discuss some fundamental features of human organization that constrain effective strategic response. First, in any human organization disagreements are likely to occur over the existence of problems and their possible solutions. This is because people develop different perceptions and values based on their experiences, interests, and whether they stand to gain or lose from organizational changes (Kaufman 1985: 47–48).

Kaufman (1985:49) also viewed the entire decision-making process within organizations as problematic given, again, the role of the human factor "... if you were designing a machine to fashion effective responses to environmental challenges, you probably would not set it up to work the way most human organizations actually work ... human beings are so complex and varied that getting them to work together to arrive at decisions is a very uncertain, imperfect art."

Finally, even if organizational members can agree upon a strategy, there is the further problem of "slippage between what is decided and what actually gets done by most of the people in an organization."

These very human aspects of organizational life led Kaufman to the conclusion—also reached by other population ecology theorists—that strategic planning and adaptive responses by organizations are unlikely to be successful. Indeed, they may actually do more harm than help over the long run and on average. Therefore, according to Kaufman, organizational survival is "largely a matter of luck."

This perspective on the inability of organizations to exercise self-determination might come as unwelcome news to the hundreds of thousands of management consultants, and their willing clients, who operate with an entirely different set of assumptions about the workings of the organizational world; namely, that particular leadership and management strategies will ensure organizational success. In contrast, because the population ecology model operates with the assumption of natural environmental selection, it tends to minimize the influence of purposive action by organizational managers.

It is interesting to note that Kaufman, while discounting the efficacy of managerial action, argued that much of the environmental volatility to which organizations are subject is the result of the adaptive (but futile) actions of other organizations. Thus, in a roundabout and perverse fashion, the adaptive maneuvering of organizations contributes to the environmental turbulence that prompts the further collective groping of organizational populations. Some of the gropers die and some survive, but there is presumably no systematic relationship between the groping technique and the organizational fate.

Resource Dependence Theory

Resource Dependence and Organizational Agency

One of the most common criticisms of both contingency and population ecology theories is *environmental determinism* (Astley and Van de Ven 1983; Perrow

1986). This implies that these theories place too much emphasis on the ability of the environment to determine the internal structure and fate of organizations.

The question of environmental determinism is actually linked to a much larger debate in social theory regarding the extent to which actors in a social system—be they individuals, organizations, governments, or nation-states—have the ability to exercise "agency" to influence or alter environmental and structural constraints. The debate over structure and agency, and the recent efforts to integrate the microlevels and macrolevels of analysis, center on this fundamental issue. In the context of environmental models of organization, resource dependence theory advances an alternative to the environmental determinism of other approaches. Rather than viewing organizations as largely passive or impotent in relation to environmental forces, resource dependence theory emphasizes *proactive strategies* that can be pursued to deal with environmental constraints.

Jeffrey Pfeffer and Gerald Salancik (1978) have provided the most comprehensive elaboration of the resource dependence perspective. They lay out the underlying premises:

> To survive, organizations require resources. Typically, acquiring resources means the organization must interact with others who control these resources. In that sense, organizations depend on their environments. Because the organization does not control the resources it needs, resource acquisition may be problematic and uncertain: Others who control resources may be undependable, particularly when resources are scarce. Organizations transact with others for necessary resources, and control over resources provides others with power over the organization. Survival of the organization is partially explained by the ability to cope with environmental contingencies; negotiating exchanges to ensure the continuation of needed resources is the focus of much organizational action (1978:258).

Differentiation, the Task Environment, and Uncertainty

One of the fundamental consequences of the social division of labor is that various economic activities and the resources they generate are neither controlled by a single organizational entity nor located in a single place. Economic specialization and differentiation increase the number of organizations and the types of resources they command. The resulting interdependence among organizations gives rise to a broader range of transactions and exchanges between them. The resource dependence perspective is premised on this division of labor. Therefore, the primary challenge for organizations is to gain and secure reliable and dependable access to needed resources that exist in the environment.

The problem is not simply that organizations depend upon particular resources to carry out the job but that these resources are controlled by other organizations that have their own interests and constraints. The coordination of resource allocation is a central objective of organizations in the resource dependence model. Rather than assuming that organizations will simply adapt to their resource dependence or that the environment will select the organization best able to secure needed resources, resource dependence theory examines the process used by organizational managers to assess the environment, devise strategic responses, and restructure the organization to reduce or eliminate resource vulnerability. Thus, organizations act proactively to manage resource dependence and, in the process, they can shape and alter the very environment in which they operate.

Resource dependence theory provides a particularly powerful framework within which to situate some very specific and familiar organizational actions. To link the theory to some real organizational processes, it is important to note the environmental level at which the theory operates. The greatest focus has been on the *task environment* (Dill 1958; Scott 1981). This refers to those elements of an organization's environment that have a direct impact on the ability of the organization to carry out its specific production-related tasks. The four major sectors of the task environment include:

- *Customers* for the organization's output (buyers, consumers, clients, distributors, retailers).
- *Suppliers* of materials (human, physical, informational, and financial).
- *Competitors* (for both customers and materials).
- *Regulatory groups* (government, trade associations, labor unions).

While each of these sectors exists as an identifiable social actor in the environment of most organizations, each organization must evaluate and assess the most relevant and critical aspects of the task environments and determine whether strategic actions must be taken.

In determining what element of the environment is most critical or what action should be taken to address a particular form of resource dependence, subjective distortions can play a significant role. Karl Weick (1969) used the term *enacted environment* to describe the way human actors, usually managers, create the environment to which the system then conforms. Human actors do not react to the environment, they enact it (1969:64). Since one does not physically feel the task environment, it is socially constructed or "created" by managers on the basis of some mental model about the relevant factors that make up the environment. These mental models are heavily determined by the "focal organization" within which managers operate; that is, what one sees or creates depends on the point from which they are looking. "The question of what the environment is, is meaningless without regard to the focal organization which enacts it, or more precisely, the individuals who enact it in planning the activities of the organization" (Pfeffer and Salancik 1978:73). Therefore, as one analyzes resource dependence and strategic responses, it is important to take the perspective of the focal organization. One must consider which resources are most critical to that organization and how managers make sense of a highly complex environment based on what is often incomplete information.

We can now consider a stylized example of a focal organization—a vinyl siding producer—that illustrates some of the central concerns of resource dependence theory. The single most vital material required for the production of the vinyl panels is petroleum. A reliable supply of petroleum represents the most logical environmental concern of this company. Since it depends heavily on this resource, several possible scenarios could pose environmental threats. First, if there is only a single supplier, the vinyl producer will be in an especially vulnerable position because it must rely on a single firm to provide it with its most critical raw material. Second, the supplier might be unreliable in providing a steady and predictable supply of petroleum. Third, the supplier may take advantage of its position as the single supplier by raising the price of petroleum to levels that threaten the economic viability of the vinyl producer. Finally, it is also possible that supplies and prices will fluctuate because the supplier itself depends on several different sources (or countries) to obtain the raw material. As this example indicates, the overarching concern in situations of resource dependence is *uncertainty*. It is difficult for a firm to plan production over the long run or to develop long-term marketing strategies when the cost and supply of its leading raw material resource cannot be predicted. Fluctuations in the price and supply of a needed resource represent the most pressing form of uncertainty.

Strategies to Manage Resource Dependence

Organizations can manage uncertainty using *buffering strategies*. For example, an organization can develop "inventories of sufficient size to permit the organization to continue operating even when supplies are scarce" (Pfeffer and Salancik 1978:108). In this way the organization purchases a large inventory of supplies at a given price. This reduces fluctuations and vulnerabilities in price and supply. It creates resource security.

Organizations can also use *bridging strategies* (Pfeffer and Salancik 1978). This involves developing relationships and formal connections with other organizations in the task environment. Bridging can include *long-term contracts* that establish supply and price over an extended period, or a *joint venture* that brings together the managerial personnel from different firms and contributes to a perception of common interests between the supplier and the producer. A further bridging strategy is the *vertical merger* or vertical integration in which the vinyl producer buys out the petroleum supplier and gains control of the critical resource. The various bridging strategies identified by resource dependence theorists anticipate the more sweeping organizational trend toward networks and alliances, the subject of the next chapter.

We can complement the hypothetical example of the vinyl producer with a real and more complicated case from the auto and steel industries. In 1999 Bethlehem Steel Corporation signed a multibillion dollar four-year contract with General Motors to deliver cold-rolled steel. This appears to be the case of a dependent auto manufacturer negotiating a bridging strategy with a strategic supplier. However, Bethlehem agreed to the deal with steel prices at a 10-year low. This suggests that GM was in the more powerful position with less dependence on resources vis-à-vis its steel suppliers. As *Business Week* described it, this reflects "how powerful steel buyers are and how eager to please steel makers have to be" ("An Ironclad Deal with GM." *Business Week,* March 8, 1999, p. 36). As it turned out, the cost for steel suppliers of locking into the low price was compensated by a reduction in uncertainty. As Bethlehem's CEO explained, the upside is stability in the business plan. "With a clear picture of revenues, steelmakers can plan a transition to higher tech ways of making the high-quality steel that customers demand." A further interesting twist involves the way Bethlehem can use the long-term contract to strengthen its bargaining position with another organization in its environment—organized labor. Upcoming negotiations with the United Steel Workers of America might produce union concessions when Bethlehem reveals that its long-term revenue stream is tied to relatively low steel prices. This could produce a much tougher stance in the labor talks.

Money: The Ultimate Resource

In *The Power Structure of American Business* (1985), Beth Mintz and Michael Schwartz addressed some additional dynamics central to the resource dependence perspective. Their analysis begins with a consideration of arguments about managerial control and autonomy. In the 1960s and 1970s, an intense debate took place over who controlled the modern corporation. Earlier, the *managerialism thesis* (Berle and Means 1932; Burnham 1941) had argued that the increasing size and complexity of the modern corporation requires a greater reliance on professionally trained managers. Thus, power, control, and decision making would shift from the entrepreneurial owner to the professional manager and would be based on professional and technical knowledge rather than property ownership. It was assumed that this shift toward professional management would produce a more "soulful" corporation that would be less single-mindedly fixated on maximizing profit and more prone toward a wider range of social and ethical considerations and objectives. The modern corporation would now be managed by socially responsible and professionally trained experts who would exercise discretionary decision-making power.

But how can managers exercise this kind of power and freedom in the context of a resource dependence framework that assumes organizations and their managers must adapt to and devise methods for dealing with external environmental entanglements? Mintz and Schwartz used a resource dependence perspective to challenge the managerialism thesis. They began with the principle that some organizations are more resource dependent and control more valuable resources than other organizations. An organization's level of dependence on others, and the value of the resources it possesses, will determine the extent to which the organization can exercise discretion or whether it is limited by constraint. *Discretion* refers to the "ability to make relatively independent strategic decisions about the firm." *Constraint* refers to the "existence of external forces in the environment which must be considered and assessed before discretionary decisions can be made." Constraints limit discretionary decision making.

The two major forms of constraint are mutual deterrence and hegemony. *Mutual deterrence* exists when the action of one firm produces predictable responses from other competing firms that render the original action unsuccessful. An example is the decision of a firm to slash prices to increase market share. In a competitive setting, competing firms will follow suit and also slash their prices. While consumers may benefit from such price competition, the competing firms gain nothing. It is "destructive competition."

Hegemony refers to an interorganizational relationship in which one corporation is more powerful than, and less dependent upon, a second firm. Therefore, it can make decisions that advance its interests, forcing the second firm to adapt or comply with its decision. This second firm is unable to nullify the effects or exercise any mutual deterrence. Hegemony can be exercised when a firm is the most powerful party in a relationship and dependence is not mutual. For example, there are many small firms whose sole economic activity is producing a component for a larger corporation. The large corporation is the primary or sole customer for the smaller firm's output. The small firm is in a highly dependent position and is likely to have little choice but to adapt to and comply with the wishes of its primary customer.

Hegemonic asymmetrical relations are also based on an organization's control of a valued strategic resource. In attempting to locate the primary source of power in the intercorporate network, Mintz and Schwartz directed their attention to finance capital. Their "financial hegemony thesis" argues that banks control a strategic resource that allows them to exercise hegemony over other organizations in the intercorporate network. Therefore, organizations that depend on banks to finance their operations cannot always exercise discretion.

Why and how do banks exercise this hegemonic influence? Financial institutions control a universally needed resource—money. It is the single most fluid resource. It is the means by which other resources are obtained. Since all corporations need liquid capital, the resource is unique and strategic.

Further, banks gain hegemonic leverage when corporations turn to them during periods of economic stress and crisis. Corporations are often in desperate circumstances and thus willing to make concessions to banks in exchange for a loan. As a condition for issuing the loan, banks may demand a particular interest rate, repayment schedule, or even a position on the corporation's board of directors. Mintz and Schwartz were particularly interested in the last concession. They noted that financial institutions are disproportionately represented on the boards of the largest U.S. corporations and they emphasized the power of banks to secure a seat on the corporate board as a condition for a loan. Since banks have a direct interest in the ability of the corporation to repay the loan, they also have a desire to influence corporate policy in ways that ensure this outcome. A seat on the board can provide decision-making influence. This arrangement will have a direct bearing on managerial discretion. While decision-making power may have shifted from the individual owner to the professional manager, the manager is still heavily constrained to maximize the short-term profit of the firm and repay the financial institutions. To place this in a resource dependence framework, resource dependence on finance capital undermines the discretion of management and forces it to pursue short-term profit-maximizing strategies or strategies consistent with the interests of finance capital even though managers may prefer alternative strategies.

The case of Braniff Airlines provides a particularly striking example of this process (Mintz and Schwartz 1985:33–34). In the late 1970s, the U.S. airline industry was hit with rising fuel prices, overcapacity, and federal deregulation. This resulted in increased costs, reduced operating revenues, and increased competition. A prevalent strategy to deal with these pressures was to shift to more fuel-efficient aircraft. The purchase of aircraft, however, required significant infusions of finance capital.

Braniff decided to borrow funds to purchase new fuel-efficient aircraft while it also expanded service into the most lucrative routes. Unfortunately for Braniff, the strategy was unsuccessful. Demand for air travel continued to decline and competitors countered with their own strategies to retain lucrative market share. The cash crunch intensified. Braniff was not only unable to repay initial loans, but was having difficulty borrowing additional funds. In 1979 the banks began to take an active role in corporate decision making at Braniff. This included vetoing a stock issue, demanding the sale of a portion of Braniff's aircraft fleet, canceling a number of routes, and, finally, removing the chief executive officer. As Mintz and Schwartz (1985:34) concluded:

> In this way, Braniff became a prototypical case of bank control . . . The logic of bank intervention is clear: to protect an existing investment, the banks became

involved in Braniff's decision-making process. This is hardly surprising if we note the $100 million exposure of the banks. With an investment of this size, bank officials would be irresponsible if they failed to take an active interest in the affairs of the company. As the crisis deepened, this interest matured into concern that Braniff would default; it was therefore transformed into active intervention.

The active intervention, however, was unable to turn Braniff around. The airline downsized dramatically through the 1980s and filed for bankruptcy in 1989.

Institutional Investors and Resource Dependence

A second more recent study of corporate America reveals another form of managerial constraint and the powerful influence of interorganizational dependence. Michael Useem examined the relationship between publicly held corporations and institutional investors in his book *Investor Capitalism* (1996).

Publicly traded companies that sell their shares on the stock market have seen a significant shift in the composition of their shareholders. Individual investors are holding a steadily smaller percentage of shares, while the percentage of shares held by institutional investors is rising. Today, public and private pension funds, banks, insurance companies, and mutual funds dominate stock market activity and hold the largest blocks of stock shares. The corporations are now highly dependent on large institutional investors who exercise considerable influence over the corporations held in their portfolios. Useem argued that managerial capitalism has been replaced by "investor capitalism."

Prior to the rise of the large institutional investors (e.g., Calpers, Fidelity, TIAA-CREF, Aetna), stock ownership was dispersed among a wider range of smaller individual investors. These investors might have held the stock for personal reasons related to a long-term commitment to the company, a belief in the product, family tradition, or for purely economic gain. If the performance of the company was deemed unsatisfactory, the individual investor could hold the shares ("loyalty") or it could unload the shares ("exit") on the stock market. This was the basic logic driving the corporation-investor relationship.

However, as the proportion of shares became increasingly concentrated in the hands of large institutional investors, "loyalty" and "exit" (Hirschman 1970) were not always satisfactory options. Institutional investment fund managers have their own set of constraints. They need to post a decent performance and return for their shareholders. When fund managers hold a large block of shares, it is not always easy to "exit" or sell off the shares. If a company is underperforming, it will be difficult to find a buyer for a large block of shares at a satisfactory price. For this reason, institutional investors have turned to the third option: "voice."

> The traditional Wall Street rule is that an investor sells stock rather than confront poorly performing executives. As institutions become significant shareholders, however, they are modifying the rule. Now, when a large investor is dissatisfied

with a company's top management, it often retains much of the holding but presses for improved performance. If results are not forthcoming, it lobbies the directors, votes against management, or even seeks new management—as the executives of the Bank of Boston, Kmart, Morrison Knudsen, Philip Morris and W. R. Grace learned to their dismay. The disgruntled investor might sell some of its stock in keeping with the Wall Street rule, but it is also more likely to speak up rather than cash out (Useem 1996:6).

The voices of institutional investors are primarily interested in short-term performance and steady economic returns for their mutual fund holders and pension members. The viability of their operations depend on these bottom-line considerations. There is something highly ironic about this development. Much of the criticism of corporate America is based on the claim that managers are more interested in short-term profits than long-term investments. Corporate managers are constantly criticized for closing plants and factories, downsizing their operations, moving facilities from one location to another, and shifting capital from one investment activity to another—with little regard for the social and human consequences. Many of the critics are the same people who plow a large portion of their paychecks into mutual and pension funds. These funds represent the financial interests of a large percentage of the U.S. population who, of course, want their financial assets to expand rather than contract. In a perverse fashion, financial resources and a desire for financial security provide the material foundation and rationale for institutional investors to demand that companies produce short-term results. These results may be based on the very managerial strategies and tactics that fundholders find socially irresponsible. Like the research of Mintz and Schwartz, Useem found that "short-termism," often assumed to be an inherent characteristic of American managerial action, is instead heavily shaped by interorganizational resource exchanges and external environmental pressures.

The resource dependence perspective is one of the most powerful theoretical models for providing a framework in which to analyze environmental constraints and entanglements. These models are based on the fundamental resource interdependencies that characterize interorganizational systems.

Environmental Influences on Public-Sector Organizations

The relationship between environmental pressures and internal processes provides a useful framework for comparing public- and private-sector organizations. It is often argued that public-sector organizations face greater pressures for representativeness, accountability, and responsiveness than private-sector firms. The range of legitimate demands placed on public-sector organizations may also be greater in the public than private sector. Thus, internal administrative structures will be heavily influenced and constrained by these external forces. Robert Golembiewski's (1985:13–42) analysis of public organization and organizational development yields the following set of observations about environmental influence:

1. Public organization provides a large number of opportunities for "multiple access to multiple authoritative decision-makers"; that is, policy-making processes are designed to be influenced by a range of constituencies that represent a wide range of views.

2. The pressures for accountability and the fear of the political and legal repercussions of decisions result in administrative behavior that is highly cautious and constrained by multiple layers of approval. This can also encourage a culture that generates the "Dr. No Syndrome"— "it often becomes all too easy to fall into the habit of generating reasons why actions cannot work, should not be undertaken, will be objected to by certain power figures, real or alleged, and so on and on" (Golembiewski 1985:36).

3. The goals and objectives of the public organization may be imposed by "multiple external authorities" such as the legislative and judicial branches of government.

4. External agencies are also more likely to mandate the administrative and managerial practices in public organizations.

5. Given the political environment in which public-sector organizations operate, personnel often combine career administrators with temporary short-lived political appointees. The entry of political appointees can result in a rapid change in organizational priorities for the purpose of short-term political gain.

6. Budget constraints and public oversight of employee salaries and compensation diminish the range of incentives that can be used to encourage inventiveness, risk taking, and extraordinary work effort.

7. Finally, the bureaucracy that characterizes and epitomizes the public-sector organization is largely the product of externally imposed requirements for accountability and rationality in public service. In this sense, adaptation to environmental demands may not be the most efficient action but one which is required for the ongoing flow of public funds and support.

Institutional Theory

It is difficult to place institutional theory within a single organizational approach, such as the environment, because institutionalist analysis has been employed by a wide variety of disciplines and theorists and has, accordingly, taken on a wide variety of meanings and usages (see Scott 1995; chap. 1). To narrow the scope, this section will concentrate on the institutional theory of organizations as conceptualized, analyzed, and researched by sociologists.

Organizations as Institutions

Within sociology, an *institution* is defined as "an established order comprising rule-bound and standardized behavior" and *institutionalism* is the "process, as well as the outcome of the process, in which social activities become regularized and routinized as stable, social-structural features" (Jary and Jary 1991).

At the most basic level, institutional theory places organizations in the same category as other social institutions such as the family and political system. This theoretical treatment of organizations becomes significant when this conceptualization is contrasted with the economic or bureaucratic model that views organizations as uniquely and formally rational instruments for the realization of clearly defined objectives. Once an organization is viewed as an institution, it takes on the sociological baggage that renders it less rational, less formal, and less single-mindedly goal directed. Calling organizations "institutions" means that they are not simply black boxes that produce goods and services but human organizations driven by emotion and tradition.

A prime example of this type of organizational analysis is provided in the work of Philip Selznick (1949; 1957), one of the founders of institutional theory. As a student of Robert Merton, Selznick was heavily influenced by the idea of "unintended consequences" and "goal displacement." Selznick (1948) noted that while organizations are purportedly "rationally ordered instruments for the achievement of stated goods . . . and the structural expression of rational action," they "never succeed in conquering the nonrational dimensions of organizational behavior." This happens because "rational action systems are inescapably embedded in an institutional matrix." In this sense, viewing organizations as institutions means that organizations have a history, a culture, a set of values, traditions, habits, routines, and interests. These aspects of all human organization produce patterns of activity that depart from the rational means-ends calculus of formal bureaucratic theory.

When Selznick used the term *institutionalization,* he was referring to the organizational policies and practices that become "infused with value beyond the technical requirements of the task at hand." He argued that "the test of degree of institutionalization is the readiness with which an organization's structure or procedures is given up or changed in response to new circumstances or demands." Within institutions there is a value for and attachment to procedures and methods independent of their ability to advance the objectives of the organization. Thus, one measure of institutionalization is the extent to which the methods become as important as the objectives.

The Institutional Environment

To relate this perspective to the subject of this chapter—the environment—it is necessary to consider where particular routines and practices originate. John Meyer and Brian Rowan offered one answer in their now classic article (1977). They stated that it is not only organizations that undergo institutionalization but also the environment in which they operate. The *institutional environment* is "characterized by the elaboration of rules and requirements to which individual organizations must conform if they are to receive support and legitimacy from the environment (Scott and Meyer 1983:140). Thus, "organizations are driven to incorporate the practices and procedures defined by prevailing rationalized concepts of organizational work and institutionalized in society" (Meyer and Rowan 1977:340).

The precise rules and practices to which an organization must conform depend upon the type of organization, its primary function and activity, and the kind of task environment in which it operates. These determine the organization's "population" or "field." The institutionalized rules and procedures of an organizational field must be incorporated into the formal structure of an organization if it is to be viewed as a legitimate member of that field. While these aspects of the organization's formal structure may promote productivity and efficiency, it is the way they confer legitimacy that contributes to the survival prospects of the organization (Meyer and Rowan 1977:340).

This perspective has been applied to the study of "management fashions" (Abrahamson 1996). The production and proliferation of management fads and trends, embraced and discarded in rapid succession by most corporations, are driven by institutionalized normative pressures for firms to demonstrate a commitment to progress and rationality. Organizations, therefore, are constantly seeking out and employing management methods and techniques that will presumably improve performance and efficiency. For example, quality circles have been widely discussed and implemented and also have the valuable feature of containing, within the term, both the progressive objective ("quality") and the instrumental means to achieve it ("circles") (Abrahamson 1996:261). Institutional pressures are also revealed in surveys of corporate managers who consistently express support for and the desire to implement the latest management techniques in spite of past failures and structural obstacles (Applegate 1995).

Institutions of higher education provide another prime example of the institutional process. Most colleges and universities, if they are to be viewed as legitimate institutions of higher education, must organize the learning and teaching process in a particular fashion. Students must complete a certain number of credits and choose a major in a predefined discipline. The university must be divided into academic and professional schools and place faculty in established academic departments and disciplines. Grade point averages must be used to rank students and determine who can stay and who must leave. Teaching must take place in a classroom, information should be transmitted through the lecture mode, and instructors should have a Ph.D. The presence of these standard operating procedures is how people determine the seriousness and rigor of the organization. When institutions deviate from these traditional patterns, they threaten their legitimacy and viability.

Meyer and Rowan referred to these institutionally enforced practices and procedures as *rationalized myths*. They are rationalized to the extent that most organizational members believe them to be the most efficient and appropriate means to achieve a particular goal or mission. They are myths because attachment to these procedures is based more on tradition and conformity than empirically demonstrated effectiveness. As Meyer and Rowan noted, organizations adopt them "ceremonially." This points to an interesting paradox. On the one hand, conformity to institutionalized rules produces support and legitimacy. On the other hand, this conformity may encourage practices that conflict with the efficient realization of organizational objectives. Organizational survival, however, depends on both of these potentially contradictory conditions: legitimacy and productive efficiency.

Meyer and Rowan's analysis directs us to the *symbolic significance of organizational structure and forms.* Organizational structures and practices possess a socially shared meaning that communicates conformity, legitimacy, and a desire for acceptance. In this version of institutional theory, organizing the way others have organized and doing the same things as other established organizations are key to being regarded as a legitimate player. In turn, these symbolic actions have real consequences for the resource flow. For example, customers may be reluctant to do business with an organization that is "different" or "deviant." Banks may be reluctant to loan capital to firms that do not conduct business according to established and preconceived notions of appropriate practices and structure. Further, the ability to receive governmental support or accreditation may depend upon conformity with established conventions and procedures. In sum, according to Meyer and Rowan:

> Organizational success depends on factors other than the efficient coordination and control of productive activities. Independent of their productive efficiency, organizations which exist in highly elaborated institutional environments and succeed in becoming isomorphic with these environments gain the legitimacy and resources needed to survive (1977:352).

This argument can be compared and contrasted with other environmental theories. While this rendition posits the necessity of a match or fit between the organization and the environment, it is not simply a matter of congruency between internal structure and niche or implementing mechanisms for the direct requisition of resources. Instead, the match with the environment revolves around the symbolic importance of adopting and conforming to established and institutionalized practices and procedures.

A useful distinction is drawn between the *institutional environment* (as defined above) and the *technical environment*. The latter is defined as the environment "within which a product or service is exchanged in a market such that organizations are rewarded for effective and efficient control of the work process" (Scott and Meyer 1983:140). This definition is the more familiar aspect of the environment in which productive efficiency plays the key role in determining organizational success.

A point for students to consider is whether conformity with the institutional environment necessarily precludes the ability to also meet the demands of the technical, or task, environment. While there may be tension or a contradiction—and clearly there is an important difference between institutional and technical demands—there is no reason to assume that the two pressures cannot converge. For example, the automobile industry has faced enormous institutional environmental pressure to implement Japanese-style production methods oriented on quality. These have become the "litmus test of managerial competence" for the biggest U.S. automakers (Babson 1996:82). At the same time, there is substantial evidence to indicate that conformity to these production practices has advanced the productivity and efficiency of automakers vis-à-vis the technical environment.

Institutional Isomorphism

Meyer and Rowan's reference to *isomorphism*—meaning a single form or shape—anticipates a further theoretical argument of institutionalist theory focusing on the mechanisms that explain similarity among organizations within the same field or population (DiMaggio and Powell 1983). They referred to these mechanisms as mimetic, normative, and coercive.

Mimetic forces refer to the tendency for organizations to imitate the procedures and structures of those organizations that are exemplary models, carry high prestige, or have successfully adapted to the environment. Japanese management techniques are a prime example.

Normative pressures operate to channel organizational behavior and procedures in appropriate, expected, and legitimate directions. The examples from higher education apply here.

Coercive mechanisms imply some formal consequences for failure to conform with particular operating procedures and structures. An example would be the regulatory requirements for an industry.

Each of these mechanisms can serve to create organizational fields and populations that are highly homogeneous in their operating assumptions, formal structures, and day-to-day operations. Thus, the observed level of institutionalization may be the product of more than simply a desire to appear legitimate. It may be due to powerful normative systems supporting the appropriate organizational practices (normative); legal requirements that are enforced by the state (coercive); or the quasi-rational assessment of efficient organizational procedures and a systematic effort to institute those proven methods within an organization (mimetic).

Institutional Pillars

Perhaps the most systematic effort to sort through the various meanings of institutionalism is found in the work of W. Richard Scott (1995). Scott's definition of institution distinguishes between the different institutional emphases used in his conceptual framework. "Institutions consist of cognitive, normative, and regulative structures and activities that provide stability and meaning to social behavior. Institutions are transported by various carriers—cultures, structures, and routines—and they operate at multiple levels of jurisdiction." Table 9–2 presents Scott's organizing scheme.

The three "pillars" of institutions represent the varying emphases of institutional theorists. The *regulative* pillar stresses explicit and formal pressures

TABLE 9–2 Scott's Model of Institutional Pillars and Carriers

	Pillar		
	Regulative	*Normative*	*Cognitive*
Distinguishing Criteria			
Basis of compliance	Expediency	Social obligation	Cognitive
Mechanisms	Coercive	Normative	Mimetic
Logic	Instrumentality	Appropriateness	Orthodoxy
Indicators	Rules, laws, sanctions	Certification, accreditation	Prevalence, isomorphism
Basis of legitimacy	Legally sanctioned	Morally governed	Culturally supported, conceptually correct
Carrier			
Cultures	Rules, laws	Values, expectations	Categories, typifications
Social structures	Governance systems, power systems	Regimes, authority systems	Structural isomorphism, identities
Routines	Protocols, standard procedures	Conformity, performance of duty	Performance programs, scripts

Adapted from Table 3.1 and Table 3.2 in W. Richard Scott, *Institutions and Organizations* (Thousand Oaks, CA: Sage, 1995), pp. 35, 52.

on organizations and behaviors that are often backed up by sanctions of punishment and reward. Governmental regulations and requirements are the most obvious examples. The *normative* pillar influences organizations and behavior on the basis of social obligation and expectations about the appropriate way to organize and carry out activities. The *cognitive* pillar shapes organizations and behavior through common understanding and taken-for-granted assumptions and premises. The "carriers" of these institutional patterns are cultures, social structures, and routines. Together, these institutional pressures contribute to the stability of organizational operations and the conformity of standard operating procedures.

Institutional Analyses of U.S. Corporate Strategy

The many insights of institutionalist theory can be further elaborated by turning to the question of how corporations attempt to control both their own operations and the environments in which they are situated. Neil Fligstein's (1990) historical analysis of the corporate landscape in the United States from 1880 to 1980 is characterized by the institutionalist logic while it also incorporates a dynamic component to explain transformations in corporate strategies.

Fligstein's central theoretical tool is the *conception of control* which refers to the "perspective on how firms ought to solve their competitive problems and is collectively held and reflected in their organizational fields" (Fligstein 1990:12). This is a normative conception that permeates the institutional environment of large corporations. Fligstein enumerated four major conceptions of control over the past 100 years:

1. Direct control of competition.
2. Manufacturing control.
3. Sales and marketing control.
4. Finance control.

Each of these conceptions implies a particular set of strategies and structures.

Under the direct control of competition, firms engaged in aggressive and predatory pricing and trade practices along with efforts to establish cartels and monopolies. The manufacturing conception of control brought about a shift from competitive practices that were deemed illegal to strategies designed to stabilize production processes and extend control over supply and distribution networks. This included the vertical integration of production units. The sales and marketing conception of control focused on the demand side of production. The key challenge was to find, create, and retain markets through sales and advertising strategies. The fourth and currently dominant finance conception of control is based on maximizing rates of return through the use of financial mechanisms such as mergers and corporate restructuring.

In the context of institutionalist theory, it is important to emphasize that there is no required relationship between the shift from one conception to another and the move toward a more rational or efficient organizational structure and strategy. The conceptions are shaped by changing economic environmental conditions (e.g., the Great Depression of the 1930s), regulative efforts by the state (e.g., antitrust legislation), competing forces within an organization (e.g., manufacturing versus marketing and sales), and the prevalent conception of what constitutes organizational success.

Once a particular conception is institutionalized among organizational fields, it serves as a benchmark and model independent of its empirically verified relationship to economic performance. For example, within the financial conception of control, success was measured on the basis of growth achieved through, among other means, acquisitive conglomerates. Fligstein (1990:18–19) noted that:

> [T]he conglomerate strategy of merging unrelated firms to achieve growth spread through the population of the larger firms. Yet most economic studies show conglomerates did not earn higher profits than samples of similar size firms that were not pursuing that strategy.

The popularity of the strategy was based on the spectacular rates of growth, and increased status to the firm, produced by mergers. As competitors began to emulate this strategy, it took on the status of an institutionalized myth. It was assumed to be the best way to do business (Fligstein 1990:19).

More recently, another numbers game has driven corporate strategy and behavior. While the financial conception of performance continues to be employed, corporations now are fixated on a new measure of success—earnings growth. As this becomes the yardstick for corporate performance and the primary investment criteria used by Wall Street analysts, creative financial accounting practices play a larger role in corporate strategies.

Through the 1990s observers noted an increasing tendency to enhance future earnings prospects by taking one-time charges on expenses related to research and development or acquisition and mergers, or on revenues related to long-term contracts. Rather than spreading the expenses or revenue over the appropriate time period, the accounting technique of one-time charges provides a distorted but more positive picture of earnings growth potential. *Business Week* reported on these increasingly common, but highly questionable, financial practices, and pointed to some of the environmental pressures fueling these tactics.

> Throw in an eight-year bull market in which earnings growth came to be the only measure many investors looked at, and add the pressure those market forces have created on managers to make the numbers look as good as possible. If anyone had

set out to invent a system in which the means, motives, and methods to encourage companies to stretch earnings all came together perfectly, they couldn't have done a better job . . . companies desperate to keep up earnings and stock prices will practice even more aggressive accounting. ("Who Can You Trust?", *Business Week,* October 5, 1998, p. 136.)

A fundamental feature of institutional theory is the argument that organizations develop an attachment to a particular practice, routine, or , in this case, "conception" that does not necessarily represent the best means to achieve given ends. The prevailing finance conception has encouraged strategies of acquisition, merger, and manipulative accounting practices in the service of measurable growth. That this organizational strategy is misdirected and contradicts the best available evidence on the most effective means to organizational success is the subject of Jeffrey Pfeffer's *The Human Equation* (1998) in which he wrote:

> Over the past decade or so, numerous rigorous studies conducted both within specific industries and in samples of organizations that cross industries have demonstrated the enormous returns obtained through the implementation of what are variously called high involvement, high performance practices. . . But even as these research results pile up, trends in actual management practice are, in many instances, moving in a direction exactly *opposite* to what the growing body of evidence prescribes.
>
> Rather, than putting their people first, numerous firms have sought solutions to competition challenges in places and means that have not been very productive— treating their businesses as portfolios of assets to be bought and sold in an effort to find the right competitive niche, downsizing and outsourcing in a futile attempt to shrink or transact their way to profit. . . (Pfeffer 1998:xv).

Institutional Stability and Change

It should now be apparent that much of the argument behind institutional theory revolves around the assumption that organizations do not exercise free will nor do they continually change and transform themselves. Instead, as institutions, they are constrained by standard operating procedures, values, and premises that regularize patterns of behavior, increase predictability, and enhance legitimacy. This aspect of institutionalization is often emphasized in organizational accounts that highlight the problems of inflexibility and inertia in the face of changing conditions, demands, and circumstances. An underlying assumption of this perspective is that the process of institutionalization facilitates persistence, endurance, and stability.

Institutional theory plays on our knowledge of and familiarity with organizational habits, routines, and sacred practices. We know they are pervasive and often bothersome, and institutional theory helps us understand the source of these rigidities. On the other hand, we also know that organizations change. They regularly restructure, reengineer, revise, and discard procedures and methods. Therefore, let's now consider some of the ways that an institutional model can help make sense of the tension and change that characterize all organizational forms.

One way to approach this issue is to consider the counterprocess to institutionalization—deinstitutionalization. Christine Oliver defined *deinstitutionalization* as "the process by which the legitimacy of an established or institutionalized practice erodes or discontinues" (1992:564).

In identifying the various factors that contribute to the deinstitutionalization of organizational practices, Oliver (1992) distinguished between *intraorganizational* and *environmental* determinants (see Table 9–3). Pressures may arise *within* the organization as new members are recruited, performance declines, power alignments shift, goals are more clearly defined, or the organizational structure is transformed owing to diversification or mergers. These rather common events can conceivably threaten, or at least call into question, institutionalized patterns of organization and behavior and stimulate change.

External *environmental forces* may also facilitate deinstitutionalization. These might include increasing competition or environmental turbulence, changes in government regulations, shifts in public opinion, dramatic events or crises, and changes in task environment relationships. Again, each of these are rather common elements of interorganizational life and therefore must be considered significant counterforces to the tendency toward institutionalized stability.

TABLE 9–3   Determinants of Deinstitutionalization

Intraorganizational Factors	Environmental Factors
Changes in political distributions	**Competitive environmental pressures**
Increasing workforce diversity	Increasing resource competition
Performance crises	Increasing innovation
Changes in functional necessity	**Social environmental pressures**
Increasing goal clarity	Changing government regulations
Reassessment of ends and means	Changes in public opinion
Changes in social consensus	**Random external occurrences**
Turnover and succession	Disasters or dramatic unexpected changes
Weakening socialization	
Diversification, mergers, and alliances	
Changes in constituent relations	
Shifts in resource dependence	
Shifts in task environment relations	

Adapted from Table 2 in Christine Oliver, "The Antecedents of Deinstitutionalization," *Organization Studies* 13(1992), p. 579.

A second criticism of institutional theory concerns the relative neglect of the human factor as an active agent possessing interests and intentions. Human actors are the ultimate carriers of regularized patterns of behavior, routines, traditions, and values. Instead of focusing simply on "institutional forces" or "regulatory pressures," it is important to identify the actors that support institutionalized patterns of behavior and the interests that are served by their perpetuation. Equally critical, and also often ignored, are those groups or factions that have an interest in altering the institutionalized arrangements. In the context of deinstitutionalization and delegitimation, particular actors or groups within the organization may challenge long-standing practices. Thus, they serve as deinstitutionalizing "change agents."

Paul Colomy (1998) recently argued that "human agency" must reenter the analysis of institutional change and that the study of change requires examining the role of "institutional entrepreneurs" (Eisenstadt 1980). These are individuals and groups who have an interest in transforming the normative, cognitive, and regulative aspects of institutions. Institutional entrepreneurs can delegitimize and deinstitutionalize organizational systems. According to Colomy, they organize their activities around a "project" that involves not only a preference for alternative arrangements and procedures but also a strategy that must operate within the context of existing institutional constraints. These projects call into question existing goals, assumptions, habits, and routines while simultaneously framing these criticisms within an acceptable "vocabulary of motives." "Entrepreneurs draw on an institutionalized problem-solving frame available to innovators advancing a broad array of programs. . . Entrepreneurs frequently rely on established cultural systems for standards to critically evaluate institutionalized practices. . ." (Colomy 1998:272–73).

This is a classic example of how institutionalized norms and cultures both shape and are used as resources by those actors interested in challenging or transforming the organization. Institutional entrepreneurs conduct their own kind of institutionalist analysis by identifying the "rationalized myths" and the methods and procedures that are inefficient and ineffective. Existing arrangements are discredited while the proposed techniques are glorified. Colomy argued that "in most instances the delegitimation of existing practices and the legitimation of alternative arrangements are complementary processes" (Colomy 1998: 276).

Given the power of the institutionalization process in establishing norms, routines, and practices, and the human attachment to these organizational patterns, the change agents are likely to confront significant opposition and resistance to change. Just as these institutional entrepreneurs have an interest in altering and transforming the arrangements, there will be organizational members and coalitions that have an equally intense interest in preserving them. In this context, organizational conflict and tension revolves around the competing institutional visions of human actors. Colomy employed Karl Polanyi's

(1944) notion of a "double movement" to describe the common opposition to organizational change by those who have some interest in defending the existing order. One movement proposes change and a second, "reactionary," movement seeks to preserve existing practices and arrangements. Change, depending on the organization and the members involved, can typically threaten material resources, job security, prestige, and identity.

Colomy's "micro corrective" to institutional theory points to the importance of including the role of human agency and interests in the analysis of institutionalization and deinstitutionalization. Once the "correction" is made, it is easier to view the organization as one characterized by alternative institutional visions as well as conflict, tension, and change.

The Political-Economic Environment

Consideration of a "macro" environmental approach will enable us to examine some of the broad conditions shaping the behavior of economic organizations. At the most general level, the political-economic environment includes all those conditions of existence that make economic production profitable and possible. At this level of environmental analysis, no specific organizational population or field is being identified. Instead, the *political-economic approach* identifies conditions that shape and facilitate the economic activities of "capital." *Capital* refers to the collective aggregate category that includes privately held productive property ("the means of production") in the form of businesses, firms, corporations, or industries that produce commodities for profit. The political-economic approach is heavily influenced by Marxist theory; therefore, an important dynamic of this model is the social relationship between capital (the capitalist class) and labor (the working class).

The Capacity to Produce and the Capacity to Consume

Two broad and absolutely fundamental environmental conditions are necessary for capitalist growth and accumulation. These have been referred to as the "capacity to produce" and the "capacity to consume" (Amin 1976; DeJanvry 1981). The *capacity to produce* refers to the political-economic conditions that allow and encourage investment by private capitalists. For capitalist development and accumulation to occur, those who control capital resources must feel confident that investments in physical capital and human labor will yield a profit. If such confidence is lacking, there will be little investment and weak growth. These are known as "supply-side" conditions, or incentives, that must be in place if capitalists are going to invest, produce, and supply a market with commodities.

The *capacity to consume* refers to the conditions that ensure that the commodities produced will be consumed and purchased. This is the "demand side" of the economy. Firms must have a sufficient demand for their products to realize a profit. Someone must buy the goods produced. The two capacities point to the very broad environmental conditions that will ensure investment and the realization of profit.

A fundamental contradiction or tension is built into these dual requirements. On the one hand, the capacity to produce suggests that costs, such as wages, should remain low so that capitalists will be encouraged to invest with the anticipation of profit. On the other hand, the capacity to consume suggests that wages should be high so that the population has the income or buying power to purchase the commodities produced. This paradox, the dual requirements for low wages on the supply side and high wages on the demand side, are linked in neo-Marxist theory to economic crises and the global expansion of capitalism.

The Social Structure of Accumulation

Efforts to identify the broad political-economic conditions fostering capital accumulation are associated with the *regulationist school* (Aglietta 1979; Amin 1994). This approach links the domination of a particular industrial organizational model to historically specific class relationships, economic norms, and forms of governmental intervention. One regulationist model is the *social structure of accumulation* (Gordon, Edwards, and Reich 1982).

> By social structure of accumulation we mean the specific institutional environment within which the capitalist accumulation process is organized. Such accumulation occurs within concrete historical structures: in firms buying inputs in one set of markets, producing goods and services, and selling those outputs in other markets. These structures are surrounded by others that impinge upon the capitalist accumulation process: the monetary and credit system, the pattern of state involvement in the economy, the character of class conflict, and so forth. . . These social structures of accumulation define successive *stages* of capitalist development (Gordon, Edwards, and Reich 1982:9).

Organization theorists use the concept of the social structure of accumulation to explain the historical phases of capitalist accumulation and development. They assume that capitalism is a constantly evolving and dynamic system of production alternating between periods of growth and stagnation. These "long swings" are explained by the exploration, consolidation, and decay of social structures of accumulation.

During the *exploration* phase, which is prompted by a sustained period of stagnation, capitalists begin to experiment with new methods of production and organization. The construction of new institutions for organizing production and managing labor relations—providing a foundation for a renewed phase of profitability and accumulation—is the *consolidation* phase. During this period, a particular social structure of accumulation is institutionalized.

Inevitably, however, the economic boom fades as profitable opportunities within a social structure of accumulation begin to diminish and a period of *decay* re-emerges (Gordon, Edwards, and Reich 1982:10).

The Fordist model, discussed in Chapter 6, fits this framework. This industrial organizational model emerged during an "exploratory stage" when the U.S. economy shifted toward mass production and developed assembly line techniques of production. The consolidation of Fordism was established during the period from the end of World War II to the 1970s. The decay began as the Fordist model was challenged by foreign competition and alternative production systems.

Geographic and Cross-National Variations in Organizational Environments

While the social structure of accumulation model was developed to examine the *temporal* variations in capital accumulation (that is, from one historical period to the next) much of the literature on the political economic environment of organizations has been cross-national or comparative. The comparative political economic literature points to an often overlooked aspect of the organizational environment—the extent to which environmental conditions vary *spatially* or *geographically.*

Recall that resource dependence theory assumes that organizational strategies and change are determined by efforts to gain access to and reduce dependence on environmental resources. If resource availability varies across geographic units, a logical organizational strategy entails the relocation of production facilities to a more hospitable environment.

Firms might relocate to production areas that allow easier access to suppliers and markets (task environment) or regions where costs are lower, regulations fewer, and labor cheaper (political economic environment). These features of the political economic environment are often referred to as the "business climate." It is assumed that this climate varies from one geographic location to another. Therefore, these variations may play a role in the spatial mobility and geographic location of organizations (Jaffee 1988).

Thus, if the social structure of accumulation is conceptualized as a set of political-economic environmental conditions that vary *not only over time but also across geographic units* (cities, countries, states, nations), the process of "exploration" might also involve the shifting of capital assets and productive facilities from one location to another—that is, from a less favorable to more favorable social structure of accumulation. This can take place both within a nation (from one state or region to another) or across national boundaries.

Returning now to the *temporal dimension* of the social structure of accumulation, one might argue that the greatest shift of assets and facilities or search for new and alternative production locations will occur during periods of decay and exploration. Using the social structure of accumulation in both a spatial and temporal context allows for a further elaboration of organizational responses to environmental forces (namely, geographic capital mobility) and the likely timing of the most intense level of this activity (during periods of economic crisis and stagnation).

These ideas about the political economic environment prompt three questions: Why would organizations shift their operations? Where would they shift them? When might the greatest shifting take place? One way to address these questions is to argue as follows: Organizations depend on and are influenced by resource conditions in their environment that can determine their level of profitability; some of these resources vary geographically and thus prompt an examination of alternative locations that might be more cost effective; this search and subsequent mobility might be most intense during periods of economic crisis.

A recent example of this dynamic occurred in Sweden. A number of major international corporations headquartered in Sweden, most notably Ericsson Telecommunication, have started moving segments of their operations to other European countries. *Business Week* reported in 1998 that "Sweden's astronomical tax rates, restrictive labor laws, and supergenerous welfare programs have long made it a tough place for business. Unless that country's business climate improves, more jobs, capital, and talented workers could flee." ("Swedish Companies May Vote with Their Feet," *Business Week,* October 19, 1998, p. 60.) More specifically, high taxes make it difficult to recruit managerial and technical staff; rigid work rules hamper efforts to restructure and downsize; and there is anxiety over possible government policy to shorten the workweek. Together, these environmental constraints increase the likelihood of the movement of capital to more hospitable political-economic climates.

It should be emphasized that these analyses of organizational strategy make a number of assumptions about the bases of organizational behavior and the consequences of particular political economic conditions. First, firms are motivated primarily by cost-related environmental conditions and act in a rational calculative manner in shifting capital resources and facilities to minimize costs and maximize benefits. This is akin to the notion of *homo economicus*—that humans base their decisions and behavior on rational self-interest and material gain—but applied to organizational behavior and strategy. Therefore, just as sociological analyses of human behavior include a moral and normative dimension that emphasizes the social factors influencing behavior (e.g., obligation and loyalty), so must these forces also be considered in the analysis of organizations.

This means that the conception of the organization as a footloose, purely profit-maximizing, entity must be complemented with a conception of the organization as *embedded* in a larger social and institutional environment. This environment entails more than simply a set of transactions that enhance or detract from profit but instead offer a set of long-term social relationships that involve obligation, trust, and reciprocity. If organizations are situated in this kind of environmental landscape, they become more firmly wedded to a particular location and may be less likely to relocate.

The concept of *embeddedness* (Granovetter 1985) can be applied to counter the conception of an organization as a purely self-interested, opportunistic actor. It introduces the role of social relationships and cultural norms that give rise to trust, commitment, and obligation. Embeddedness is an important concept for understanding organizational networks, alliances and coalitions, and the larger normative constraints on organizations (Romo and Schwartz 1995).

A second assumption built into the political-economic analysis of organizational mobility is that certain environmental conditions are necessarily costly. However, social welfare and labor market institutions may indeed have unintended consequences that ultimately enhance organizational performance. Pfeffer (1998) argued in his study of successful organizations that institutional constraints requiring firms to retain and bargain with labor (in countries like Sweden) force firms to develop "high road" strategies that ultimately maximize worker productivity and exploit the diverse capacities of the human resource.

Business Systems as Organizational Environments

Business systems are another way to think about the institutional and political-economic environment (Whitley 1991, 1992, 1994). These can be thought of as "distinctive ways of organizing economic activities and resources in market economies." In relation to a nation's institutional environment, business systems are "relatively cohesive and stable ways of ordering firm-market relationships that develop interdependently with dominant social institutions (1994:175). In this framework, the institutional environment is not viewed as a set of resources or constraints that prompt particular strategic responses, but as sets of cultural, financial, and state-market conditions that shape intraorganizational and interorganizational structures and practices. In the context of a comparative cross-national analysis, the business system model prompts the question: How do societies dominated by different social institutions develop distinctive ways of organizing and controlling economic activities which structure the sorts of firms that become established, and how do they cooperate and compete (1994:175)?

Richard Whitley delineated three components of business systems that tend to vary across capitalist economies: (1) the characteristics of the firm as units controlling economic resources, (2) the extent of market relations among organizations (the interorganizational dimension), and (3) the forms of authority and control within organizations (the intraorganizational dimension).

TABLE 9–4   Components and Characteristics of Business Systems

---

1. Characteristics of the firm
How decentralized is economic power?
What is the relationship between property-rights' owners and management?
How self-sufficient are economic actors?
How diverse are the activities and resources controlled by firms?

2. Market relations among firms
How prevalent are long-term, reciprocal obligations among firms?
How significant are intermediary organizations in coordinating relations?
How dependent are market relations on personal ties?

3. Forms of authority and control within organizations
How impersonal are authority relations?
How much distance is there between superiors and subordinates?
How centralized is coordination and control?
How integrated and interdependent are activities and resources?
How specialized are roles, tasks, and authority?
What is the nature of the employment relationship?

Source: Richard Whitley, 1994. Table 1 "Dominant Forms of Economic Organization in Market Economies," *Organization Studies* 15, no.2 (1994), p. 157.

For each of these components, there are a set of characteristics or questions that can be posed (see Table 9–4).

The three components represent fundamental aspects of organizational analysis. The second and third components—relations among and forms of control within organizations—align with the interorganizational and intraorganizational framework presented in this text. For the present purpose, the components and questions are designed to stimulate thought about the relationship between national institutional arrangements and business systems. For example, if we consider the first question—how decentralized is economic power?—the answer might be that decentralization is associated with particular national institutional structures. As it happens, most observers associate decentralization with Anglo-Saxon and, specifically, U.S. political-economic institutions. Whitley classified Anglo-Saxon societies as high on the decentralization measure and argued that the institutional differentiation and pluralism associated with Anglo-Saxon societies tend to yield "decomposed" or "partitional" business systems involving greater market-based interaction (1994:173).

Similarly, Chris Tilly and Charles Tilly wrote:

> *Markets* predominate where the state fosters decentralization and deconcentration, where product markets are relatively competitive (with easy entry), and where there are relatively few preexisting relations among businesses. The classic example, of course, is the United States. U.S. antitrust laws for decades discouraged business collaboration and, to a lesser extent, brake concentration (Tilly and Tilly 1998: 127).

Likewise, Louis Pauly and Simon Reich (1997), in their research on national structures and corporate behavior, labeled the dominant economic ideology in the United States as "free enterprise liberalism," which is embodied in economic institutions characterized by decentralized open markets, unconcentrated fluid capital markets, and an antitrust tradition. These institutional characteristics in turn produce distinctive national forms of corporate behavior. Some of the interorganizational consequences of these political-economic environmental conditions will be the subject of the next chapter.

Summary

1. Much of the intraorganizational literature focuses on the internal structures of organizations and attempts to determine the one best way to organize. The environmental approach introduces the role of external forces and pressures that lie outside the organization but shape and influence internal structural arrangements and processes.

2. Contingency theories seek to determine the relationship between the environment (e.g., stable versus turbulent) and the most appropriate internal organizing scheme. What may be a successful structural arrangement for one organization may be a less successful scheme for another, depending on particular environmental conditions and demands.

3. Population ecology theory applies a biological or organic metaphor to the analysis of organizational populations. Birth and death, success and failure, are tightly connected to ecological characteristics that shape the carrying capacity of organizational populations and resource availability.

4. In contrast to contingency and population ecology theory, which tend to assume that the environment determines the fate of organizations, resource dependence theory highlights the proactive capacity of organizations. In this perspective, organizations are constrained by their dependence on organizations that control needed resources, but they also have the ability to develop strategies to manage and minimize this dependence. Resource dependence theory also points to the asymmetric interorganizational relationships and the strategic value of particular resources.

5. Institutional theory analyzes organizations as human institutions characterized by values, habits, routines, and traditions. This perspective challenges the rational goal-directed image of organization and introduces a picture of organizations driven by myths, symbols, and the desire for social legitimacy.

6. The environmental approach to organization can also include the macro political-economic conditions that shape organizational behavior and strategy. In the political-economic perspective, one might consider the conditions that encourage capital investment and the consumption of goods and services. Government policies that impact the costs of production (e.g., tax rates, labor laws) also play a key role. These macro conditions also vary across nations. National "business systems" influence the variation in the internal organization of firms and their strategic behavior.

10 INTERORGANIZATIONAL DYNAMICS: MARKETS, HIERARCHIES, AND NETWORKS

Rather than dwindling away, concentrated economic power is changing its shape, as the big firms create all manner of networks, alliances, short and long-term financial and technological deals—with one another, with governments at all levels, and with legions of generally (although not invariably) smaller firms who act as their suppliers and subcontractors.
Bennett Harrison, *Lean and Mean,* New York: Basic Books.

This chapter will consider a number of central questions in organization theory related to the structural and spatial relationship among organizations. Continuing our discussion and analysis of interorganizational dynamics, we confront the strategies organizations use to gain access to resources, organize their relationship with other firms, control environmental uncertainty, and locate activities across geographic space. Addressing these issues will take us from the literature on markets and hierarchies to the work on the globalization of production.

The common theme in all of this work is the recurring tension between the differentiation of production activities, or the social division of labor, and the coordination and integration of these interdependent activities. Some of the most exciting work in organization theory today is grappling with this persistent tension.

The Markets and Hierarchies Approach

Chapter 2 introduced the "social division of labor" to describe the differentiation of economic activities across organizations and firms. This can be thought of as a case of specialization. Firms devote their resources and energies to their core competencies or capabilities. Specialization and differentiation of economic activities create interorganizational dependence. Organizations must turn to other organizations to secure the resources they need, but do not themselves control or produce. This raises a central question: What is the most cost-effective way to gain access to the resources needed for production?

Markets and Transaction Costs

The last chapter considered some corporate strategies suggested by resource dependence theory to deal with this problem, such as bridging and buffering. Here, a slightly different approach is taken, beginning with the idea that all resources can potentially be obtained through *market transactions*. In this scenario, a wide range of organizations own and control resources that are bought and sold in a market. The market is the arena where organizations—the buyers and sellers—meet. In these market transactions, price is the primary determinant of supply and demand. If an acceptable price is established, the supplier sells and the demander buys the required resource. After the market exchange, the relationship is terminated.

The economist Ronald Coase raised the question in his now famous article, "The Nature of the Firm" (1937), of whether this is the best way to access resources. He directed attention to the *transaction costs* that are incurred with market exchange. These costs of conducting business arise in a market when (1) the parties are driven by self-interest and (2) there is uncertainty about the quality, reliability, and long-term availability of the needed resource. If firms are driven by self-interest, one firm alone cannot rely on the good will of other firms but must establish contracts to ensure that all parties meet their obligations. Negotiating, writing, and enforcing contracts is costly. If there is uncertainty, firms must collect information on the value, price, quality, and availability of resources. This is also a costly process. A firm, or organization, may decide to reduce these costs by producing the resource itself or acquiring the firms that do. This would be an alternative to obtaining it through the market. Once the activities are controlled by a single organization, market transactions are replaced by directives and commands. Transaction costs associated with obtaining information about prices, or establishing contractual obligations, are eliminated.

This abstract discussion of firms and markets can be illuminated with a few examples. Some writers have argued that the relationship between an owner and a worker could be conducted as a simple market transaction. The owner purchases the labor services of a worker in a market whenever those services are needed. In this example, the owner may have some capital facilities, like machines and a factory, and the worker possesses labor power. They could negotiate on a daily basis about hours and wages, determine a fair price, maybe write up a contract, and then commence a certain production process.

This represents a market transaction between an owner who "demands" and a worker who "supplies" labor services. Alternatively, the firm could hire a worker as a "permanent" employee at a set wage and, once the worker is hired, direct and command the worker to do this or that without having to negotiate on the price and terms of the labor service. This would presumably reduce the transaction costs associated with negotiating and bargaining. In this example, an *externalized* market transaction is replaced by *internalized* control and command.

Another simple example can be represented by a craftsperson and a toolmaker. A craftsperson can purchase the tools in the market when needed. Alternatively, the craftsperson might simply hire a toolmaker as a permanent employee and internal provider of the hardware. The toolmaker will then make tools as part of his or her job for the craftsperson's firm.

In both of these examples, it is important to emphasize that the move to the firm establishes an employment relationship. From a Marxist perspective, it establishes a social class relationship that will inevitably entail exploitation of the worker by the owner, or the toolmaker by the craftsperson/capitalist. Replacing a market transaction with administrative fiat or a social class relationship parallels, in many respects, the rise of the factory system presented in Chapter 3. It raises the issue of management, the supervision of workers, and the agency problem.

Hierarchies and Transaction Costs

In this chapter our primary interest is in the relationship between interdependent production units or organizations rather than between individuals within an organization. Coase's conceptual framework can be extended to address the interorganization dynamic. The most significant application is found in the work of Oliver Williamson (1975; 1985), most notably in his *Markets and Hierarchies* (1975).

Williamson employs a transaction-cost logic to explain the nature of relationships between firms, and the kinds of organizational structures that might arise to deal with these relationships. What makes his analysis especially interesting is the use of additional organizational theories and concepts with which we are now familiar. These include the environmental conditions of certainty/stability compared with uncertainty/instability (see Chapter 9) and the human factor condition of bounded rationality (see Chapter 5).

Williamson's model and argument is best explained with reference to a hypothetical example. Let's begin with two organizations called Autos Inc. (AI) and Parts, Inc. (PI). AI manufactures automobiles. PI produces parts or components for automakers like AI. AI buys parts from PI that it uses to build and assemble automobiles. This transaction might take place in a market. When AI wants parts, it meets with PI and negotiates an agreeable price.

AI pays PI money, PI hands over the parts, and the two parties go their separate ways. This resembles a kind of one-time market transaction, similar to walking into a store, finding a product at an agreeable price, purchasing the product, and terminating the "relationship." This is called a "spot market" transaction. There are no extended obligations or relationships between buyer and seller. In this scenario, market transactions may, according to Williamson, be the most cost-effective means to obtain needed resources.

However, Williamson noted a common fact of organizational life; that is, many if not most transactions are not one-time exchanges but long-term arrangements. Returning to AI and PI, suppose that AI needs a variety of parts and components from PI over an extended period of time, in certain quantities, delivered at different times, and meeting particular specifications. Because the future cannot be predicted with any certainty, the relationship between AI and PI is now much more complicated than a spot market transaction. AI and PI will now have to sit down and establish how much, for how long, in what size and shape, and at what price. A delivery schedule will also be needed. All of this will likely require the writing of contracts that stipulate the conditions and terms of the relationship.

An environmental variable—certainty/stability versus uncertainty/instability—can now be introduced. If AI knows exactly what the demand for its automobile models will be over a five-year period (certainty/stability), it can order the exact quantity and specification of parts that will be used for that duration. But what if the environment for AI is much more uncertain? Rather than stability, there is a great deal of instability in the demand for automobiles. Further, a variety of models will have to be developed over the five-year period to meet rapidly shifting consumer tastes. Moreover, the kinds of parts needed will also change as innovations or product designs are brought to the manufacturing process. Based on this increasingly complicated and uncertain environment, it is almost impossible for AI to establish, with any level of confidence, a rational long-term contract that can stipulate, in writing, everything that is needed.

This is a case of Simon and March's bounded rationality running headlong into Lawrence and Lorsch's contingency theory. More specifically, *as the environment becomes increasingly uncertain, rationality becomes increasingly bounded.* Bounded rationality is based on the fact that humans can neither have full knowledge about nor anticipate future events. The inability to predict the future in an uncertain environment means that contracts must contain an increasing number of contingency clauses. There is also a greater likelihood that the contract will need to be rewritten or broken because of changing conditions. All of this requires more time, energy, lawyers, meetings, and possible legal actions to enforce or escape from contracts that, over time, are no longer in the interest of one of the two parties. Thus, transaction costs steadily increase.

A second environmental variable that comes into play is what Williamson referred to as "small numbers." In this situation PI is the only, or one of a few, suppliers of the parts needed by AI. This places AI in a highly dependent position vis-à-vis PI. Under this condition, according to Williamson, PI is likely to exercise "opportunism"; that is, PI will take advantage of its relatively stronger bargaining position to extract concessions from AI, increase its price, or try to impose its own terms on the transaction. To summarize, *as the environmental condition of small numbers increases, the likelihood of opportunistic behavior also increases.* Bounded rationality also plays a role here since imperfect information provides the opportunity for one firm to take advantage of another.

The question now posed is: Does it make sense for AI to secure needed resources from other firms, in particular PI, using market transactions? Is there a less costly alternative? Under environmental conditions of uncertainty and small numbers, Williamson believed it is more cost-effective to use hierarchical command rather than market exchange. In our example, this means that AI would buy up PI and make it a part of AI. PI is now a parts-producing unit within the AI corporate organization. Parts and components are now produced as needed, when needed, with the correct specifications and quality requirements. None of these things have to be negotiated contractually. Parts components are produced and delivered on command. This reduces transaction costs and may increase profit.

What Williamson described as a *hierarchy* is more commonly known as *vertical integration.* This is the process of joining sequentially related and interdependent production units and processes under the control of a single organizational authority system. Note that the integrative or hierarchical "solution" is a way to manage the fundamental fact of differentiated but interdependent production units. Williamson saw the cost of market transactions between the different specialized organizations as the problem with differentiation. With the hierarchy, the value of having independent firms specializing in their core competencies is sacrificed for greater integration and control of the different activities. The costs associated with market transactions are replaced by the costs of hierarchical administration. Thus, vertical integration will make sense when the cost of hierarchical administration is less than the cost of market transaction (Teece 1976).

The practice of vertical integration has a long history in American industry. It has been documented most comprehensively in the work of Alfred Chandler (1962). The hypothetical example of the auto industry is more than a coincidence as Chandler devoted considerable space to the case of General Motors. The logic of vertical integration applies well to this industry. Many of the arguments associated with transaction cost theory, advocating the vertically integrated form, were formulated by Chandler. In particular, Chandler identified the problems faced by large firms such as General Motors, which needed to establish economies of scale. To ensure a steady supply of needed parts and inputs, as well as sufficient marketing and distribution of the final product, the firm would extend ownership control backward and forward. Ownership extended backward to parts suppliers because they could not be relied upon to make the necessary capital investments nor assume the risk required to achieve scale economy. Ownership extended forward because the products, once produced, required a reliable marketing and distribution network if the goods were to be sold. These were some of the primary reasons, according to Chandler, for the rise of the vertically integrated firm.

Chandler is also known for his analysis of the multidivisional structure (multidivision form, or M-Form). The establishment of this organizational structure stems less from vertical than *horizontal integration*. This involves the merging of firms engaged in similar lines of production. In the case of the auto industry, for example, one firm would buy out or merge with several independent car producers. The auto firm could then produce a more diverse number of models. The different models would represent the multiple decentralized divisions existing within the larger centralized hierarchy of a single firm.

Problems with the Vertically Integrated Hierarchy

In each of these cases—vertical and horizontal integration—the organizational strategy is aimed at managing and controlling the interorganizational environment. Both forms are also consistent with the logic of resource dependency theory and the strategy of bridging (Pfeffer and Salancik 1978).

Before considering alternatives to the vertically integrated firm, it is worth examining some of the criticisms of this strategy. One obvious criterion on which to evaluate the hierarchy is cost. Presumably, the rationale for instituting the vertically integrated structure is to reduce costs, specifically transaction costs. Is it conceivable that this arrangement can actually increase transaction costs? Perrow (1986:241–46) identified a number of possibilities. First, it is possible that transaction costs will increase if, after buying out the supplier, you now have to establish market transactions and contracts with the firms that supplied the supplier. In the example of AI and PI, PI is likely to have an assortment of organizations upon which it depended for various resources. These transactions must now be handled by AI. The net number of market transactions might therefore increase.

Second, suppose AI experiences a sharp downturn in demand and no longer needs to produce the PI parts since it is unable to sell its automobiles. In the past, PI would have to bear the costs of a termination of production and idle facilities in the parts sector. Under the hierarchy, AI is now saddled with this unused capacity and must bear the cost of slack demand. In both of these examples, the vertically integrated solution increases costs to the firm.

Third, it is conceivable that PI will operate less efficiently under the hierarchical arrangement. PI is no longer in a competitive environment which might have stimulated efficiency and innovation. As part of the vertically integrated structure, PI operates with what is essentially a guaranteed market. Further, the managerial and production workers in the PI unit may have a weaker commitment and attachment as a result of exercising less autonomy and discretion over the direction of the firm.

Finally, a more general criticism of the hierarchical solution is the problem of administrative costs. As an increasing number of pieces are added to the organization, management must integrate them structurally and socially. Administrative coordination of the new production or distribution units requires management, supervision, coordination, and planning. Workers in the new production unit may also require training, socialization, and cultural indoctrination. Labor costs also increase. All of this adds costs—in time, personnel, and administration.

Taken together, these critical observations indicate that vertical integration is not an unequivocally cost-reducing strategy. Like a great deal of management strategy, it poses the familiar dilemma of trade-offs. Does the reduction in transaction costs from internalizing transactions compensate for the increase in new transaction and administrative costs? Ironically, this dilemma is compounded by the very informational limits on human rationality that suggest the hierarchy in the first place—bounded rationality. It is often impossible to anticipate the costs of hierarchy. Future conditions can potentially negate the intended gains.

Between Market and Hierarchy: Theoretical Rationales

Socially Embedded Economic Action

Several other critical analyses of the market versus hierarchy, or transaction cost, model also suggest a fundamentally different way of posing the problem. The first was advanced by the sociologist Mark Granovetter (1985) in his well-known piece, "Economic Actions and Social Structure: The Problem of Embeddedness." Granovetter argued that Williamson's model, and the choice between market or hierarchy, is based on empirically inaccurate views of behavior taken from sociological and economic theory. These assumptions about human motives and behavior provide the rationale for the hierarchical solution, but are they accurate or warranted?

At one end of the spectrum, economic theory assumes that humans are self-interested and profit-maximizing creatures. Accordingly, people and firms enter and transact in markets with the objective of getting the best possible deal by any means possible. In this environment, suppliers and distributors are driven by selfish interests. They will take advantage of any opportunity to maximize economic gains. The parts supplier will jack up prices if it believes it is the only source of parts. The parts supplier may also produce cheap and low-quality parts if it believes you will not know the difference. A distributor is driven by the same motives. It might offer you a lower price for your finished goods if it believes you have no alternative outlet. The distributor might also try to cut costs in marketing and promoting your products. In this kind of market environment, there can be little trust. All kinds of legal contractual mechanisms will have to be established to ensure that suppliers and distributors meet their obligations. However, contracts cannot specify every possible contingency and they cannot provide an ironclad guarantee that firms will act in your best interests.

Granovetter labeled this the *undersocialized conception of economic behavior.* This conception assumes that humans and organizations will cheat, lie, steal, and engage in opportunistic behaviors in the pursuit of material gain. It also assumes that economic actors have not been "socialized" in the sense of internalizing moral, ethical, and social values that would constrain such selfish behavior. If a firm subscribes to this undersocialized view, it will be driven to establish all kinds of contractual safeguards to ensure that suppliers and distributors meet their obligations. As a consequence, transaction costs will rise and market transactions will appear increasingly unattractive.

However, the vertically integrated solution is also based, according to Granovetter, on an equally fallacious assumption. He labeled this the *oversocialized conception of economic behavior.* This conception assumes that organizations can control and program all human activities that fall within the legal boundaries of the firm. He found this to be equally problematic. The extreme assumptions of undersocialized actors in markets and oversocialized actors in the vertically integrated firm create the appearance of a solution in hierarchies. People and organizations cannot be trusted to do the right thing in markets, so they must be controlled and socialized by vertically integrated authority.

Granovetter argued against both the under- and oversocialized conceptions of behavior. His alternative approach is captured by the concept of *embeddedness.* This means that the behavior of people and their organizations is constrained, shaped, and influenced by social relationships that can generate norms of obligation, trust, and reciprocity. In this view economic behavior lies more realistically somewhere between the undersocialized market and the oversocialized hierarchy. While Granovetter viewed humans as having the freedom and capacity to act and make choices (closer to the market but further from the hierarchy), these actions are always embedded in social relationships, norms, and institutions (closer to the hierarchy but further from the market) that constrain purely self-interested behavior. All of this suggests that hierarchies are neither required nor a solution because market behavior is always socially constrained and hierarchies are incapable of exerting complete effective control. Furthermore, in the real world, relationships between firms are not governed by pure opportunism nor do they require hierarchical coordination.

Dynamic Transaction Costs

A second approach to the markets and hierarchies questions also suggests a third path toward managing the social division of labor. Richard Langlois and Paul Robertson (1995) advanced what they called a "dynamic theory of the boundaries of the firm." It is dynamic and less static than the transaction-cost approach because it assumes that degrees of uncertainty and bounded rationality vary over time. If this is true, then the arguments supporting hierarchy and vertical integration may also be less compelling at one point in time than another.

Much of Langlois and Robertson's theory rests on the notion that hierarchy is based largely on insufficient information and knowledge about other firms. Lack of information about the motives, quality of goods and services, and long-term reliability of other firms encourages the vertically integrated structure. It is a way to control uncertainty and ensure the integration of production in the absence of confidence in one's trading partners (the suppliers and distributors).

Langlois and Robertson made the important distinction between ownership integration and coordination integration. Generally, *ownership integration* is the assumed outcome of hierarchy. One firm buys up another firm, owns its assets, and presumably integrates its production activity into its own. *Coordination integration* implies coordinating the activities of legally independent entities. Langlois and Robertson correctly emphasized that ownership does not automatically create tight coordination, cooperation, or structural and social integration. It is conceivable that higher levels of collaboration and cooperation can exist between two legally independent firms. This suggests that control and certainty can be established without resorting to a vertically integrated arrangement.

Langlois and Robertson based the likelihood of the nonhierarchical outcome on the information gathering and learning process. They wrote:

> [O]ne cannot have a complete theory of the boundaries of the firm without considering the process of learning in firms and markets. The reigning transaction-cost theories of vertical integration provide illuminating snapshots of possible responses to momentary situations but they do not place those responses in the context of the passage of time (1995:30).

Over time, organizations are able to learn about other firms, develop relationships, gain confidence and, in turn, reduce transaction costs associated with incomplete information. Consistent with the logic of their model, Langlois and

Robertson referred to *dynamic transaction costs* as the "costs of persuading, negotiating, coordinating, and teaching outside suppliers" (p. 35). These costs can decrease substantially over time and therefore reach the point in which a "market" transaction is more effective and potentially less costly than vertical integration. As knowledge and information spread, and as uncertainty is reduced, market-based transactions become more attractive. This suggests that, over the long run, vertical disintegration may become an increasingly common tendency (Langlois and Robertson 1995:43).

Granovetter and Langlois and Robertson offered interesting arguments that would lead to expectations of alternatives to pure market or pure hierarchical arrangements between organizations. For Granovetter, the emphasis is more sociological, focusing on trust and obligation in social relationships. For Langlois and Robertson, the analysis is grounded in a more microeconomic approach to information and decision making. However, the arguments are not mutually exclusive, and both are likely to play a role in existing and emerging interorganizational configurations.

To Vertically Disintegrate or Not to Vertically Disintegrate: GM and Delphi

The calculus and trade-offs involved in the organizational decision to vertically integrate or disintegrate are nicely posed in Malcolm Salter's (1996) analysis of General Motors and its parts division, Delphi Automotive Systems. GM has a long history, chronicled in the work of Chandler (1962) and others (Sloan 1972), of vertical integration and the acquisition of upstream parts and components producers. At the time of Salter's writing, Delphi was a wholly owned subsidiary of GM producing a variety of automotive components—chassis, interior and lighting, electric, energy and engine management, steering, and thermal. With more than 170,000 employees in 31 countries, and over $26 billion in sales, Delphi represented a huge and critical unit in the GM production chain. The high level and long-term dependence on parts and components would suggest the appropriateness of this vertically integrated (or hierarchical) approach. On the other hand, the trend toward—and rationale driving—the lean and flexible approach adopted by many of GM's more successful competitors might encourage spinning off (or disintegrating) the Delphi operation. The options facing GM at that time related directly to several larger theoretical questions which Salter (1996:3) posed.

> To what extent is vertical ownership superior to external contracting as a way of governing exchanges between suppliers and end-product manufacturers?

What competitive advantage does vertical ownership offer that external contracting with suppliers does not?

What forces tend to encourage vertically integrated firms to contemplate divesting formerly owned operations?

What barriers exist to changing the ownership and governance of formerly integrated operations, and how can these barriers be overcome?

In addressing these questions, Salter introduced some additional factors and considerations that have not yet been discussed here. The first involves *scale advantages.* If an integrated supplier, by virtue of the huge and constant demand for its parts, can achieve significant cost savings, the end-product manufacturer, in this case GM, might be hesitant to allow these scale economies to be shared with competing auto firms. Thus, the parts unit would be retained within the administrative hierarchy of the larger firm. On the other hand, if GM has a significant number of other parts producers of comparable size and scale to which it might turn for components, the case for divesting the parts unit would be strengthened. The number of large-scale parts producers has increased, while the market for GM products has decreased. The GM product line has also become increasingly fragmented. Thus the advantages associated with scale economy have diminished. This led Salter to conclude that the scale economy argument does not support retaining the vertically integrated arrangement with Delphi.

A second factor is the importance of *coordination and technology transfer.* If there are special coordinating processes required between the supplier and manufacturer, or distinct technology and knowledge sharing, a tight, ownership-integrated linkage may be required. On the other hand, if coordination and information sharing can be accomplished through some intermediate arrangement (between market and hierarchy), the need for vertical integration is weakened. Salter argued that coordination of information and technology is not only established between GM's competitors and its suppliers *without vertical integration,* but that Delphi itself has established such relationships with non-GM manufacturers. Thus, integration and coordination does not require formal hierarchical ownership.

A third consideration in deciding about vertical disintegration is *switching costs* and *"hold up."* Does the supplier produce such a manufacturer-specific asset that the manufacturer would be unable to locate an alternative supplier, if necessary? How great would be the costs of switching to an alternative supplier? Would switching costs be so significant that the original supplier can leverage its privileged position, exercise opportunism, and increase selling prices? These considerations are directly related to the problem of "small numbers" discussed previously. On this criteria, Salter also believed that the evidence indicates an increasing number of high-quality alternative suppliers who could produce to GM specifications. Thus, the need to own and control the supplier is diminished.

A fourth and final factor we can consider is *proprietary knowledge* and *end-product differentiation.* If the supplier controls special proprietary knowledge about a particular set of components or component systems, and these effectively differentiate the final product from that of the competition, vertical ownership of the supplier would be strategically advantageous. On the other hand, if the components and their features are widely available from other suppliers, these component systems will not serve to differentiate the end product or translate into any major market advantage; again, there will be less need for formal ownership and control.

In the case of Delphi, Salter saw a number of minor advantages in Delphi's modular systems, such as cockpits and doors, that arrive as fully assembled units. The supply of these units reduces manufacturing assembly time. However, this advantage is not entirely unique to Delphi and, therefore, it can be accessed or nurtured through other suppliers. This factor, considered alongside the others, led Salter to conclude that

> [T]he limited opportunities for end-product differentiation do not seem to outweigh the substantial financial gains of divestiture, and the economic case for reversing GM's long-standing vertical ownership of a broad array of component suppliers looks stronger than ever before. Delphi is another prime candidate for divestiture and should be considered such by GM's most senior strategists (1996:33).

In 1996 these were prescient words. Two years later, GM officially announced that it would be spinning off Delphi Automotive Systems Corporation as an independent company effective January 1, 1999. This represented a "dramatic shift" from the legacy of vertical integration. GM executives indicated that the move would make it easier to develop relationships with other automakers that had been reluctant to work with a wholly owned GM parts supplier. The spin-off would also make it easier for GM to use independent and potentially lower-cost suppliers for parts and components.

Another significant factor that came into play in the GM decision was GM's relationship with the United Auto Workers (UAW). The UAW strongly opposed the divestiture of Delphi because Delphi workers were represented under the general collective bargaining agreement with GM and were paid the same wages as automobile assembly plant workers. The UAW viewed the spin-off as part of a larger effort by GM to outsource a greater proportion of parts production to nonunion suppliers. There was also fear that Delphi, as an independent firm, would close several of its U.S. plants that it considers uncompetitive or unprofitable. In its future negotiations with GM, the UAW will request that GM insist on UAW-based standards in its continued contractual agreements with Delphi suppliers. Since the formal breakup, Delphi has secured $4 billion in new contracts with GM as well as $2 billion with non-GM firms.

Vertical Disintegration and Alternative Arrangements

The theoretical arguments for alternatives to the market or hierarchical relationship have been given a major nudge by real-world events. As documented in Chapter 6, organizations are moving in the direction of leanness. This suggests a trend from hierarchical organization and toward vertical disintegration. In this chapter, our interest lies in the impact of this trend on the larger external environment of the organization and subsequent interorganizational relations. Several issues shall be considered. First, why the shift toward leanness? Second, what kind of interorganizational form will result from the process of vertical disintegration?

Why Disintegrate?

The first question has already been considered in some detail. It begins with the argument that the vertically integrated, Fordist-style form, whatever its past or static cost advantages, is today a structural liability. It is a highly rigid and inflexible arrangement in what has become a highly uncertain and turbulent economic environment.

There is an irony here. The environmental characteristic that at one time supported vertical integration—uncertainty—is now used to argue for vertical *dis*integration. Are organizational theorists confused, or has something changed? Probably both. But what may have changed most dramatically is the type of uncertainty, or dynamism, in the contemporary environment. It rewards *economies of scope* as much as, if not more than, *economies of scale.* The ability to produce a wide range of different products for diverse markets and to innovate rapidly in product designs and process technology are hindered by the vertically integrated structure. The coordination of, and costs sunk in, production units becomes less advantageous when designs, models, markets, and production techniques are changing rapidly. For these reasons, less vertically integrated structures emerge as corporations shed units and divisions, and focus on core competencies. However, vertical disintegration comes with a greater number of externalized transactions that must be established. Does this return us to the market-based transaction approach or is there an alternative?

Embedded Networks

Most theorists believe many industrial organizations now occupy a middle ground between markets and hierarchies that will be referred to as *embedded networks* (Gereffi and Hamilton 1996). This term connotes aspects of interorganizational relations that defy the market-hierarchy duality. Network relations imply some structural interdependence; embeddedness implies that the relations are situated in a social normative context. More specifically, Gary Gereffi and Gary Hamilton (1996:24-25) defined embedded networks as

> the patterns of relationships among economic participants; some of these may be heads of firms, others owners of capital, others possessors of labor, and yet others skilled in the use of special technologies . . . participants interrelate in ways that are, in addition to their economic content, patterned by relations that have a societal content as well. The content may be legal, sociological, political, or, more likely, some combination of these.

An embedded network is the most general way to describe the myriad interorganizational arrangements that defy the market-hierarchy duality and which have become increasingly common. Embedded networks can include temporary alliances, arrangements, or agreements designed to combine the core competencies and capacities of different firms for the purpose of research, design, and production for a particular market. The network is characterized by cooperation, collaboration, and the sharing of information. Thus, it is unlike a pure market transaction.

On the other hand, the firms participating in the network are legally independent production units. The network strategy is a particularly appropriate adaptation to the demand for the rapid deployment of economic resources to meet changing environmental conditions. Firms can produce for and participate in a wide range of markets—enhancing economies of scope—without the enormous investment that would be required to establish all the necessary forms of production and expertise in a single corporation. The network reduces the problem of sunk costs in capital, inventory, and labor.

Competitive Advantages of the Network Form

Recall from Chapter 6 the comparison between the "just-in-case" and "just-in-time " approaches. Under the old just-in-case approach, firms would integrate vertically to control resources "just-in-case" they were needed or difficult to obtain. Under the network system, resources are accessed and brought together "just-in-time" to respond to particular market opportunities. After the opportunities have been exploited, the network may dissolve with individual members forming new networks or later reforming old networks to pursue a new project.

In an aptly titled article, "Neither Market nor Hierarchy," Walter Powell (1990) argued that networks represent a "distinct form of coordinating activity" that can be compared with the market and hierarchy arrangements. A comparison of Powell's central elements is shown in Table 10–1. Most generally, the network combines the flexibility of independent nonvertically

TABLE 10–1   Markets, Hierarchies, and Networks

Features	Organizational Form		
	Market	*Hierarchy*	*Network*
Normative basis	Contract-property rights	Employment relationship	Complementary strengths
Means of communication	Prices	Routines	Relational
Methods of conflict resolution	Haggling—legal contractual enforcement	Administrative fiat	Norm of reciprocity—reputational concerns
Degree of flexibility	High	Low	Medium
Amount of commitment among parties	Low	Medium to high	Medium to high
Tone or climate	Precision and/or suspicion	Formal, bureaucratic	Open-ended, mutually beneficial
Actor preferences or choices	Independent	Dependent	Interdependent

Source: Table 1, in Walter Powell, "Neither Market nor Hierarchy: Network Forms of Organization," in Barry M. Staw and Larry L. Cummings, eds., *Research in Organizational Behavior* (Greenwich, CT: JAI Press, 1990), p. 300.

integrated firms in a market with the tighter connections found in hierarchies. As Powell (1990:303) explained it:

> Networks are "lighter on their feet" than hierarchies. In network modes of resource allocation, transactions occur neither through discrete exchanges nor by administrative fiat, but through networks of individuals engaged in reciprocal, preferential, mutually supportive actions. Networks can be complex: they involve neither the explicit criteria of the market, nor the familiar paternalism of the hierarchy.

Manuel Castells (1996) offered another version of this argument. He argued that the difficulty in breaking into new markets, and keeping up with technological changes, has encouraged greater cooperation and networking. It allows the sharing of costs and risks, and a greater capacity to stay technologically current.

> In other words, through the interaction between organizational crisis and change and new informational technologies a new organizational form has emerged as characteristic of the information/global economy: the *network enterprise* (Castells 1996:168–71).

In Castells's analysis, information technologies play a key role. They facilitate the rapid transmission of information between firms—through computer networks and telecommunication systems—and permit the integration of differentiated production units. One of the key attributes of the successful network is its *connectedness*—"its structural ability to facilitate noise-free communication between its components"—and *consistency*—"sharing of interests between the network's goals and the goals of its components" (Castells 1996:171). Connectedness and consistency correspond to our concepts of structural and social integration, respectively. Connectedness implies communication and coordination while consistency implies shared goals and objectives.

Connectedness and consistency also facilitate another advantage of networks and alliances: the exchange of information and knowledge. Some forms of knowledge can be accessed without necessarily creating an alliance with other firms. This is *migratory knowledge* (Badaracco 1991). "It can move very quickly and easily because it is encapsulated in formulas, designs, manuals, or books, or in pieces of machinery. If an individual or organization with the appropriate capabilities gets the formula, the book, the manual, or the machine, it can get the knowledge" (1991:9).

Other forms of knowledge, more accurately described as *embedded knowledge,* "resides in relationships, usually complex social relationships. A team, a department, or a company sometimes 'knows' things that none of its individual members know, and some of its knowledge cannot be fully articulated" (1991:10).

Embedded knowledge cannot be easily codified or formalized in written documentation. It exists in processes and emerges synergistically. If firms want to gain access to this knowledge, they must form more than a simple transaction, or product link, and instead establish what Joseph Badaracco termed a *knowledge link.* These are "alliances through which a company sought to learn or jointly create new knowledge and capabilities . . . Many of these alliances reflect the special character of embedded knowledge . . . For one organization to acquire knowledge embedded in the routines of another, it must form a complex, intimate relationship with it" (1991:12). Thus, in Badaracco's formulation, strategic alliances are based on the desire to establish knowledge links in order to gain access to embedded forms of knowledge. Or, as Powell (1990:304) put it, "The open-ended, relational features of networks . . . greatly enhance the ability to transmit and learn new knowledge and skills."

In considering alliances, the analysis of interorganizational relations can be extended to include not only interdependent firms connected in a production chain but also alliances between competing firms. These are becoming increasingly common. For example, IBM and Toshiba compete in the laptop computer market, but they also have formed a strategic alliance to develop and produce a key component of this product—the liquid crystal display (LCD) monitors. Think of this as a *horizontal alliance* or a form of horizontal cooperation. David Teece (1992:12–13) discussed the rationale for this arrangement:

> [I]nnovation and commercialization of new products and processes are often high cost activities. The scale and scope of assets needed will often lie beyond the capabilities of a single firm. This cooperation—both horizontal and vertical—may be the only viable means for moving forward. In addition, cooperation will reduce

wasteful duplicate expenditures on research and development. Innovation also entails significant risk. . . Indeed, when risk is particularly high because the technology being pursued is both expensive and underdeveloped, cooperation may be the only way that firms will undertake the needed effort.

Teece (1992) has been a strident advocate for strategic alliances that advance innovation and technological progress (Jorde and Teece 1990). It is worth noting that political-economic environmental forces influence the likelihood that these cooperative corporate arrangements will occur. Most notable are the legal policies that either encourage or restrict the formation of alliances between firms in the same industry. Teece argued that "antitrust policy in the United States is likely to remain a barrier to innovation because it has the capacity to stifle beneficial forms of interfirm cooperation" (1992:23). This is one of the central environmental factors in the U.S. business system that tends to promote decentralized relationships among firms in comparison to other industrialized nations (Whitley 1994).

Alliance Capitalism: The Rise and Demise of the Keiretsu

Highly successful organizational arrangements tend to serve as models for other organizations. The process of mimicry and replication has played a significant role in the rise of network and alliance interorganizational structures. Again, as was the case with various *intra*organizational strategies such as lean production and quality circles, the Japanese industrial organization has served as a model.

Michael Gerlach's (1992) study of Japanese business enterprise identified a distinct form of capitalism based on the particular interorganizational arrangement employed by the largest Japanese corporations. He used the term *alliance capitalism* to describe the institutional pattern of relationships between corporations and other organizational actors. At the center of this capitalist system is the *keiretsu,* an intercorporate alliance characterized by "institutionalized relationships among firms based on localized networks of dense transactions, a stable framework for exchange, and patterns of periodic collective action" (Gerlach 1992:3).

The Japanese keiretsu possess several distinct traits. First, the alliance enterprises are connected by *affiliational ties* that promote preferential exchange. However, there is no singular chain of command as one might find in a hierarchy or vertically integrated firm. Relationships between affiliated organizations within the keiretsu exist in the space between the market and the hierarchy.

Second, the relationship between firms has developed over a long period. This engenders informal but strong mutual normative obligations that facilitate trust, reciprocity, and continuous interaction. High trust and shared norms reduce the need for contractual compliance and enforcement and, in turn, transaction costs. The relationship between firms in this scenario fits the model of the "normative clan" (Ouchi 1980). It is characterized by informal relations, familial-like interactions, a common culture, trust and loyalty, obligation and responsibility, and a moral dimension.

Third, the relationships between the member firms of the keiretsu are characterized by *multiplexity*. Interorganizational linkages extend beyond production-related transactions and include "overlapping transactions" in the form of equity investments and personnel interlocks. Equity investment takes the form of *cross-shareholding* (or interlocking shares). Each company within the keiretsu is a shareholder and debt holder of other firms in the group. This arrangement is viewed as advantageous because it solidifies common interest, takes pressure off firms to achieve short-term profit at the expense of long-term investment, and reduces the likelihood of a hostile takeover. This serves to further strengthen and consolidate economic ties among the firms.

Fourth, the firms in the keiretsu make up an *extended network* comprised of a family of affiliated firms that share information and equity capital.

Last, the interorganizational alliance is infused with *symbolic significa-tion* based upon a common culture, organizational mission, and set of objectives that further preclude the need for legal contractual arrangements. According to Gerlach, these distinctive features of the keiretsu have contributed to the economic success of the Japanese organization and larger economy.

The best known Japanese keiretsu is Mitsubishi (see Figure 10-1). As one of the largest industrial groups in the world, it reported revenue of $115 billion in 1999. The core of Mitsubishi lies in its 36 factories and 15 research facilities. Approximately one-third of the firms engage in "process manufacturing"—the production of materials such as cement, chemicals, plastics, and synthetic fibers—that supply the manufacturing units. Another third are devoted to "fab-rication manufacturing"—the production of products such as automobiles, computers, and air conditioners. The remaining organizational units are engaged in various "circulation activities" such as financial management, banking and investing, insurance, and marketing.

Mitsubishi's organizational arrangement was described in *Business Week*.

> The Mitsubishi group is not a single corporate entity with a central "brain." The cross-shareholdings, interlocking directorates, joint-ventures, and long-term busi-ness relationships—all underpinned by common educational and historical links—create a family of companies that do not depend on formal controls, but rather recognize their mutual interests . . . In a keiretsu no single company pre-dominates. Since one core member of a keiretsu rarely owns more than 10 percent of another, it doesn't do business with another unless it makes economic sense. . . But the financial cross-holdings among companies in a keiretsu do weave a dense

FIGURE 10–1

The Mitsubishi Group

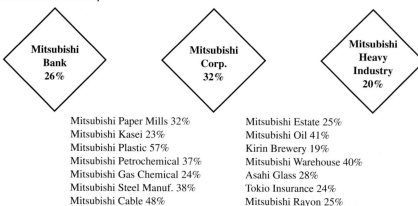

Mitsubishi Paper Mills 32%   Mitsubishi Estate 25%
Mitsubishi Kasei 23%   Mitsubishi Oil 41%
Mitsubishi Plastic 57%   Kirin Brewery 19%
Mitsubishi Petrochemical 37%   Mitsubishi Warehouse 40%
Mitsubishi Gas Chemical 24%   Asahi Glass 28%
Mitsubishi Steel Manuf. 38%   Tokio Insurance 24%
Mitsubishi Cable 48%   Mitsubishi Rayon 25%
Mitsubishi Metal 21%   Mitsubishi Electric 17%
Mitsubishi Aluminum 100%   Mitsubishi Trust and Banking 28%
Mitsubishi Mining & Cement 37%   Mitsubishi Motors 55%
Mitsubishi Construction 100%   Nikon Corp. 27%
Nippon Yusen 25%   Mitsubishi Kakoki 37%

Note: Percentages refer to shares of each company held by other members of the group.
Source: *Business Week,* September 24, 1990, p. 99.

fabric of relationships that can be exploited when mutually beneficial. In effect, companies in the keiretsu enjoy a family safety net that encourages long-term investment and high-tech risk taking. ("Mighty Mitsubishi Is on the Move." *Business Week,* September 24, 1990, p. 98.)

One of the major aspects of the keiretsu alliance is the privileged position of member firms in the supply of parts and components to the manufacturing units. This is not only the case within Japan but also for Japanese transplants. For example, Mitsubishi's Diamond-Star Motors, located in Illinois, receives the air-conditioning units from Mitsubishi Heavy Industries, starters from Mitsubishi Electric, springs from Mitsubishi Steel, and ball bearings from its affiliated firm of United Globe Nippon. Many of these suppliers have set up facilities in the United States to serve the just-in-time needs of the manufacturing unit.

Mitsubishi is an example of a *horizontal* or *intermarket keiretsu* that manufactures a wide range of functionally unrelated products and materials. *Vertical keiretsu,* such as Toyota, include a network of suppliers and distributors that exist in a hierarchical relationship with an industry-specific manufacturing unit. Several vertical keiretsu can exist within a single horizontal keiretsu.

In 1990, *Business Week* wrote of "mighty Mitsubishi" as an "international dynamo" and the keiretsu as "a distinctively Japanese form of capitalism with built-in advantages over independent Western companies" based on the characteristics cited above. Eight years later, when Japan experienced its worst recession in the post–World War II period, the keiretsu was viewed as both an organizational liability and a source of economic crisis. The tight and familiar relationship among keiretsu firms is now deemed problematic: "The web of personal connections in politics is reproduced in corporate practices. In the notorious keiretsu system of cross-shareholdings, related companies hold shares in each other, propping up stock values. Banks belonging to the keiretsu keep lending to weak members" (1998a). A 1998 report on Japan's economic crisis listed the keiretsu as one of Japan's "crumbling pillars":

> They used to provide cheap capital, steady management, reliable partners, and friendly shareholders for big Japanese companies. But the system has dulled Japan Inc.'s competitiveness and created unsustainable levels of debt. ("Japan: Wanted: A New Economy." *Business Week,* November 30, 1998, p. 66.)

The system of cross-shareholding that provided low-cost capital for long-term projects is being abandoned to free up funds. The chairman of Mitsubishi now describes the shareholding arrangements as a "waste of precious capital." Keiretsu members are also trying to break out of agreements with other alliance partners.

One especially dramatic indication of the erosion of the keiretsu-style alliance can be seen in the rise of outsourcing with non-keiretsu companies. In 1998 Mitsubishi announced it was outsourcing its U.S. cellular phone production to a California-based firm with production facilities in Georgia.

The tightening financial pressure on Japanese firms has also prompted a greater openness to external partnerships. A growing number of U.S. firms are forging alliances with Japanese keiretsu. Toshiba and IBM are sharing the cost of a memory chip facility; GM's Delphi parts division supplies components to Toyota; Mitsubishi and Caterpillar are jointly designing excavating equipment (" Keiretsu Connections," *Business Week,* July 22, 1996, p. 52). These are additional examples of both vertical and horizontal alliances.

These newly formed strategic partnerships suggest that the alliance structure remains a viable interorganizational form. The keiretsu is just one version of an alliance configuration, but it may be an insufficiently flexible arrangement because of its long-term obligations and commitments within the keiretsu. The insular keiretsu structure, protected from market pressures, may have also discouraged efforts to contain costs. These are some of the now widely noted unintended negative consequences of the keiretsu system. However, one must be careful not to overgeneralize from the temporary Japanese economy crisis. The keiretsu is likely to reemerge as a global organizational model, albeit in a somewhat modified form.

The Spatial Dimension

Thus far, the discussion of differentiation and integration has been confined to the relationships among firms and production units; that is, what is the best interorganizational structure? Should interdependent production units exchange in markets, combine into a vertically integrated hierarchy, or form a network alliance? Much of the criteria on which to base a decision rests with the relative cost advantages of the various strategies.

Bringing Geography Back

However, cost advantages and disadvantages are due not only to the *structural configuration* of production units but also to the *spatial configuration*. This refers to the geographic location of economic activities that are sequentially or mutually interdependent. Should they be concentrated in close proximity or dispersed to take advantage of geographic variations in costs? A familiar tension reasserts itself at this level as well. How will geographically (rather than structurally or administratively) differentiated units be integrated into a productive, efficient, and cost-effective process?

Historically there has been a desire to concentrate related and associated organizational activities spatially. This would address two major considerations: transportation costs and communication. The movement of physical components of a production process from one location to another will be less expensive if the different activities are in close proximity. Similarly, the integration and coordination of activities will be easier if the organizations are able to interact and communicate on a regular basis.

Each of these factors produces tendencies toward what economic geographers describe as *agglomeration*—the geographic concentration of economic activity. This widely cited phenomenon involves not only the clustering of firms connected by a single production process, but also firms that may provide some service (e.g., financial information) or retailers attempting to gain access to the income stream generated by the primary economic sector. Agglomeration also can include firms interested in sharing knowledge and ideas. The concentration of human population in urban areas is a by-product of this agglomeration process.

At the other end of the spectrum is the geographic *dispersal* of economic activity. Related production activities may take place in different geographic areas because some of the activities depend on an immobile natural resource (e.g., iron ore), attempt to exploit particular political-economic advantages that can affect cost (e.g., labor costs and the business climate), or develop in a remote location for historically accidental reasons (e.g., the firm's owners just happened to live in Maine). Recent trends suggest a greater overall dispersal of economic activity driven primarily by the political-economic advantages but also facilitated by

FIGURE 10–2

Spatial and structural organizational configurations

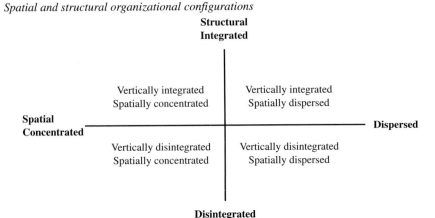

emerging information technologies (Castells 1996). This process has been variously described as disagglomeration, deterritorialization, or globalization.

In cross-classifying the spatial and structural configuration of organizations, four possible interorganizational arrangements emerge (see Figure 10–2). The upper left-hand quadrant combines a vertically integrated structure with geographically concentrated production activity. The upper right-hand quadrant describes firms that retain hierarchical control over production units but disperse the units across geographic space. The lower right-hand quadrant illustrates vertical disintegration combined with geographic dispersion while the lower left-hand quadrant shows vertically disintegrated production that is geographically concentrated. Each of these four structural-spatial combinations will be considered.

Vertically Integrated and Spatially Concentrated

Fordism was characterized as a vertically integrated structure that also sought to geographically concentrate sequentially interdependent activities. One notable example is Ford's River Rouge industrial complex. In 1915 Henry Ford acquired a 2,000-acre site on the Rouge River in Dearborn, Michigan. This site became the most fully integrated automobile manufacturing facility in the world. Every production unit required in the production of a car was located on the site, including a blast furnace, an open hearth mill, a steel rolling plant, a glass plant, a devoted power plant, and the assembly line. It was once described as "the greatest industrial domain in the world."

The fully integrated production system was designed to ensure that all aspects of the manufacturing process would fit together smoothly, including such minute details as screw threads and nut and bolt sizes. The objective was to eliminate the wasted time and excess cost due to incompatible components, defects, and rework. Total control and integration of the upstream and downstream production and distribution requirements were a means to accomplish this objective. Spatial proximity also eliminated transportation costs and ensured direct and immediate communication between the production units.

Prior to the construction of the River Rouge complex, the Detroit region had been established as a major steel producer, supplying steel not just to automakers but also to shipbuilders and stove makers. As a hub of steel production with access to the Great Lakes transportation system, the region generated powerful agglomeration effects.

Vertically Integrated and Geographically Dispersed

Why Disperse Geographically? What kind of logic would encourage a more dispersed or "disagglomerated" configuration of related economic activities? We can begin with a simple example taken from economic geography (Clark 1981). Suppose we have a vertically integrated computer company that is engaged in two primary activities—(1) research and development of new products and software, and (2) the manufacturing and assembly of personal computers. Because the firm owners were educated at the Massachusetts Institute of Technology (MIT), they decide to start their business which they called COMPTECH close to their college stamping grounds in the Boston area. COMPTECH'S central office, research and development operations, and assembly facility are all located in an organizational complex just outside Boston. The economic activities are spatially concentrated. Long-term strategic planning, however, suggests these activities should be geographically dispersed. What is the rationale for this proposal?

First, and most important, the two primary activities of COMPTECH have very different organizational and labor market requirements. Research and development employs highly educated and technically skilled engineering and computer science workers. These employees exist in relatively small numbers given the scarcity of credentials and skills. However, they are most likely to be found, and to live in greater numbers, in regions that have major technical research universities, such as Boston with MIT. The Boston area also possesses the lifestyle amenities that would attract qualified personnel from other locations.

The computer assembly operation, on the other hand, might be located most cost effectively in a different geographical area. There is no shortage of the semiskilled labor required for the assembly operation. The skills are not scarce, nor does the labor force exist in "small numbers." Therefore, it might be more economical to find a location where supply greatly exceeds the demand.

Retaining COMPTECH'S assembly unit in the Boston metropolitan area has a number of additional disadvantages. First, the cost of living is higher in metropolitan areas, which tends to push up wage costs. Second, the high salaries, generous benefits, and job security provided to the research and development employees may influence the demands made by the assembly workers. This *"demonstration effect,"* often reported in regional economies, results in efforts and negotiations by lower-paid workers to obtain the levels of compensation provided to more highly skilled employees. The demonstration effect is strengthened when the different groups of workers exist in geographic proximity to one another. A third potential disadvantage, from the perspective of production costs, is the strength of labor unions and the tradition of labor militancy in Massachusetts.

For each of these reasons, COMPTECH decides to relocate the assembly operation to North Carolina. This geographic location may possess several advantages from the perspective of COMPTECH'S owners. Labor is cheaper, the cost of living is lower, the demonstration effect is eliminated, unions are weak or nonexistent, and there is no legacy of worker militancy. The end result of the geographic shifting of the assembly operation is a *spatial division of labor* (Massey 1984) within a single firm. In this particular case, the geographic distribution of economic activities is based on a calculation of labor-related cost differences in research and development compared with manufacturing activities.

More generally, this example recalls an earlier discussion of the political-economic environment and the spatial variation in social structures of accumulation (Chapter 9). These spatial variations in standards of living, regulations, legal requirements, and social class relations can influence the geographic configuration of the social division of labor within and among organizations.

Globalization.   There is no reason to limit the spatial option to the national level. Even wider variations and cost advantages exist globally. The global distribution of production activities is a further instance of spatial dispersion. While production has always taken place in different parts of the globe, the globalization of today is presumably a qualitatively distinct interorganizational development. Peter Dicken (1992:1) distinguished between *internationalization* and *globalization:*

> [E]conomic activity is becoming not only more internationalized but . . . it is becoming increasingly globalized . . ."Internationalization" refers simply to the increasing geographical spread of economic activities across national boundaries— as such it is not a new phenomena. "Globalization" of economic activity is qualitatively different. It is a more advanced and complex form of internationalization which implies a degree of *functional integration between internationally dispersed economic activities* (emphasis added).

Dicken added that the traditional patterns of exchange between industrialized and less developed nations, such as the exchange of raw materials and agricultural products for manufactured goods, have given way to a "highly complex, kaleidoscopic structure involving the *fragmentation* of many production processes and their *geographical location* on a global scale in ways which slice through national boundaries" (1992:4). Or, as Philip McMichael (1996:90–91) explained, "Instead of countries specializing in an export sector (manufacturing or agriculture), production sites in countries specialize in a constituent part of a production process spread across several countries." The capacity for spatial dispersion is enhanced today because "shifts in technology, transportation, and communication are creating a world where anything can be made anywhere on the face of the earth" (Thurow 1996:9).

All of this suggests a social division of labor that is increasingly spatially differentiated beyond national borders. If we return to the logic of the upper right-hand quadrant of Figure 10–2 and extend geographic horizons across the globe, we can consider some organizational techniques employed by transnational corporations.

The first, *global Fordism,* indicates a vertically integrated ownership structure with facilities and factories distributed in different parts of the globe. The shift from the upper left-hand to the upper right-hand quadrant corresponds to a chronological movement from a vertically integrated firm that is spatially concentrated to one that is spatially dispersed across national boundaries. The vertically integrated configuration, coupled with Fordist production techniques but situated in a location aimed at cost advantages, conforms with the early notions of a *spatial fix* (Harvey 1982). This strategy was used by Fordist-style firms in the 1970s and 1980s to contain costs and reestablish shrinking profit rates by moving facilities and factories to low-wage production sites. This has already been described as a "low road" organizational strategy but one that does *not* entail significant innovations in productivity enhancements or production processes. Instead, this is driven purely by cost considerations and the search for cheap, unregulated, social structures of accumulation.

The global Fordist strategy is visible in the use of wholly owned maquiladora plants located along the U.S.-Mexican border. The maquiladoras are the assembly plants located on the Mexican side of the U.S.-Mexico border that are able to import components and materials duty-free and export final products to the U.S. and Canada under preferential tariff rates. Production is labor-intensive—typically manufacturing and assembly—with cheap labor the primary cost advantage. Other organizational activities, such as research and design, are located elsewhere. The Mexican maquiladora offers transnational firms some additional "advantages" such as lax environmental regulations and weak enforcement of labor and occupational health and safety provisions. Transnational corporations taking the "low road" approach might be attracted to these features.

A second and related technique that falls under the vertically integrated, spatially dispersed, category is *foreign direct investment.* In this case, corporations buy up firms in other countries or they establish a branch or subsidiary operation in that country. In either case, some piece of the vertically integrated hierarchy is geographically dispersed.

Foreign direct investment can conceivably be directed toward any location in the world. Maquiladora facilities are one form of direct investment that benefits from particular advantageous arrangements in tariffs, taxes, and duties. Bilateral agreements between Mexico and the United States, extended with the passage of the North American Free Trade Agreement (NAFTA), have stimulated and are designed to attract further direct investment by transnational corporations.

Another measure stimulating the spatial dispersion of production is the *export processing zone.* These are designated areas or regions, usually within a less developed nation, that are explicitly designed to attract export-oriented direct foreign investment by offering incentives such as the duty-free importation of components, exemptions from legislative regulations, and the provision of physical infrastructure. In China, for example, the Shanghai Jinqiao export processing zone boasts a favorable geographic location, complete infrastructure, consultation services, and tax incentives. Again, the most common activity in these zones is labor-intensive assembly and manufacturing. The finished products are usually destined for export markets in the developed industrial nations.

As production has become increasingly globalized, and vertically integrated firms have become spatially dispersed, new concepts have emerged to describe these organizational arrangements. One of the most useful and widely employed concepts is the global commodity chain (Gereffi 1995). *Global commodity chains* (GCCs) are transnational production systems that link firms and networks around the economic processes of developing, manufacturing, and marketing specific commodities (Gereffi 1995:113).

The four main dimensions of GCCs are:

1. A value-added chain of products, services, and resources linked together across a range of relevant industries.

2. A geographic dispersion of production and marketing networks at the national, regional, and global levels, comprised of enterprises of different sizes and types.

3. A governance structure of authority and power relationships between firms that determine how financial, material, and human resources are allocated and flow within a chain.

4. An institutional framework that identifies how local, national, and international conditions and policies shape the globalization process at each stage in the chain (Gereffi 1995:113).

Global-level commodity chains are by definition spatially dispersed. Item 3, however, pertains to variations in the structural characteristics. The vertically integrated unit is one type of governance structure that controls and directs the geographically far-flung units of production. This pattern of coordination conforms most closely with *producer-driven commodity chains* which are large transnational industrial enterprises that coordinate and control a production system through the administrative headquarters of the enterprise (Gereffi 1995:115). Producer-driven commodity chains can include a vertically (ownership) integrated structure or a partially or fully disintegrated structure with a lead manufacturer, such as an automotive or aircraft firm, directing the production of international subcontractors or entering into strategic alliances with other firms.

Vertically Disintegrated and Spatially Dispersed

As commodity chains have become increasingly disintegrated, we can shift our attention to the lower right-hand quadrant of Figure 10–2. There, a vertically disintegrated structure combines with spatially dispersed links in the production chain. The disintegrated-dispersed arrangement takes a wide variety of forms. These can include producer-driven commodity chains that rely more on subcontractors than subsidiaries, cross-national strategic alliances, and the wide variety of flexible networks joining vertically and horizontally related firms.

The other major form of commodity chain—*the buyer-driven commodity chain*—can also be included here. Buyer-driven commodity chains are led by large retailers and brand-name merchandisers who arrange for production among an array of decentralized producers, usually in less developed nations, who produce or assemble a final product that meets the specification of the retailer or merchandiser (Gereffi 1995:116).

The major players in buyer-driven commodity chains are the familiar athletic footwear companies such as Nike and Reebok, apparel companies like The Gap and Liz Claiborne, and retailers like Wal-Mart Stores that purchase large quantities of the bonded merchandise.

What is distinctive about the buyer-driven commodity chain is that the central companies do not own or control any production facilities. They devote their energy toward product design, marketing, and integrating the firms into the chain. The actual production of sneakers, a garment, or a toy is carried out in independent factories overseas. These buyer-driven companies that only design and market the products are often referred to as "hollow corporations" because they do not engage in the core manufacturing process that creates the product with which they are most closely associated.

These firms are akin to the "commercial" or "merchant" capitalists who buy cheap and sell dear. They are totally detached from the conditions or methods of production. As long as they can obtain what they need at a low price, they remain largely indifferent to working conditions or manufacturing processes employed to produce the goods. The "industrial capitalists" in this system are the local entrepreneurs in less developed nations who own the factories, organize the production process, and produce the final product.

This represents a significant change in the nature of global capitalism. More importantly, the most powerful and profitable links in the production chain are not the industrial units that manufacture the product, but the commercial units that design, brand, and market the goods. In buyer-driven commodity chains this is where the greatest value is added and profits are realized. The manufacturing link of the chain, on the other hand, is highly labor intensive and highly competitive. These factors make it a likely candidate for global outsourcing and place enormous downward pressure on costs, which are primarily labor.

The net result of this global arrangement is the well-documented "slave wage" rates and substandard working conditions in many global factories producing sneakers, toys, and clothing. It also raises the issue of who is ultimately responsible for these conditions: the buyers (merchant/commercial capitalists) who do not own or control the factories but order and purchase the goods? the domestic capitalists in less developed nations who own and manage the firms? or the governments in these countries who fail to institute and enforce labor and employment standards?

In the United States and elsewhere, labor and consumer campaigns and boycotts of major buyer-driven firms place pressure on the network of independent subcontractors to improve labor conditions (Gereffi and Hamilton 1996). A number of organizations, such as the Fair Labor Association, have formed to monitor wages and working conditions in these global factories ("Sweatshop Reform: How to Solve the Standoff," *Business Week,* May 3, 1999, p. 186–90).

Vertically Disintegrated and Spatially Concentrated

The final quadrant in the two-dimensional analysis from Figure 10-2 combines disintegrated companies or independent specialized firms with spatial concentration. This arrangement can be the product of vertical disintegration along with the desire or necessity to stay geographically close to former suppliers and distributors. It can result from a very unique set of agglomeration forces that cannot be replicated or easily relocated. It can also be due to a decision by vertically disintegrated and spatially dispersed organization to return to a more geographic concentrated environment. Each of these will be considered in turn.

Structurally Embedded Concentration.   A vertically integrated firm may decide to eliminate and shed various units (disintegrate) but keep transactions with other firms in a concentrated geographic area. A firm may have long-standing ties with a particular region or community. The firm may also have long-standing ties with particular suppliers and distributors in the region who are highly trusted, reliable, and not easily replaced. In this scenario, business decisions about the spatial location of facilities are "structurally embedded" (Romo and Schwartz 1995). Instead of basing interfirm relationships purely on comparative costs associated with different geographic locations, such "relationships congeal into long-term dependencies that constrain the migration behavior" (Romo and Schwartz 1995:880).

Again, one can see how the concept of embeddedness is used to offer an alternative to a strict market or cost-based decision-making calculus. While these actions may seem economically irrational, they are designed more for the purpose of reducing uncertainty than reducing cost. Suppliers and distributors that are "known quantities" and have established a record of reliability are often preferable to lower-cost but unknown quantities.

There is also the issue of establishing just-in-time (JIT) inventory and delivery systems that benefit from close proximity to suppliers and distribution networks. The just-in-time system has already been discussed as it pertains to the internal organization of production, but equally, if not more, critical is its relationship to suppliers who are expected to deliver parts and components as needed or "just in time."

The objective of the just-in-time system is to ensure that all materials, resources, and other elements required for production will be available at the necessary place and time for immediate deployment. This system eliminates the cost and management of inventory stockpiles. It also places pressure on the production process and personnel to eliminate errors and waste. The reason this system might encourage some spatial coordination is that it requires close coordination between suppliers and customers. In addition, with deliveries of supplies occurring—often several times daily—transportation time and cost become major considerations. One might wonder whether these challenges could be handled by returning to the old-fashioned vertically integrated and spatially concentrated industrial complex. However, it is widely assumed that a disintegrated JIT arrangement provides many of the same benefits without the costs and financial obligations associated with formally managing the integrated units.

The various arguments for and against disintegration and dispersion point to the fundamental and ongoing tension between differentiation and integration. Differentiated and specialized production activities must be integrated and coordinated to constitute a single articulated production process. Tight vertical integration enhances coordination but is costly and prohibits flexibility. Disintegration enhances flexibility but sacrifices tight coordination. Now the just-in-time production system seems to require high levels of coordination. But firms have not returned to the old vertically integrated solution. Rather, embedded networks are formed as a way to transact, exchange, and coordinate independent firms. Some of the activities might be conducted most cost effectively in particularly advantageous geographic locations that spatially disperse the network. However, the network may employ just-in-time supply and distribution systems that would benefit from geographic concentration. These various pros and cons make it difficult to settle on a final interorganizational arrangement. There are tendencies and countertendencies that encourage a wide range of possible configurations.

Agglomeration and Milieus of Innovation.   The territorialization of economic activity and the geographic clustering of organizations may also result from powerful agglomeration forces. These forces can extend beyond the obvious functional and resource dependencies that might characterize, for example, the gravitation of auto parts producers to the Detroit region. They can include the less formal or tangible exchanges that are common in fields of rapid innovation and take place between people and firms facing similar problems and challenges. One example are the *milieus of innovation* common in the information technology sector. Silicon Valley in California is the prime case. Castells (1995:56) described the key elements:

> [T]he development of the information technology revolution contributed to the formation of the milieus of innovation where discoveries and application would interact, and be tested, in a recurrent process of trial and error, of learning by doing; these milieus required . . . spatial concentration of research centers, higher education institutions, advanced technology companies, a network of ancillary suppliers of goods and services, and business networks of venture capital to finance start-ups. Once a milieu is consolidated, as Silicon Valley was in the 1970s, it tends to generate its own dynamics and to attract knowledge, investment, and talent from around the world.

It is important to point out that the spatial clustering in this milieu of innovation consists of independent firms, start-ups, entrepreneurs, venture capitalists, and spin-offs. Rather than involving firms that are sequentially integrated in a production chain, the milieu of innovation first involved firms that were interested in advancing a basic technology—the semiconductor—and then developing myriad applications of this technology. The milieu facilitates processes of learning, exchanging tacit knowledge, diversification of applications, and informal information flows. Firms and individuals seek to expose and embed themselves in this organizational and cultural environment. This is one example of a positive externality, or external economy, that attracts firms, provides cost-free benefits, and reinforces spatial concentration and agglomeration.

Those who have closely studied interorganizational relations in Silicon Valley believe that sustained economic viability and innovation of the region has been based on the gradual shift toward greater collaborative networks both regionally and globally (Gordon and Kimball 1998; Castells 1998).

> The most striking development since the [mid-to-late] 1980s has been the absolute *centrality of collaborative partnerships* in the innovation process. Strategic alliances have become nearly ubiquitous as a region legendary for its embodiment of Schumpeterian individualistic entrepreneurialism has shifted, in the space of a decade, to more collective forms of innovation organization. Entrepreneurialism has shifted its focus from one organizational principle—self sufficiency, aggressive competition, and proprietary technologies—to a radically different principle: participation in collaborative production chains, interfirm cooperative networks, and open standards (Gordon and Kimball 1998:14).

This description of the dynamics of Silicon Valley indicates that a dense geographic concentration of organizations can exist under both a highly competitive or highly cooperative interorganizational relationship. The shift from the former to the latter is consistent with the more general trends outlined for interorganizational dynamics.

The two primary activities in the milieu of innovation are product conception and research and development. A dispersed spatial division of labor may still apply because the actual production of semiconductors, wafers, and technical devices can be located elsewhere. In the case of Silicon Valley, production takes place both locally and offshore, and the division of labor between assembly and production versus research and development manifests itself in sharp differences in working conditions, wages, and salaries (Fuentes and Ehrenreich 1983).

Concentrating Manufacturing and Research.   We can now consider some of the arguments for a greater spatial concentration of these different activities. One rationale for geographic concentration hinges on the distinction between product and process technology (Thurow 1992) and the necessity to tighten the link between the innovative and production activities. *Product technology* refers to the activities of research and development, product design, and application. *Process technology* refers to the development and application of technologies used in the production process. Activity in the milieu of innovation is devoted primarily to product technology; process technology is relegated to the assembly and manufacturing units.

According to Richard Florida and Martin Kenney (1990) organizations should pursue a strategy of *structural flexibility* that involves a more tightly linked and integrated relationship, both structurally and geographically, between development and manufacturing. This allows for a more rapid flow of information and interaction between product design and process technology. Rather than confining innovation and research and development exclusively to product design, they also should be applied to production processes. Synergies between innovation and production are more likely to occur when the activities are in closer physical proximity. Together, they should contribute to higher levels of efficiency, productivity, and quality. Presumably, this will also facilitate the ability to retool production facilities more rapidly based on changes in product markets and customer needs.

David Angel (1989) provided similar arguments in his analysis of the semiconductor industry. According to Angel, the necessary conditions for maintaining competitive advantage rest on the notion of *continuous innovation*. This has been difficult to achieve because research, development, and design tend to be driven by different pressures than production and assembly. The latter are driven by cost considerations while the former are driven by technological innovation and creative synergy. This has resulted in a segmented and spatially divided production system with "innovation and product development in high-tech complexes, routinized high-volume fabrication facilities dispersed in low-wage sites outside metropolitan areas, and labor-intensive assembly in low-wage locations offshore" (Angel 1989:12). A problem of "manufacturability"—design proceeds without sufficient input from production engineers—has been created by this tripartite spatial and international division of labor. This makes it difficult to codevelop new products and new production techniques. Reconnecting the functionally integrated units would also encourage greater contacts and interaction with major end users and customers.

This organizational logic suggests that high-technology industry would be engaged in a reintegration and desegregation of production and research facilities, giving rise to a greater concentration of organizational units in a single geographic location or region. This contradicts the general trend toward the spatial dispersion of organizational units and functions. However, these potentially new forms of functional integration do not necessarily require ownership integration as much as coordination integration (Langlois and Robertson 1995) through vertically disintegrated alliances and networks. This is more consistent with recent interorganizational developments.

Recent Developments: Supply Chains and Real Options

The analysis of the structural and spatial dimensions of the social division of labor has uncovered a variety of trends and logics. Over the past 10 years, there seems to be a concentrated effort by most firms to structurally disintegrate. This results in outsourcing and a greater number of interfirm transactions that must be managed. A return to a more differentiated and disintegrated social division of labor places even greater pressure on the functional integration and coordination of interdependent activities. "Getting lean" has meant relying on other organizations to carry out functions formerly controlled by the firm. While management consultants advocate the shedding of peripheral activities, it is not without its downside. Some predictable problems with outsourcing have been reported. "An errant supplier can delay a key product launch and anger customers . . . Some companies have found themselves locked into long-term contracts with outside suppliers that are no longer competitive" ("Has Outsourcing Gone Too Far?", *Business Week,* April 1, 1996, p. 28).

While each of these difficulties are the precise reason for the erection of vertically integrated hierarchies, there is little evidence that firms are reversing the disintegration process. Instead, the emphasis is on managing these interfirm relations. This has spawned a new industry: *supply chain planning and management* (Fisher 1997; Poirier 1999; Ross 1997). The supply chain is

> a network of facilities that procure raw materials, transform them into intermediate goods and then final products, and deliver the products to customers through a distribution system (Lee and Billington 1995:43).

In managing and planning this chain, organizations seek to realize the seemingly timeless goal of getting resources in the right quantities, at the right place, at the right time, and at the lowest cost. This is, again, an organizational challenge that stems directly from the tension between differentiation and integration.

In relating organization theory to management practice, the emphasis here has been on the contradictions, tensions, and trade-offs inherent in any decision about organizational strategy. Much of the current theory and practice has rested on the assumption that flexibility in an uncertain world requires an organization that is lean and devoted to its core competencies. This process of vertical disintegration is a direct reflection of this principle.

However, if there are perpetual tensions and trade-offs, this strategy cannot be unequivocally successful. As is common in organization and management studies, an increasingly popular theory now argues for a diametrically opposed strategy. This is called *real options theory* (Amran and Kulatilaka 1998).

Real options is an approach to corporate finance that has significant implications for the structure of the organization. Rather than shedding all units, or avoiding heavy investments in the sunk costs of long-term projects, this perspective argues for a systematic assessment of these options. An uncertain environment offers opportunity as well as peril. When things change rapidly, it is best to have some options available to exploit the uncertainty. These options can come in the form of investment projects in certain activities that might, at time one, appear to have greater costs than benefits. At time two, however, under a different set of conditions—which are constantly changing anyway—the options can provide an opportunity to provide enormous benefits.

The following example was reported in *Business Week:*

This June, Envon Corp. will open three gas-fired power plants in northern Mississippi and western Tennessee that are inefficient—deliberately so. They will generate electricity at an incremented cost 50 percent to 70 percent higher than the industry's best. Most of the time, the production costs of these spanking new plants will be too high to compete.

Envon hasn't gone crazy. By building less efficient plants, it saved a bundle on construction. It can let the plants sit idle, then fire them up when prices rise. Last June 25, the price of a megawatt-hour of electricity in parts of the Midwest soared—briefly—from $40 to an unprecedented $7,000. With such volatility, Envon executives figured they can make money from their so-called peaking plants even if they operate only a week or so per year ("Exploiting Uncertainty," *Business Week,* June 7, 1999, p. 118).

Real options represents a "just-in-case" rather than "just-in-time" logic; that is, because of the possibility that a highly profitable opportunity will emerge, it is important to have the resources on hand just in case. This approach introduces a high-risk, speculative edge to corporate decision making. This option is unlikely to be adopted by a wide number of firms because it requires a resource base and level of security that most firms do not possess. It is an interesting development and example of the contradictory theories and strategies that can emerge from the same empirical reality.

Summary

1. The social division of labor and economic specialization between production units poses the fundamental organizational problem of how to control and gain access to required resources. The traditional choice has been between *market* transaction or vertically integrated *hierarchy.* More recently, a third intermediate option has gained in theoretical prominence and strategic importance. This is the *network* or *alliance* among interdependent organizations.

2. One of the prime examples of the network model is the Japanese *keiretsu.* This intercorporate configuration includes a large number of independent but affiliated firms that exchange resources and share stock ownership. Once touted as singularly responsible for Japanese economic dynamism, the keiretsu are now regarded as problematic with the crisis in the Japanese economy. The organizational arrangement, once a model for the rest of the world, is now in the process of radical restructuring.

3. In addition to the *structural configuration* of interdependent production units, there is the equally important *spatial configuration*. This refers to the geographic distribution and location of production activities. As firms shift production to new locations or enter into transactions with firms across the globe, geographic differentiation and dispersal increase. This prompts the development of means to functionally integrate the geographically dispersed but interdependent activities.

4. The cross-classification of the structural configuration (vertically integrated or disintegrated) and spatial configuration (concentrated or dispersed) yields four interorganizational arrangements. While there has been a clear shift toward the vertically disintegrated and spatially dispersed option (or quadrant), some countertendencies suggest the existence of an emerging logic of structural disintegration alongside relative spatial concentration in certain economic sectors.

THE FUTURE OF ORGANIZATION AND POSTMODERN ANALYSIS

11

The problem with our times is the future is not what it used to be.

Paul Valéry, *French poet (1871–1945)*

It is customary to devote the final chapter to a review of the main points in the text. I shall depart from this custom. Instead of repeating all the main points and arguments repeated at the end of each chapter, I shall close with a topic that points us toward the future, not the past. This involves the issue of the postmodern approach to organizational studies, a topic that allows us to evaluate and assess the relationship between the intraorganizational and interorganizational levels used to organize the material in this text as well as the future relevance of the central organizational tensions that have been emphasized. In this way, the key themes in the book can be reviewed in the context of an emerging mode of analysis.

Modernist and Postmodernist Approaches

A developing point of comparison in organization studies revolves around the distinction between modernist and postmodernist organization theory (Hatch 1997; Clegg 1990; Berquist 1993). However, the vast majority of existing organizational and management literature is, by definition, modernist. This denotes a particular grand or metaconceptualization of organization that is also, for the most part, transmetaphorical; that is, the modernist approach is based on a set of global assumptions about what constitutes an organization. These characterize most organizational theories and metaphors. What are some of the key elements of this modernist approach?

280

First, the modernist model conceptualizes organizations as bounded definable entities. It is assumed that organizational boundaries distinguish the internal processes from environmental or external processes. Organizations are viewed as mechanical systems. They combine factors of production—or inputs—within the boundaries of the organization and produce a product or service—or output—that is sent into the environment. In short, the organization has an "inside" and an "outside."

A parallel image is the organization as the proverbial "black box." It secures inputs, engages in some processes, and produces outputs. The distinction between the internal organization and the external environment in modernist organization studies informs our division of theoretical literature into intraorganizational and interorganizational levels.

A second and closely related assumption concerns the notion of differentiation. Modernist approaches assume that positions, tasks, and departments can be differentiated into meaningful and clearly distinct categories that correspond to real activities. The discussion of differentiation throughout this text is founded on this assumption.

Third, modernists are heavily influenced by "modes of rationality" (Clegg 1990). This mode of theorizing assumes that organizations are instruments designed to accomplish definable goals and that formal structures are the means to ensure goal-directed behavior. Accordingly, organizational behavior can be explained using the rational discourse that links formal means with intended ends. A corollary assumption is that organizational members act on the basis of a definable self-interest, or bounded identity, as a worker, manager, or owner. In the modernist approach, differentiation, roles, and interests explain purposive action.

How does postmodernism challenge these modernist tenets? Before a clear answer can be provided to this question, a distinction between two postmodernist positions must be made. Martin Parker (1992) identified two strands in postmodern writing on organization (and society generally) that he referred to as postmodern epistemology and post-modern periodization (the hyphenation is used to distinguish the two positions).

Postmodern epistemology addresses the question of how we know what is real or how we come to understand the world around us? This strand of postmodernism rejects the entire modernist method for understanding organization. It questions the modernist assumption that there are perceivable, observable, and definable structures that can be described, classified, or modeled. It also rejects the notion that human subjects act on the basis of any rationally defined interest or unitary identity. Thus, according to postmodern epistemology, organizations are subjective constructions based on images, language, and rhetoric. The essence and meaning of organization is constantly shifting, depending on the perspective of the observer. In this view, any claim to descriptive validity about the shape or purpose of organizations is simply an attempt to "privilege" one particular perspective over another—a form of epistemological imperialism.

Post-modern periodization, on the other hand, would evaluate the modernist conception of organization using a modernist epistemology that assumes organizations represent an observable empirical reality. Rather than reject modernism on epistemological grounds, the post-modern approach would challenge modernist claims about organizational structure because they are no longer applicable to, nor do they accurately describe, contemporary and emerging organizational forms. Post-modern periodization employs the epistemology of modernism as a means to evaluate and critique modernist assumptions about organizational structure.

This approach assumes an empirical organizational reality that can be observed and described. However, the reality has changed dramatically so one must reconceptualize organizations. The post-modern periodization strand will be the most useful for the purposes of this chapter. It will allow us to make statements based on empirical observations about the changing organizational world.

Post-Modern Condition and Identity

The post-modern literature tends to be big on description and small on explanation. There is no shortage of descriptive narratives outlining postmodern features of contemporary life. However, it is difficult to find comprehensible explanations identifying the sources of this new social world. As a way to better understand some of the central aspects of post-modern society, two useful concepts—time-space compression (Harvey 1989) and the saturated self (Gergen 1991)—will be considered.

David Harvey (1989) attempted to explain the post-modern condition (or sensibility) in the context of the larger political-economic process of *time-space compression.* The underlying premise of his thesis is that our conceptualization of time and space varies historically, depending on the way people organize productive activity (see also Berman 1982; Bell 1973). For example, the rise of the factory system reshaped our conception of time to revolve around the beginning and end of a workday measured by clock time. This differed from more traditional conceptions of time driven by the rhythms of nature. At the present time, time and space compression, a continuing process under capitalism, has entered an accelerated phase. Harvey defined it variously as follows:

> It has also entailed a new round of . . . "time-space compression" in the capitalist world—the time horizons of both private and public decision-making have shrunk, while satellite communication and declining transport costs have made it increasingly possible to spread those decisions immediately over an ever wider and variegated space (1989:147).

I use the word "compression" because a strong case can be made that the history of capitalism has been characterized by a speed-up in the pace of life, while so overcoming spatial barriers that the world sometimes seems to collapse inwards upon us . . . As space appears to shrink to a "global village" of telecommunications and a "spaceship earth" of economic and ecological interdependencies—to use two familiar and everyday images—and as time horizons shorten to the point where the present is all there is (the world of the schizophrenic), so we have to learn to cope with an overwhelming sense of compression of our spatial and temporal worlds (1989:240).

Some further explication is in order. It is important to understand the relationship between the system of capitalism and time-space compression because many organizational consequences stem from this connection. As this relationship pertains to the *time dimension,* capitalist organizations are driven to reduce the amount of time between capital investment in production and the realization of profit through the sale of commodities. The reduction of this "turnover time" is a principle objective of capitalist organizations. This is manifested in the increasingly rapid deployment of capital to capture market opportunities and the equally rapid retooling of production for new product models and markets.

The *spatial element* refers to the desire of capital to break down geographic obstacles to investment opportunities and markets. The profitability of capitalist organizations is based on the ability to access remote locations for the production and sale of goods. The post-modern period is said to be characterized by an acceleration of both time and space compression. This is fueled by the development of telecommunication and information technologies (Castells 1996) and heightened levels of competition. These are the macrolevel forces that shape emerging approaches to organizational structure and analysis.

At the microlevel, Kenneth Gergen (1991) argued that we are also seeing a qualitatively new self, or identity, that he labeled the *saturated self.* The postmodern era exposes humans to a greater variety of experiences, a broader range of roles and social relationships, and a wider assortment of different cultures and perspectives. As a result, according to Gergen, an authentic, independent, and bounded self-identity is eroded and replaced by a fragmented and saturated self.

More than ever before, thoughts and actions are informed by multiple perspectives and values. It is increasingly difficult to establish a single best way to approach any question or problem. The saturated self can be seen as the microincarnation of the macrolevel processes of time and space compression. It, too, is fueled by the technologies that connect us to others and contribute to information overload. Time compression tends to create a blurring of role boundaries and multiple role performance within a narrower time frame. Communications technologies (e.g., e-mail and cell phones) make it increasingly difficult to spatially segregate or develop boundaries around our roles and identities. Physical distance, historically one of the most potent segregators, can no longer provide an adequate excuse for the segmentation of role responsibilities.

Together, the observations of Harvey and Gergen can provide a basis for generalizing the post-modern conditions to organizational dynamics. We can now turn to some of the organizational implications.

Organizational Implications of Post-Modernism

The following list of organizational features, many discussed in earlier chapters, are representative of a shift from the modernist to post-modernist organization. (For more extensive detail on them, see Castells 1996; Harvey 1989; Berquist 1993; Hirschhorn 1997; Clegg 1990.)

1. *The rapid shifting of financial and productive resources across borders and from one location to another.* This is part of the larger phenomenon of the flexible deployment of resources and spatial dispersion. It signals the transient, temporary, footloose nature of economic production and organizational presence.

2. *The philosophy and practice of just-in-time resource utilization.* This is designed to reduce turnover time in the quest for rapid returns on investment. Resources are purchased only when needed, which ensures that what is invested at the point of production will contribute to the realization of profit at the point of consumption.

3. *The different working arrangements associated with flexibility.* Flextime, temp service, outsourcing, subcontracting, and telecommuting reflect dramatic shifts in how people conceptualize work time and the workplace. It contributes to the demise of a fixed identity anchored in a single organization or lifelong career. There is no longer a sharp differentiation between work, home, and leisure. As a consequence, these segregated identities began to erode.

4. *The virtual organization as placeless, timeless, and seemingly boundaryless.* Each of these aspects defies the modernist conception of an organizational entity that has some permanent shape and presence. A virtual organization cannot be sensed empirically in the conventional fashion. It is not a physical thing located in a fixed place. It is increasingly difficult to say when someone enters and leaves an organization.

5. *The pastiche of organizations, firms, consultants, and subcontractors that form organizational networks and alliances.*

This further blurs the boundaries and makes it increasingly difficult to distinguish where one organization "ends" and another "begins" or the "inside" from the "outside" of the organization. As different organizations meld into one another, unitary goals or objectives are also diluted with secondary, alternative, competing, and subsidiary objectives.

6. *Projects rather than careers.* Work processes organized around projects produce a continuous shifting of roles and relationships within the organization. This defies the modernist notion of a patterned social structure. Instead, the organization is designed to continually create and re-create temporary and emergent "social structures." Thus, the differentiation and specialization of organizational positions gives way to "dedifferentiation." This poses a major challenge to the long-standing tension between the differentiation of parts and their integration into an organizational whole. The emerging practice of multitasking, multiskilling, multiple careers, and multiple projects consistent with a saturated self may require an entirely different kind of integration strategy.

7. *The demise of the personal office.* The office on wheels, and "hot-desking" are emerging practices that obliterate modernist conceptions of time and space in the organization.

8. *The practices of managing uncertainty (rather than eliminating it), and developing enlarged rationalities.* This reflects an acknowledgment of chaos rather than order, and multiple rather than unitary objectives of organization. Clearly defined goals, the hallmark of the rational model, are replaced by multiple and paradoxical goals and demands.

9. *If there is a saturated self, there is also a saturated organization.* The bounded function and identity of organizations are also eroding. For example, what was once a "telephone company" is now a "communications service company" involved in managing information networks, providing technology, consulting on organizational designs, and, increasingly less significant, providing telephone service. According to Larry Hirschhorn (1997:2), "The leaders and members of an enterprise can no longer depend on an enduring definition of their business based on a specific product or encounter. As an enterprise takes on broader business objectives, it increasingly *negotiates* the meaning of its business with its customers, competitors, and partners."

10. *Individual roles and identities become less solid and more transient.* As organizational members shift across positions, tasks, and

projects, formal structures and job descriptions become increasingly less relevant. As a consequence, authority is less impersonal.

"If individuals are to bring their strivings and passions to their work (as their bosses desperately want), they must now rely more on internalized images of themselves—on an emotional appreciation of who they are, who they wish to become, and what they can contribute specifically to an enterprise. *They have to rely in greater measure on their personal authority*" (Hirschhorn 1997:9).

11. *The multitude of competing perspectives, experiences, roles, and identities.* These serve to generate a postmodern epistemological stance in the human factor of production. As the self becomes more saturated, it is increasingly difficult to adjudicate between competing claims of knowledge and authority. Rather than one best way, there are multiple plausible alternatives; rather than a single source of authority, there are competing sources. This text has emphasized the difficulty in attempting to control and manage the human factor. This may be accentuated in the context of a postmodern sensibility that entails shifting, rather than fixed, sources of knowledge and authority.

BLUR: Post-Modernism Popularized

Analysis of the post-modern organization is not confined to the groves of organizational theory. It has also penetrated the popular management and business press. One particularly powerful presentation is Stan Davis and Christopher Meyer's *BLUR: The Speed of Change in the Connected Economy* (1998). The term *blur* describes the post-modern sensibility of transience and impermanence. Nothing is fixed or permanent; everything is moving and shifting. Blur includes the time and space dimensions. Davis and Meyer also described the changing nature of organizational outputs ("offers"). More specifically, the idea is captured in the following equation (1998:5):

BLUR =	Speed × Connectivity × Intangibles
Speed:	Every aspect of business and the connected organization operates and changes in real time.
Connectivity:	Everything is becoming electronically connected to everything else: products, people, companies, countries, everything.
Intangibles:	Every offer has both tangible and intangible economic value. The intangible is growing faster.
BLUR:	The new world in which you will come to live and work.

"Speed" captures the time, and connectivity the space dimensions of post-modern compression. "Intangibles" describe the changing essence of organizational outputs or offers.

Dedifferentiation is a central dynamic of blur. There is a dedifferentiation between product and service. At one time a product was a tangible object purchased by a customer. Service either came with the product or it was a separate and distinct activity. Today the two are combined, or "bundled," into hybrid forms variously described as "productized services" or "servicized products." The book you are reading is an example of this kind of offering. Not only is there the physical object of the book, but also the ongoing service provided through the website. This creates a continuous relationship between the buyer (reader) and the seller (author and publisher).

Otis elevators, for example, are equipped with communication devices designed to automatically trigger service calls (Davis and Meyer 1998: 24–25). Similarly, automobile antitheft devices transmit signals to a central service switchboard indicating the location of the automobile.

Dell computers epitomize the hybridization of two strategies that were formerly viewed as incompatible: "mass customization" (see Pine and Pine 1992). A mass market is reached over the Internet while customers are able to mix and match whatever features they desire. This combines the cost advantages of scale economy in a mass market with the ability to meet the distinct individual needs of customers. Such paradoxical demands, hybridizations, and dedifferentiations are presumably a defining feature of postmodern organization.

There is also a dedifferentiation between the buyer and the seller, or the organization that provides the offering and the customers in the environment who purchase the goods. The clearly defined boundaries and roles of the two parties are eroding. An exchange or transaction, a fundamental concept of organizational theory, has customarily been based on a sharp role distinction between buyer and seller. In the post-modern context, every seller is a buyer and every buyer is a seller.

Davis and Meyer wrote that the buyer-seller relationship involves the exchange of economic, informational, and emotional value. While the economic exchange is the most familiar—money for goods—even this has become blurred as "sellers" pay "buyers" for their business using rebates, prizes, and frequent flyer miles (Davis and Meyer 1998: 52–55).

Informationally, the unilateral flow of product information from seller to buyer has given way to bilateral exchanges. Buyers provide information to sellers on their lifestyle, product preferences, and consumption patterns which in turn drive product development and marketing strategies. Sellers provide information to buyers on related products and other buying opportunities. The online bookseller, Amazon.com, uses information on buyers' book preferences to suggest additional titles under the heading: "Customers who bought this book also bought . . . " Buyers can also post book reviews as a service to other customers.

Emotionally, sellers spend as much time selling an image or feeling as they do a product. Likewise, buyers return these efforts with loyalty and attachment to a brand name. Together, the mutual exchange of economic, informational, and emotional value signals a departure from the modernist notion of the differentiated roles of buyer and seller.

In many ways, blur is simply a metaphor for the dedifferentiation, boundaryless, accelerated time, and compressed space elements that make up the post-modern organization. Davis and Meyer argued that organizational success requires that one embrace and incorporate the chaos and turbulence that characterize rapid economic change. The final chapter of their book is a prescriptive inventory titled "50 Ways to Blur Your Business and 10 Ways to Blur Yourself." Rather than devise methods to buffer and segregate the organization from the uncertainty of the market environment, the message is to transform the organization so that it resembles the market environment.

> The organization web must run by the principles of the economic web . . . Your organization cannot be a set of little factions in a planned economy. It must be run by the rules of the economic web, managed by the market, displaying increasing returns, and forming evanescent alliances. Since you can't define the boundaries of your connected organization from the outside, you shouldn't define them from the inside either. That's why the distinction between "intranet" and "extranet" is a step backward. It's like putting a blockage in every capillary, it's unconnected and therefore unhealthy (Davis and Meyer 1998:118–19).

If Davis and Meyer have indeed seen the future, the long-standing distinction between the intraorganizational and interorganizational levels may soon be extinct.

Fragmented Humans and Dedifferentiated Structures

This chapter concludes with a consideration of the postmodern implications for the central organizational tensions outlined in Chapter 2 and elaborated throughout the text.

Organizations will continue to be peopled by and depend upon human laborers who exert physical and mental energy. The question for the postmodern era is no different than the question for prior eras: How will organizations be able to extract this energy from human subjects who are able to reflect consciously on their roles and activities and who have the capacity to resist? Does this perpetual organizational challenge take on a new character under the postmodern condition?

According to postmodern commentators the human factor—the self—has undergone a transformation in the direction of fragmentation and saturation. Humans are not less conscious under this new regime but more conscious and reflective about their self, their identity, and their increasingly blurred roles. If the organization employs a "whole person," as argued in Chapter 2, it is more than the formal working role and the informal nonworking role. Rather, it is a human who might be developing multiple identities and roles at work, employing multiple sensemaking perspectives, and occupying positions of authority and subordination simultaneously.

The multifaceted self will also be less predictable. From the perspective of management, it will become increasingly difficult to develop strategies of social control based on the assumed needs and interests of employees. With multiple roles and identities come multiple standards for evaluating the quality of the employment relationship and, in turn, the bases for deciding under what conditions employees will willingly exert their physical and mental energies. Under such conditions, no single strategy of control can hope to mobilize all employees or galvanize compliance over an extended period of time.

Organizing opposition to management will be increasingly difficult for similar reasons. The distinct categories of worker and management become blurred with each other and with other roles and identities. Multiple attachments and interests conspire against a clean and unambiguous bifurcated model of labor versus management. Standardized organizational analyses based on occupational positions, class interests, and political conflicts will become progressively problematic and inadequate.

While all of this suggests a highly unpredictable organizational landscape, the fundamental dynamic is still operative; that is, models of organization and management strategies will continue to be based on certain assumptions about the human factor. These will continue to produce unintended consequences and unanticipated reactions based on the inadequacies of the assumptions. If it is true that the human factor is becoming less rather than more predictable—because of the saturated and fragmented self—the consequences will also be less predictable. Contemporary management literature attempts to incorporate this dynamic in the terminology of its titles—chaos, paradox, blur, disorganization.

Organization theorists are also subjecting the long-standing relationship between differentiation and integration to a radical reassessment. Let's return to the distinction between the technical and social division of labor. At the intraorganizational level, technical divisions of labor, supported by bureaucratic formalization of the labor process, were traditionally assumed to be the best means to greater efficiency and effective control of labor. Under postmodern organizational forms, technical differentiation gives way to deformalization, multiskilling, and multitasking. While these changes are often interpreted as more advanced methods of work intensification and labor extraction, they pose new challenges for social integration. Attachment to the objectives of the organization are engendered less through formal compliance than normative attachment. The rise of strong corporate cultures, and the culture paradigm, reflect this trend.

The social division of labor at the interorganizational level, depicting distinct production units and activities, is also breaking down. While structural differentiation (Smelser 1963) was viewed as the leading indicator of socioeconomic development and modernization, this is now giving way to the dedifferentiation and blurring of functions and responsibilities. There is much greater interaction among the formerly distinct units within an organization (e.g., research and development, manufacturing, sales and marketing) through "rugby" and project style organizational models. There is also the rise of alliances, partnerships, and networks among firms that are not only legally independent but market competitors. As a consequence, vertical forms of integration based on command and control are being replaced by horizontal forms of integration based on collaboration and cooperation. It is important to note that the concept of dedifferentiation is not universally applicable here. Vertical integration, now viewed as a modernist relic, involved its own mode of dedifferentiation by assuming control over a variety of differentiated functions within a single organizational entity. More recently, the shedding of units and the return to core competencies signal a return to specialized differentiation as well as a need to manage expanding interorganizational interdependencies. In this context, it is not so much that dedifferentiation takes place among firms but that the forms of differentiation are being managed through relatively unique horizontal or network integration strategies. These strategies tend to blur the boundaries and support notions of boundary dedifferentiation.

In short, the postmodern organizational landscape must still contend with the enduring and central organizational tensions. Human participants must be motivated to exert mental and physical energy. Human tasks and production units must be defined, coordinated, and integrated. The tensions generated by these transactions continue to arise. What is constantly changing, perhaps now in a postmodern and radical fashion, are the means and methods used to manage these tensions.

BIBLIOGRAPHY

Abrahamson, Eric. 1996. "Management Fashion." *Academy of Management Review* 21(1):254–85.

Adler, Paul S., and Bryan Borys. 1996. "Two Types of Bureaucracy: Enabling and Coercive." *Administrative Science Quarterly* 41:61–89.

Aeppel, Timothy. 1997. "Missing the Boss: Not All Workers Find Idea of Empowerment as Neat as It Stands." *The Wall Street Journal,* September 8: A1, A10.

Aglietta, Michel. 1979. *A Theory of Capitalist Regulation: The U.S. Experience.* London: NLB.

Alderfer, Clayton P., and K. K. Smith. "Studying Intergroup Relations Embedded in Organizations." *Administrative Science Quarterly* 27:35–65.

Aldrich, Howard. 1979. *Organizations and Environment.* Englewood Cliffs, NJ: Prentice Hall.

Alexander, Jason Hansen, and Joseph W. Grubbs. 1998. "Wired Government: Information Technology, External Public Organizations, and Cyber Democracy." *Public Administration and Management* 3(1). Online journal at http://www.pamijicom.

American Management Association. 1999. " 'Stalling' Elements: The 2000% Solution." *American Management Association.* Online document at http://www.amanet.org/research/specials/sstalling.htm.

Amin, A. 1994. *Post-Fordism: A Reader.* Oxford: Blackwell.

Amin, Samir. 1976. *Unequal Development.* New York: Monthly Review Press.

Amran, Martha, and Nalin Kulatilaka. 1998. *Real Options: Managing Strategic Investment in an Uncertain World.* Cambridge: Harvard Business Press.

Angel, David P. 1989. *Restructuring for Production: The Remaking of the U.S. Semiconductor Industry.* New York: Guilford Press.

Appelbaum, Eileen, and Rosemary Batt. 1994. *The New American Workplace: Transforming Systems in the United States.* Ithaca, NY: ICR/Cornell University Press.

Applegate, Lynda. 1995. "Managing in an Information Age: Organizational Challenges and Opportunities." Harvard Business School Paper No. 9-196-002.

Aram, John D. 1976. *Dilemmas of Administrative Behavior.* Englewood Cliffs, NJ: Prentice Hall.

Argyle, Michael. 1953. "The Relay Assembly Test Room in Retrospect." *Occupational Psychology* 27:98–103.

Argyris, Chris. 1993. *Knowledge for Action: A Guide to Overcoming Barriers to Organizational Change.* San Francisco: Jossey-Bass.

———. 1990. *Overcoming Organizational Defenses.* Boston: Allyn and Bacon.

———. 1982. *Reasoning, Learning and Action.* San Francisco: Jossey-Bass.

———. 1964. *Integrating the Individual and the Organization.* New York: John Wiley.

Aronowitz, Stanley. 1973. *False Promises: The Shaping of American Working Class Consciousness.*

Ashby, William Ross. 1960. *An Introduction to Cybernetics.* London: Chapman and Hall.

Ashkenas, Ron; Dave Ulrich; Todd Jick; and Steve Kerr. 1996. *The Boundaryless Organization: Breaking the Chains of Organizational Structure.* San Francisco: Jossey Bass.

Astley, W. Graham, and Andrew H. Van de Ven. 1983. "Central Perspectives and Debates in Organizational Theory." *Administrative Science Quarterly* 28:245–73.

Avolio, Bruce J., and Bernard M. Bass. 1994. *Improving Organizational Effectiveness Through Transformational Leadership.* Thousand Oaks, CA: Sage.

Babson, Steve. 1996. "A New Model Ford?" In Paul Stewart, ed. *Beyond Japanese Management: The Find of Modern Times?* Portland, OR: Frank Cass.

Bacharach, Peter, and Edward L. Lawler. 1980. *Power and Politics in Organizations.* San Francisco: Jossey-Bass.

Badaracco, Joseph L. 1991. *The Knowledge Link: How Firms Compete through Strategic Alliances.* Cambridge: Harvard Business School Press.

Barker, James R. 1993. "Tightening the Iron Cage: Control in Self-Managing Teams." *Administration Science Quarterly* 38:408–37.

Barley, Stephen, and Gideon Kunda. 1992. "Design and Devotion: Surges of Rational and Normative Ideologies of Control in Managerial Discourse." *Administration Science Quarterly* 37:363–99.

Barley, Stephen, G. Meyer, and D. C. Gash. 1988. "Cultures of Culture: Academics, Practitioners, and the Pragmatics of Normative Control." *Administrative Science Quarterly* 33:24–60.

Barnard, Chester. 1938. *The Functions of the Executive.* Cambridge: Harvard University Press.

Barnatt, C. 1995. "Office Space, Cyberspace, and Virtual Organization." *Journal of General Management* 20(4): 78–91.

Barzelay, Michael. 1992. *Breaking through Bureaucracy.* Berkeley: University of California Press.

Bass, Bernard M. 1997. *Transformational Leadership.* Mahwah, NJ: Lawrence Erlbaum Associates.

Bateson, Gregory. 1979. *Mind and Nature.* New York: Bantam.

Baum, Joel A. C. 1996. "Organizational Ecology." In Stewart R. Clegg, Cynthia Hardy, and Walter R. Nord, eds. *Handbook of Organization Studies.* Thousand Oaks, CA: Sage.

Becker, Frank, and Fritz Steele. 1995. *Workplace by Design: Mapping the High Performance Workscape.* San Francisco: Jossey-Bass.

Bedeian, Arthur G. 1984. *Organizations: Theory and Analysis.* 2nd ed. New York: Dryden Press.

Bell, Daniel. 1973. *The Coming of Post-Industrial Society.* New York: Basic Books.

Bendix, Reinhard. 1956. *Work and Authority in Industry: Ideologies of Management in the Course of Industrialization.* New York: John Wiley.

Berle, Adolph, and G. Means. 1932. *The Modern Corporation and Private Property.* New York: Macmillan.

Berman, Marshall. 1982. *All That Is Solid Melts into Air.* New York: Penguin.

Berquist, William. 1993. *The Postmodern Organization.* San Francisco: Jossey-Bass.

Blau, Peter. 1955. *The Dynamics of Bureaucracy.* Chicago: University of Chicago Press.

Blau, Peter, and Marshall Meyer. 1971. *Bureaucracy in Modern Society,* 2nd ed. New York: Random House.

Blauner, Robert. 1964. *Alienation and Freedom: The Factory Worker and His Job.* Chicago: University of Chicago Press.

Bohm, David. 1990. *On Dialogue.* Ojai, CA: David Rohm Seminars.

Boswell, Terry. 1987. "Accumulation Innovations in the American Economy: The Affinity for Japanese Solutions to the Current Crisis." In Terry Boswell and Albert Bergeson, eds. *America's Changing Role in the World System.* New York: Praeger.

Bowles, Samuel, and Herbert Gintis. 1990. "Contest Exchange: New Microfoundations for the Political Economy of Capitalism." *Politics and Society* 18:165–222.

_____. 1989. *Democracy and Capitalism.* New York: Basic Books.

_____. 1982. "The Crisis of Liberal Democratic Capitalism: The Case of the United States." *Politics and Society* 11(1):51–93.

Braverman, Harry. 1974. *Labor and Monopoly Capital: The Degradation of Work in the Twentieth Century.* New York: Monthly Review Press.

Brown, J. A. C. 1954. *The Social Psychology of Industry.* New York: Penguin.

Bryman, Alan. 1996. "Leadership in Organizations." In Stewart R. Clegg, Cynthia Hardy, and Walter R. Nord, eds. *Handbook of Organizational Studies.* Thousand Oaks, CA: Sage.

Burnham, James. 1941. *The Managerial Revolution.* Bloomington: Indiana University Press.

Burns, Tom, and G. M. Stalker. 1961. *The Management of Innovation.* London: Tavistock.

Burrell, Gibson, and Gareth Morgan. 1979. *Sociological Paradigms and Organizational Analysis.* London: Heinemann.

Calas, Marta B., and Linda Smircich. 1996. "From 'The Women's' Point of View: Feminist Approaches to Organizational Studies." In Stewart R. Clegg, Cynthia Hardy, and Walter R. Nord, eds. *Handbook of Organization Studies.* Thousand Oaks, CA: Sage.

Calhoun, Craig. 1982. *The Question of Class Struggle.* Chicago: University of Chicago Press.

Carey, Alex. 1967. "The Hawthorne Studies: A Radical Criticism." *American Sociological Review* 32:403–16.

Castells, Manuel. 1996. *The Rise of the Network Society.* Malden, MA: Blackwell.

_____. 1998. "The Real Crisis of Silicon Valley: A Retrospective Perspective." *Competition and Change* 3:107–43.

Chandler, Alfred. 1962. *Strategy and Structure.* Cambridge: MIT Press.

Chawla, Sarita, and John Renesch, eds. 1995. *Learning Organizations: Developing Cultures for Tomorrow's Workplace.* Portland, OR: Productivity Press.

Chung, Kae H., and Leon C. Megginson. 1981. *Organizational Behavior: Developing Managerial Skills.* New York: Harper and Row.

Clark, Gordon. 1981. "The Employment Relationship and Spatial Division of Labor." *Annals of the Association of American Geographers* 71: 412–24.

Clawson, Dan. 1980. *Bureaucracy and the Labor Process: The Transformation of U.S. Industry 1860–1920.* New York: Monthly Review Press.

Clegg, Stewart R. 1990. *Modern Organizations: Organization Studies in the Postmodern World.* Newbury Park, CA: Sage.

Coase, Ronald. 1937. "The Nature of the Firm." *Economica* 4:386–405.

Cohen, Ira J. 1989. *Structuration Theory: Anthony Giddens and the Constitution of Social Life.* New York: Macmillan.

Cohen, Susan G., and Diane E. Bailey. 1997. "What Makes Teams Work: Group Effectiveness Research from the Shop Floor to the Executive Suite." *Journal of Management* 23:239–63.

Colomy, Paul. 1998. "Neofunctionalism and Neoinstitutionalism: Human Agency and Interest in Institutional Change." *Sociological Forum* 13(2):265–300.

Cooley, Charles Horton. 1962. *Social Organizations: A Study of the Larger Mind.* New York: Schocken.

Crozier, Michel. 1964. *The Bureaucratic Phenomenon.* Chicago: University of Chicago Press.

Cyert, Richard M., and James G. March. 1992. *A Behavioral Theory of the Firm.* 2nd ed. New York: Blackwell.

Dalton, Melville. 1959. *Men Who Manage.* New York: John Wiley.

Dassbach, Carl. 1994. "Where Is North American Automobile Production Headed: Low Wage Lean Production." *Electronic Journal of Sociology* Online document at http://www.socsci.mcmaster.ca/EJS/ vol1.00./Dassback.htm.

Davidow, William H., and Michael S. Malone. 1993. *The Virtual Corporation: Structuring and Revitalizing the Corporation for the 21st Century.* New York: Harper Business.

Davis, Keith. 1981. *Human Behavior at Work: Organizational Behavior.* New York: McGraw-Hill.

Davis, Stan, and Christopher Meyer. 1998. *BLUR: The Speed of Change in the Connected Economy.* Reading, MA: Addison-Wesley.

DeJanvry, Alain. 1981. *The Agrarian Question and Reformism in Latin America.* Baltimore: Johns Hopkins University Press.

Denhardt, Robert. 1981. *In the Shadow of Organization.* Lawrence: The Regents Press of Kansas.

Denison, Daniel R. 1991. "Organizational Culture and 'Collective' Human Capital." In Amitai Etzioni and Paul R. Lawrence, eds. *Socio-Economics: Toward a New Synthesis.* Armonk, NY: M. E. Sharpe.

DeSanctis, Gerardine, and Janet Fulk. 1999. *Shaping Organization Form: Communication, Connection, and Community.* Thousand Oaks, CA: Sage.

Diamond, Michael A. 1993. *The Unconscious Life of Organizations: Interpreting Organizational Identity.* Westport, CT: Quorum Books.

Dicken, Peter. 1992. *Global Shift: Transforming the World Economy.* 2nd ed. New York: The Guilford Press.

Dill, William R. 1958. "Environment as Influence on Managerial Autonomy." *Administrative Science Quarterly* 2:409–43.

DiMaggio, Paul, and Walter Powell. 1983. "The Iron Cage Revisited: Institutional Isomorphism and Collective Rationality." *American Sociological Review* 48:147–60.

Dohse, Knuth; Ulrich Jurgens; and Thomas Malsch. 1985. "From 'Fordism' to 'Toyotaism'? The Social Organization of the Labor Process in the Japanese Automobile Industry." *Politics and Society* 14(2): 115–46.

Dore, Ronald. 1986. *Flexible Rigidities: Industrial Policy and Structural Adjustment in the Japanese Economy, 1970–1980.* Palo Alto, CA: Stanford University Press.

———. 1973. *British Factory, Japanese Factory: The Origins of National Diversity in Industrial Relations.* Berkeley: University of California Press.

Downs, Anthony. 1967. *Inside Bureaucracy.* Boston: Little Brown.

Durkheim, Emile. 1933. *The Division of Labor in Society.* New York: Free Press.

Edwards, Richard. 1979. *Contested Terrain: The Transformation of the Workplace in the Twentieth Century.* New York: Basic Books.

Eisenhardt, Kathleen, and Brian Westcott. 1988. "Paradoxical Demands and the Creation of Excellence: The Case of Just-in-Time Manufacturing." In Robert E. Quinn and Kim Cameron, eds. *Paradox and Transformation.* New York: Ballinger.

Eisenstadt, S. M. 1980. *Revolution and Transformation of Societies: A Comparative Study of Civilizations.* New York: Free Press.

England, Paula, and George Farkas. 1986. *Households, Employment, and Gender: A Social, Economic and Demographic View.* New York: Walter deGruyter.

Etzioni, Amitai. 1996. "The Responsive Community: A Communitarian Perspective." *American Sociological Review 61:1–11.*

———. 1988. *The Moral Dimension.* New York: Free Press.

———. 1961. *A Comparative Analysis of Organizations.* New York: Free Press.

Etzioni, Amitai, and Paul R. Lawrence. 1991. *Socio-Economics: Toward a New Synthesis.* Armonk, NY: M. E. Sharpe.

Evan, William. 1976. *Organization Theory: Structures, Systems, and Environments.* New York: Wiley.

Ezzamel, Mahmoud, and Hugh Willmott. 1998. "Accounting for Teamwork: A Critical Study of Group-based Systems of Organizational Control." *Administrative Science Quarterly* 43:358–96.

Fantasia, Rick. 1988. *Cultures of Solidarity: Consciousness, Action, and Contemporary American Workers.* Berkeley: University of California Press.

Fantasia, Rick; Dan Clawson; and Gregory Graham. 1988. "A Cultural View of Worker Participation in American Industry." *Work and Occupations* 15:468–88.

Fayol, Henri. 1949. (1919). *General and Industrial Management.* London: Pittman.

Feenberg, Andrew. 1998. "Escaping the Iron Cage, or, Subversive Rationality and Democratic Theory." In R. Schomberg, ed. *Democratising Technology: Ethics, Risk and Public Debate.* Tilburg, Netherlands: International Centre for Human and Public Affairs.

Fiedler, Fred Edward. 1967. *A Theory of Leadership Effectiveness.* New York: McGraw Hill.

Fisher, Marshall. 1997. "What's the Right Supply Chain for Your Product?" *Harvard Business Review 75:105-117.*

Fligstein, Neil. 1990. *The Transformation of Corporate Control.* Cambridge: Harvard University Press.

Florida, Richard, and Martin Kenney. 1990. "High Technology Restructuring in the USA and Japan." *Environment and Planning A* 22:233–52.

Form, William. 1987. "On the Degradation of Skills." *Annual Review of Sociology* 13:29–47.

Fox, Alan. 1974. *Man Mismanagement.* London: Hutchinson.

———. 1971. *A Sociology of Work in Industry.* London: Collier-Macmillan.

Frank, Richard Herbert, and James D. Kaul. 1978. "The Hawthorne Experiments: First Statistical Interpretation." *American Sociological Review* 43:623–43.

Freeman, John H.; Glenn Carroll; and Michael T. Hannan. 1983. "The Liability of Newness: Age-Dependence in Organizational Death Rates." *American Sociological Review* 48:692–710.

Freeman, Richard B., and Joel Rogers. 1999. *What Workers Want.* Ithaca, NY: Cornell University Press.

Frenkel, S.; M. Korczynski; L. Donoghue; and K. Shire. 1995. "Reconstituting Work: Trends toward Knowledge Work and Info-Normative Control." *Work, Employment and Society* 9:773–96.

Fritz, Robert. 1989. *The Path of Least Resistance: Learning to Become a Creative Force in Your Own Life.* New York: Ballantine.

Fuentes, A., and Barbara Ehrenreich. 1983. *Women in the Global Factory.* Boston: South End Press.

Gereffi, Gary. 1995. "Global Production Systems and Third World Development." In Barbara Stallings, ed. *Global Change, Regional Response: The New International Context of Development.* New York: Cambridge University Press.

Gereffi, Gary, and Gary G. Hamilton. 1996. "Commodity Chains and Embedded Networks: The Economic Organization of Global Capitalism." Paper presented at the annual meeting of the American Sociological Association, New York City.

Gergen, Kenneth. 1990. *The Saturated Self: Dilemmas of Identity in Contemporary Life.* New York: Basic Books.

Gerlach, Michael. 1992. *Alliance Capitalism: The Social Organization of Japanese Business.* Berkeley: University of California Press.

Ghere, Richard K., and Brian A. Young. 1998. "The Cyber-Management Environment: Where Technology and Ingenuity Meet Public Purpose and Accountability." *Public Administration and Management: An Interactive Journal* 3 (1). online at http://www.pamij.com.

Giddens, Anthony. 1984. *The Constitution of Society: Outline of a Theory of Structuration.* Berkeley: University of California Press.

Gillespie, Richard. 1993. *Manufacturing Knowledge: A History of the Hawthorne Experiments.* New York: Cambridge University Press.

Goffman, Erving. 1961. *Encounters: Two Studies in the Sociology of Interaction.* Indianapolis, IN: Bobbs-Merrill.

Goldman, Paul, and Donald R. Van Houten. 1988. "Bureaucracy and Domination: Managerial Strategy in Turn-of-the-Century American Industry." In Frank Hearn, ed. *The Transformation of Industrial Organization.* Belmont, CA: Wadsworth.

Goldman, Steven L.; Kenneth Preiss; and Roger N. Nagel. 1997. *Agile Competitors and Virtual Organizations: Strategies for Enriching the Customer.* New York: John Wiley.

Golembiewski, Robert T. 1985. *Humanizing Public Organizations.* Mt. Airy, MD: Lomond Publications.

Gordon, David M. 1996. *Fat and Mean: The Corporate Squeeze of Working Americans and the Myth of Managerial "Downsizing."* New York: Free Press.

Gordon, David M.; Richard Edwards; and Michael Reich. 1982. *Segmented Work, Divided Workers: the Historical Transformation of Labor in the United States.* New York: Cambridge University Press.

Gordon, Richard, and Linda Kimball. 1998. "Globalization, Innovation, and Regional Development." *Competition and Change* 3:9–39.

Gortner, Harold F. 1977. *Administration in the Public Sector.* New York.

Gouldner, Alvin. 1954. *Patterns of Industrial Bureaucracy.* Glencoe, IL: Free Press.

_____. 1955. "Metaphysical Pathos and the Theory of Bureaucracy." *American Political Science Review* 49:496–507.

Graham, Laurie. 1995. *On the Line at Suburu-Isuzu: The Japanese Model and the American Worker.* Ithaca: NY: Cornell University, ILR Press.

Granovetter, Mark. 1985. "Economic Actions and Social Structure: The Problem of Embeddedness." *American Journal of Sociology* 91(3):481–510.

Gulick, Luther and L. Urwick. 1937. *Papers on the Science of Administration.* New York: Institute of Public Administration, Columbia University.

Gutman, Herbert. 1975. *Work, Culture and Society in Industrializing America.* New York: Knopf.

Guzzo, Richard, and Marcus W. Dickson. 1996. "Teams in Organizations: Recent Research on Performance and Effectiveness." *Annual Review of Psychology* 47:307–40.

Hagel, John, and Marc Singer. 1999. *Net Worth: Shaping Markets When Customers Make the Rules.* Cambridge: Harvard Business School.

Hall, Richard. 1999. *Organizations: Structures, Processes, and Outcomes.* Englewood Cliffs, NJ: Prentice Hall.

Hamilton, Richard F., and James D. Wright. 1986. *The State of the Masses.* New York: Aldine.

Hampden-Turner, Charles. 1990. *Corporate Culture: From Vicious to Virtuous Circles.* London: Hutchinson.

Handy, Charles. 1995a. "Trust and the Virtual Organization." *Harvard Business Review* 73(3):40–50.

_____. 1995b. "Managing the Dream." In Sarita Chawla and John Renesch, eds. *Learning Organizations: Developing Cultures for Tomorrow's Workplace.* Portland, OR: Productivity Press.

_____. 1994. *The Age of Paradox.* Boston: Harvard Business School Press.

Hannan, Michael T., and John H. Freeman. 1977. "The Population Ecology of Organizations." *American Journal of Sociology* 82:929–64.

_____. 1984. "Structural Inertia and Organizational Change." *American Sociological Review* 49:259–85.

Harrison, Bennett. 1994. *Lean and Mean: The Changing Landscape of Corporate Power in the Age of Flexibility.* New York: Basic Books.

Harvey, David. 1989. *The Condition of Postmodernity.* Cambridge, MA: Blackwell.

_____. 1982. *The Limits to Capital.* Cambridge, MA: Blackwell.

Haslam, Colin; Karel Williams; Sukhdeu Johal; and John Williams. 1996. "A Fallen Idol? Japanese Management in the 1990's." In Paul Stewart, ed. *Beyond Japanese Management: The End of Modern Times?* Portland, OR: Frank Cass.

Hatch, Mary Jo. 1997. *Organization Theory: Modern, Symbolic, and Postmodern Perspectives.* Oxford: Oxford University Press.

Heckscher, Charles, 1994. "Defining the Post-Bureaucratic Type." In Charles Heckscher and Anne Donnelon, eds. *The Post-Bureaucratic Organization.* Thousand Oaks, CA: Sage.

Heckscher, Charles, and Anne Donnelon, eds. 1994. *The Post Bureaucratic Organization.* Thousand Oaks, CA: Sage.

Hersey, Paul, Ken Blanchard, and Dewey E. Johnson. 1996. *Management of Organizational Behavior.* 7th ed. New York: Prentice-Hall.

Hirschhorn, Larry. 1997. *Reworking Authority: Leading and Following in the Post-Modern Organization.* Cambridge: MIT Press.

Hirschman, Albert. 1970. *Exit, Voice and Loyalty: Responses to Decline in Firms, Organizations, and States.* Cambridge: Harvard University Press.

Hodge, B. J., and William P. Anthony. 1984. *Organization Theory.* 2nd ed. Boston: Allyn and Bacon.

Hodson, Randy. 1999. "Organizational Anomie and Worker Consent." *Work and Occupations* 3:292–323.

_____. 1995. "Worker Resistance: An Underdeveloped Concept in the Sociology of Work." *Economic and Industrial Democracy* 16(1):79–110.

Horkheimer, Max, and Theodor W. Adorno. 1976. *Dialectic of Enlightenment.* New York: Continuum Publishing Group.

House, R. J., and M. L. Baetz. 1979. "Leadership: Some Empirical Generalizations and New Research Directions." *Research in Organizational Behavior* 1:341–423.

Howell, David, and Edward Wolff. 1991. "Trends in the Growth and Distribution of Skills in the U.S. Workplace, 1960–1985." *Industrial and Labor Relations Review* 44:486–502.

Hoxie, Robert Franklin. 1966. (1915) *Scientific Management and Labor.* New York: A. M. Kelley.

Huseman, Richard C., and Jon P. Goodman. 1999. *Leading with Knowledge: The Nature of Competition in the 21st Century.* Thousand Oaks, CA: Sage.

Inglehart, Ronald. 1977. *The Silent Revolution.* Princeton, NJ: Princeton University Press.

Jackall, Robert. 1988. *Moral Mazes: The World of Corporate Managers.* New York: Oxford University Press.

Jaffee, David. 1988. "The Political Economic Environment and the Geographic Restructuring of Manufacturing: Theoretical Perspectives and a State-Level Analysis." In Michael Wallace and Joyce Rothschild, eds. *Research in Politics and Society,* vol. 3. Greenwich, CT: JAI Press.

James, David, and Michael Soref. 1981. "Profit Constraints on Managerial Autonomy: Managerial Theory and the Unmaking of the Corporation President." *American Sociological Review* 46:1–18.

Jarillo, J. Carlos. 1995. *Strategic Networks: Creating the Borderless Organization.* Butterworth-Heinemann.

Jary, David, and Julia Jary. 1991. *The Harper Collins Dictionary of Sociology.* New York: Harper Perennial.

Jermier, John M. 1998. "Introduction: Critical Perspectives on Organizational Control." *Administrative Science Quarterly* 43:235–56.

Jones, Gareth R. 1997. *Organization Theory: Text and Cases.* 2nd ed. New York: Addison-Wesley.

Jones, Stephen R. G. 1992. "Was There a Hawthorne Effect?" *American Journal of Sociology* 98:451–68.

Jorde, Thomas M., and David J. Teece. 1990. "Innovation and Cooperation: Implications for Competition and Antitrust." *Journal of Economic Perspectives* 4: 75–96.

Kakabadse, Andrew. 1983. *The Politics of Management.* London: Gower.

Katz, Daniel, and Robert L. Kahn. 1966. *The Social Psychology of Organizations.* New York: John Wiley.

Kaufman, Herbert. 1985. *Time, Chance, and Organizations.* Chatham, NJ: Chatham House.

Kenney, Martin, and Richard Florida. 1993. *Beyond Mass Production: The Japanese System and Its Transfer to the U.S.* New York: Oxford University Press.

_____. 1988. "Beyond Mass Production: Production and the Labor Process." *Politics and Society* 16:121–58.

Kerr, Clark. 1953. "What Became of the Independent Spirit?" *Fortune* 48 (July): 110.

Kochan, Thomas A.; Russell D. Lansbury; and John Paul MacDuffie. 1997. *After Lean Production: Evolving Employment Practices in the World Auto Industry.* Ithaca, NY: Cornell University Press.

Kolodny, Harvey; Michel Lin; Bengt Stymne; and Helene Denis. 1996. "New Technology and the Emerging Organizational Paradigm." *Human Relations* 49:1457–87.

Kunda, Gideon. 1992. *Engineering Culture: Control and Commitment in a High-Tech Corporation.* Philadelphia: Temple University Press.

Labarre, Polly. 1996. "The Organization Is Dis-Organization." *Fast Company* 3:77. Online document at: www.fastcompany.com/online.03/oticon.html.

Langlois, Richard N., and Paul L. Robertson. 1995. *Firms, Markets, and Economic Change: Dynamic Theory of Business Institutions.* New York: Routledge.

Lawrence, Paul, and Jay Lorsch. 1967. *Organization and Environment; Managing Differentiation and Integration.* Homewood, IL: Richard D. Irwin.

Lee, Han L., and Corey Billington. 1995. "The Evolution of Supply-Chain Management Models and Practice at Hewlett-Packard." *Interfaces* 25:42–63.

Lee, Robert, and Peter Lawrence. 1991. *Politics at Work.* London: Stanley Thornes.

Leiberson, Stanley, and James F. O'Connor. 1972. "Leadership and Organizational Performance: A Study of Large Corporations." *American Sociological Review* 37:117–30.

Lenin, V. I. 1965. *Collected Works.* Moscow: International.

Lewchuk, Wayne, and David Robertson. 1996. "Working Conditions under Lean Production: A Worker-Based Benchmarking Study." In Paul Stewart, ed. *Beyond Japanese Management: The End of Modern Times?* Portland, OR: Frank Cass.

Lewicki, Roy J., and Barbara Benedict Bunker. 1996. "Developing and Maintaining Trust in Work Relationships." In Roderick M. Kramer and Tom R. Tyler, eds. *Trust in Organizations.* Thousand Oaks, CA: Sage.

Likert, Rensis. 1961. *New Patterns of Management.* New York: McGraw-Hill.

Lincoln, James R., and Arne L. Kalleberg. 1985. "Work Organization and Workforce Commitment: A Study of Plants and Employees in the U.S. and Japan." *American Sociological Review* 50:738–60.

Lindblom, Charles. 1959. "The Science of Muddling Through." *Public Administration: Review* 19:79–88.

Lipnack, Jessica, and Jeffrey Stamps. 1997. *Virtual Teams: Reaching across Space, Time, and Organizations with Technology.* New York: John Wiley.

Littler, Craig. 1982. *The Development of the Labor Process in Capitalist Societies.* Exeter, NH: Heinemann.

Lutrin, Carl E., and Allen K. Settle. 1967. *American Public Administration: Concepts and Cases.* Palo Alto, CA: Mayfield.

Mannheim, Karl. 1940. *Man and Society in an Age of Reconstruction.* New York: Harcourt, Brace and World.

March, James, and Herbert Simon. 1958. *Organizations.* New York: John Wiley.

Marcuse, Herbert. 1964. *One-Dimensional Man.* Boston: Beacon.

Marglin, Steven A. 1974. "What Do Bosses Do? The Origins and Functions of Hierarchy in Capitalist Production." *The Review of Radical Political Economics* 6(2):60–112.

Marini, Frank, ed. 1971. *Toward a New Public Administration: The Minnowbrook Perspective.* Scranton, PA: Chandler.

Martin, Joanne. 1992. *Cultures in Organization: Three Perspectives.* New York: Oxford University Press.

Martin, Joanne, and Kathleen Knopoff. 1997. "The Gendered Implications of Apparently Gender-Neutral Theory: Rereading Max Weber." In A. Larson and R. E. Freeman, eds. *Women's Studies and Business Ethics.* New York: Oxford University Press.

Marx, Karl. 1964. Economic and Philosophical Manuscripts of 1844. New York: International Publishing.

_____. 1963. Early Writings. Edited by T. B. Bottomore. New York: McGraw-Hill.

Maslow, Abraham H. 1943. "A Theory of Human Motivation." *Psychological Review* 50:370–96.

Massey, Doreen. 1984. *Spatial Divisions of Labor: Social Structures and the Geography of Production.* New York: Methuen.

Mayo, Elton. 1939. *The Social Problems of an Industrial Civilization.* New York: Ayer.

_____. 1933. *The Human Problems of an Industrial Civilization.* New York: MacMillan.

McGregor, Douglas. 1966. "The Human Side of Enterprise." In Warren G. Bennis and Edgar H. Schein, eds. *Leadership and Motivation: Essays of Douglas McGregor.* Cambridge: MIT Press.

_____. 1960. *The Human Side of Enterprise.* New York: McGraw-Hill.

McMichael, Philip. 1996. *Development and Social Change.* Thousand Oaks, CA: Pine Forge Press.

McWhinney, Will. 1992. *Paths of Change: Strategic Choices for Organizations and Society.* Newbury Park, CA: Sage.

Meindl, James R.; Sanford B. Ehrlich; and Janet M. Dkevich. 1985. "The Romance of Leadership." *Administrative Science Quarterly* 30:78–102.

Merton, Robert. 1957. *Social Theory and Social Structure.* New York: Free Press.

Meyer, John W., and Brian Rowan. 1977. "Institutionalized Organizations: Formal Structure as Myth and Ceremony." *American Journal of Sociology* 83:340–63.

Meyer, Marshall. 1985. *Limits to Bureaucratic Growth.* New York: Walter deGruyter.

Meyerson, Debra; Karl E. Weick; and Roderick M. Kramer. 1996. "Swift Trust and Temporary Groups." In Roderick M. Kramer and Tom R. Tyler, eds. *Trust in Organizations.* Thousand Oaks, CA: Sage.

Milkman, Ruth. 1991. *Japan's California Factories: Labor Relations and Economic Globalization.* Los Angeles: University of California, Institute of Industrial Relations.

Miller, Delbert C., and William H. Form. 1964. *Industrial Sociology.* New York: Harper and Row.

Mintz, Beth, and Michael Schwartz. 1985. *The Power Structure of American Business.* Chicago: University of Chicago Press.

Mintzberg, Henry. 1973. *The Nature of Managerial Work.* New York: Harper and Row.

Mitroff, Ian I., and J. R. Emshoff. 1979. "On Strategic Assumption-Making: A Dialectical Approach to Policy and Planning." *Academy of Management Review* 4:1–12.

Monge, Peter, and Janet Fulk. 1999. "Communication Technology for Global Network Organizations." In Gerardine DeSanctis and Janet Fulk, eds. *Shaping Organization Form: Communication, Connection, and Community.* Thousand Oaks, CA: Sage.

Montgomery, David. 1979. *Workers' Control in America: Studies in the History of Work, Technology, and Labor Struggles.* New York: Cambridge University Press.

Mooney, James D., and Allen C. Reiley. 1939. *The Principles of Organization.* New York: Harper.

Moore, Wilbert. 1963. "Industrialization and Social Change." In Bert Hoselitz and Wilbert Moore, eds. *Industrialization and Society.* Mouton: UNESCO.

Morgan, Gareth. 1997. *Images of Organization.* Thousand Oaks, CA: Sage.

_____. 1993. *Imaginization: The Art of Creative Management.* Newbury Park, CA: Sage.

Morgan, Gareth, and Asaf Zohar. 1996. "Achieving Quantum Change: Incrementally. The Art of High Leverage Change." Online document at www.yorku.ca/faculty/academic/g.morgan/0695home.html.

Mosher, Frank. 1968. *Democracy and the Public Sector.* New York: Oxford University Press.

Mouzelis, Nicos P. 1967. *Organization and Bureaucracy: An Analysis of Modern Theories.* Chicago: Aldine.

Nkomo, Stella M., and Taylor Cox, Jr. 1996. "Diverse Identities in Organizations." In Stewart Clegg, Cynthia Hardy, and Walter R. Nord, eds. *Handbook of Organization Studies.* Thousand Oaks, CA: Sage.

Nonaka, Ikujiro, and Hirotaka Takeuchi. 1995. *The Knowledge Creating Company.* New York: Oxford University Press.

Nutt, Paul C., and Robert W. Backoff. 1992. *Strategic Management of Public and Third Sector Organizations.* San Francisco: Jossey-Bass.

Offe, Claus. 1976. *Industry and Inequality.* London: Edward Arnold.

Ogasawara, Koichi, and Hirofumi Veda. 1996. "The Changing Nature of Japanese Production Systems in the 1990s and Issues for Labour Studies." In Paul Stewart, ed. *Beyond Japanese Management: The End of Modern Times?* Portland, OR: Frank Cass.

Oliver, Christine. 1992. "The Antecedents of Deinstitutionalization." *Organization Studies* 13: 563–88.

Orlikowski, Wanda J. 1992. "Learning from Notes: Organizational Issues in Groupware Implementation." MIT Sloan School Working Paper No. 3428-92. http://ccs.mit.edu/ CCSEP134.html.

Osborne, David, and Ted A. Gaebler. 1992. *Reinventing Government: How the Entrepreneurial Spirit Is Transforming the Public Sector.* New York: Perseus Press.

Ouchi, William G. 1980. "Markets, Bureaucracies, and Clans." *Administrative Science Quarterly* 25:129–41.

Pareto, Vilfredo. 1963. *The Mind and Society: A Treatise on General Sociology.* New York: Dover.

Parker, Martin. 1992. "Post-Modern Organizations or Postmodern Organization Theory?" *Organization Studies* 13:1–17.

Parker, Mike, and Jane Slaughter. 1988. *Choosing Sides: Unions and the Team Concept.* Boston: Southend Press.

Parsons, Talcott. 1960. *Structure and Process in Modern Society.* New York: The Free Press.

Parsons, Talcott. 1956. "Suggestions for a Sociological Approach to the Theory of Organizations." *Administrative Science Quarterly* 1:63–85.

_____. 1947. "Introduction." In A. M. Henderson and Talcott Parsons, eds. *Max Weber; Theory of Social and Economic Organization.* New York: Oxford University Press.

Pauly, Louis W., and Simon Reich. 1997. "National Structures and Multinational Corporate Behavior: Enduring Differences in the Age of Globalization." *International Organization* 51(1):1–30.

Percy-Smith, Janie. 1996. "Downloading Democracy? Information and Communication Technology in Local Politics." *Policy and Politics* 24:43–56.

Perrow, Charles. 1986. *Complex Organizations: A Critical Essay.* New York: Random House.

Perrow, Charles. 1967. "A Framework for the Comparative Analysis of Organizations." *American Sociological Review* 32:194–208.

Pfeffer, Jeffrey. 1998. *The Human Equation.* Boston: Harvard Business School Press.

———. 1997. *New Directions for Organization Theory.* New York: Oxford University Press.

———. 1994. *Competitive Advantage through People: Unleashing the Power of the Work Force.* Boston: Harvard Business School Press.

Pfeffer, Jeffrey, and Gerald R. Salancik. 1978. *The External Control of Organizations: A Resource Dependence Perspective.* New York: Harper and Row.

Pine, B. Joseph, and B. Joseph Pine II. 1992. *Mass Customization: The New Frontier in Business Competition.* Cambridge: Harvard Business School Press.

Piore, Michael J., and Charles F. Sabel. 1984. *The Second Industrial Divide: Possibilities for Prosperity.* New York: Basic Books.

Poirier, Charles. 1999. *Advanced Supply Chain Management: How to Build a Sustained Competitive Advantage.* Publishers Group West.

Polanyi, Karl. 1944. *The Great Transformation.* Boston: Beacon Press.

Polanyi, Michael. 1967. *The Tacit Dimension.* New York: Doubleday.

Pollard, Sidney. 1965. *The Genesis of Modern Management.* Cambridge: Harvard University Press.

Poole, Marshall Scott. 1999. "Organizational Challenges for the New Forms." In Gerardine DeSanctis and Janet Fulk, eds. *Shaping Organization Form: Communication, Connection, and Community.* Thousand Oaks, CA: Sage.

Powell, Walter. Forthcoming. "The Capitalist Firm in the 21st Century: Emerging Patterns." In Paul DiMaggio, ed. *Firm Futures.* Princeton University Press.

———. 1990. "Neither Market nor Hierarchy: Network Forms of Organization." In Barry M. Staw and Larry L. Cummings, eds. *Research in Organizational Behavior.* Greenwich, CT: JAI Press.

Prasad, Pushkala; Albert J. Mills; Michael Elmes; and Anshuman Prasad. 1997. *Managing the Organizational Melting Pot.* Thousand Oaks, CA: Sage.

Pugh, D. S., D. J. Hickson, and C. R. Hinings. 1985. *Writers on Organizations.* Beverly Hills, CA: Sage.

Quinn, Robert E., and Kim S. Cameron, eds. 1988. *Paradox and Transformation: Toward a Theory of Change in Organization and Management.* New York: Ballinger.

Rau, William, and Paul J. Baker. 1989. "The Organized Contradictions of Academe: Barriers Facing the Next Academic Revolution." *Teaching Sociology* 17:161–75.

Rinehart, James; Christopher Huxley; and David Robertson. 1997. *Just Another Car Factory? Lean Production and Its Discontents.* Ithaca, NY: Cornell University Press.

Ritvo, Roger A.; Anne H. Litwin; and Lee Butler. 1995. *Managing in the Age of Change.* Toronto: Irwin.

Rittel, Horst W. J., and Melvin Webber. 1973. "Dilemmas in a General Theory of Planning." *Policy Sciences* 4:155–69.

Ritzer, George. 1993. *The McDonaldization of Society.* Newbury Park, CA: Pine Forge Press.

Roethlisberger, F. J., and William Dickson. 1939. *Management and the Worker.* Cambridge: Harvard University Press.

Roethlisberger, Fritz, and William J. Dickson. 1966. *Counseling In an Organization.* Boston: Harvard Business School, Division of Research.

Romo, Frank P., and Michael Schwartz. 1995. "The Structural Embeddedness of Business Decisions: The Migration of Manufacturing Plants in New York State, 1960–1985." *American Sociological Review* 60:874–908.

Ross, David Frederick. 1997. *Competing through Supply Chain Management.* London: Chapman and Hall.

Salter, Malcolm. 1996. "Reversing History: The Economics and Politics of Vertical Integration at General Motors." Working Paper, Harvard Business School, 97-001.

Saxenian, Analee. 1994. *Regional Advantage: Culture and Competition in Silicon Valley and Route 128.* Cambridge: Harvard University Press.

Sayer, Andrew, and Richard Walker. 1992. *The New Social Economy: Reworking the Division of Labor.* Cambridge, MA: Blackwell.

Scanlon, Burt, and J. Bernard Keys. 1979. *Management and Organizational Behavior.* New York: John Wiley.

Schachter, Hindy Lauer. 1997. *Reinventing Government or Reinventing Ourselves: The Role of Citizen Owners in Making a Better Government.* Albany: State University of New York Press.

Schein, Edgar H. 1992. *Organizational Culture and Leadership.* San Francisco: Jossey-Bass.

Schiesl, M. J. 1977. *The Politics of Efficiency: Municipal Government and Reform in America, 1800–1920.* Berkeley: University of California Press.

Schon, Donald. 1983. *The Reflective Practitioner: How Professionals Think in Action.* New York: Basic Books.

Schultz, Majken, and Mary Jo Hatch. 1996. "Living with Multiple Paradigms: The Case of Paradigm Interplay in Organization Culture Studies." *Academy of Management Review* 21:529–57.

Scott, W. Richard. 1995. *Institutions and Organizations.* Thousand Oaks, CA: Sage.

————. 1987. *Organizations: Rational, Natural, and Open Systems.* 2nd ed. Englewood Cliffs, NJ: Prentice Hall.

Scott, W. Richard, and John W. Meyer. 1983. "The Organization of Societal Sectors." In John W. Meyer and W. Richard Scott, *Organizational Environments: Ritual and Rationality.* Thousand Oaks CA: Sage.

Selznick, Philip. 1957. *Leadership in Administration.* New York: Harper and Row.

————. 1949. *TVA and the Grass Roots.* Berkeley: University of California Press.

————. 1948. "Foundations of the Theory of Organization." *American Sociological Review* 13:25–35.

Senge, Paul. 1990. *The Fifth Discipline: The Art and Practice of the Learning Organization.* New York: Doubleday.

Sewell, Graham. 1998. "The Discipline of Teams: The Control of Team-based Industrial Work through Electronic Peer Surveillance." *Administrative Science Quarterly* 43:397–428.

Shapiro, D.; B. H. Sheppard; and L. Cheraskin. 1992. "Business on a Handshake." *Negotiation Journal* 8(4):365–77.

Siemens Communication Limited. 1998. *Flexible Working Guide.* Online document at http://www.siemenscomms.co.ok/useful_information/telecom_guides/flexible_working_guide/fw_4.htm.

Simon, Herbert. 1997. *Administrative Behavior: A Study of Decision-Making Processes in Administrative Organizations.* 4th ed. New York: Free Press.

————. 1946. "The Proverbs of Administration." *Public Administration Review* 6:53–67.

Sims, Henry P., and Peter Lorenzi. 1992. *The New Leadership Paradigm.* Newbury Park, CA: Sage.

Singh, Jitendra V., and Charles Lumsden. 1990. "Theory and Research in Organizational Ecology." *Annual Review of Sociology* 16:161–95.

Sirianni, Carmen. 1995. "Union and Management Collaborate to Democratize Work at the Shell-Sarnia Plant." Online document at: www.cpn.org/sections/topics/work/work.html].

Sloan, Alfred P. 1972. *My Years with General Motors.* New York: Doubleday.

Smelser, Neil J. 1963. *The Sociology of Economic Life.* Englewood Cliffs, NJ: Prentice-Hall.

Smircich, Linda, and Charles Stubbart. 1985. "Strategic Management in an Enacted World." *Academy of Management Review* 10:724–36.

Snizek, William. 1995. "Virtual Offices: Some Neglected Considerations." *Communications of the ACM* 38 (September): 15–17.

Sterman, John; Nelson Repenning; and F. Kofman. 1997. "Unanticipated Side Effects of Successful Quality Programs: Exploring a Paradox of Organizational Improvement." *Management Science* 43:503–21.

Sterman, John D.; Nelson P. Repenning; Rogelio Oliva; Elizabeth Kramer; Scott Rockart; and Andrew Jones. 1996. "The Improvement Paradox: Designing Sustainable Quality Improvement Programs." Available on line at web.mit.edu/jsterman/www/5096/Summary.html

Stewart, Paul, ed. 1996. *Beyond Japanese Management: The End of Modern Times?* Portland, OR: Frank Cass.

Stodgill, R. M., and A. E. Coons, eds. 1957. *Leader Behavior: Its Description and Management.* Columbus: Ohio State University. Bureau of Business Research.

Storper, Michael, and Richard Walker. 1983. "The Theory of Labor and the Theory of Location." *International Journal of Urban and Regional Research* 7:1–41.

Sullivan, B. G. 1987. "The Challenge of Economic Transformation." In S. C. Goldberg and C. R. Strain, eds. *Technological Change and the Transformation of America.* Carbondale: Southern Illinois University Press.

Tannenbaum, R.; I. Weschler; and F. Massarik. 1961. *Leadership and Organization.* New York: McGraw-Hill.

Tausky, Curt. 1970. *Work Organizations: Major Theoretical Perspectives.* Itasca, IL: F.E. Peacock.

Tayeb, Monir H. 1996. *The Management of a Multicultural Workforce.* New York: John Wiley.

Taylor, Frederick Winslow. 1911. *The Principles of Scientific Management.* New York: Norton.

Taylor, William C. 1995. "At Verifone It's a Dog's Life (and They Love It!)" *Fastcompany,* November, p. 115. Online document at:www.fastcompany.com/online/vfone.html

Teece, David J. 1992. "Competition, Cooperation, and Innovation: Organizational Arrangements for Regimes of Rapid Technological Progress." *Journal of Economic Behavior and Organization* 18:1–25.

_____. 1976. *Vertical Integration and Vertical Divestiture in the U.S. Oil Industry: Analysis and Policy Implications.* Stanford, CA: Stanford University Institute for Energy Studies.

Tenner, Edward. 1996. *Why Things Bite Back: Technology and the Revenge of Unintended Consequences.* New York: Alfred A. Knopf.

Thompson, E. P. 1963. *The Making of the English Working Class.* New York: Vintage.

Thompson, James. 1967. *Organizations in Action.* New York: McGraw-Hill.

Thurow, Lester. 1996. *The Future of Capitalism.* New York: William Morrow.

_____. 1992. *Head to Head.* New York: William Morrow.

Tilly, Chris, and Charles Tilly. 1998. *Work Under Capitalism.* Boulder, CO: Westview Press.

Tomer, John F. 1987. *Organizational Capital: The Path to Higher Productivity and Well-Being.* New York: Praeger.

Towers Perrin. 1997. "Towers Perrin 1997 Workplace Index Reveals Growing Concerns in Employer Delivery on 'The New Deal' Contract." Online document at: www.towers.com.

Trist, Eric L. 1981. "The Socio-Technical Perspective." In Andrew Van de Ven and W. F. Joyce, eds. *Perspectives on Organization Design and Behavior.* New York: Wiley-Interscience.

Trist, Eric L., and Kenneth W. Bamforth. 1951. "Some Social and Psychological Consequences of the Longwall Method of Coal Getting." *Human Relations* 4:3–38.

Upton, David, and Andrew P. McAfee. 1997. "Computer Integration and Catastrophic Process Failure in Flexible Production: An Empirical Investigation." Harvard Business School, Working Paper, 93-074.

Ure, Andrew. 1861. *The Philosophy of Manufactures.* London: H. G. Bohn.

Useem, Michael. 1996. *Investor Capitalism: How Money Managers Are Changing the Face of Corporate America.* New York: Basic Books.

Usui, Chikako, and Richard A. Colignon. 1996. "Corporate Restructuring: Converging World Pattern or Societally Specific Embeddedness?" *Sociological Quarterly* 37:551–78.

Vallas, Steven. 1999. "Re-Thinking Post-Fordism: The Meaning of Workplace Flexibility." *Sociological Theory* 17(1):68–85.

Vallas, Steven, and John P. Beck. 1996. "The Transformation of Work Revisited: The Limits of Flexibility in American Manufacturing." *Social Problems* 43:339–61.

Victor, Bart, and Caroll Stephens. 1999. "The Dark Side of the New Organizational Forms." In Gerardine DeSanctis and Janet Fulk, eds. *Shaping Organization Form: Communication, Connection, and Community.* Thousand Oaks, CA: Sage.

Walsh, James P., and Gerardo Rivera Ungson. 1991. "Organizational Memory." *Academy of Management Review* 16:57–91.

Watson, Tony J. 1980. *Sociology, Work and Industry.* Boston: Routledge and Kegan Paul.

Weber, Max. 1947. *The Theory of Social and Economic Organization.* New York: Oxford University Press.

———. 1946. From Max Weber. Edited by Hans Gerth and C. Wright Mills. New York: Oxford University Press.

Weick, Karl. E. 1995. *Sensemaking in Organizations.* Thousand Oaks, CA: Sage.

———. 1969. *The Social Psychology of Organizing.* Reading, MA: Addison-Wesley.

Weick, Karl, and Frances Westley. 1996. "Organizational Learning: Affirming an Oxymoron." In Stewart Clegg, Cynthia Hardy, and Walter R. Nord, eds. *Handbook of Organization Studies.* Thousand Oaks, CA: Sage.

Weinberg, Gerald. 1975. *An Introduction to Systems Thinking.* New York: John Wiley.

Weisskopf, Walter A. 1971. *Alienation and Economics.* New York: E. P. Dutton.

Wells, Donald. 1993. "Are Strong Unions Compatible with the New Model of Human Relations Management?" *Industrial Relations* 48(1):56–85.

Wharton, Amy S. 1992. "The Social Construction of Gender and Race in Organizations: A Social Identity and Group Mobilization Perspective." *Research in the Sociology of Organizations* 10:55–84.

Whitley, Richard. 1994. "Dominant Forms of Economic Organization in Market Economies." *Organization Studies* 15(2):153–82.

_____. 1992. *Business Systems in East Asia: Firms, Markets and Societies.* Beverly
  Hills, CA: Sage.

_____. 1991. "The Social Construction of Business Systems in East Asia." *Organization
  Studies* 12(1):1–28.

Whitsett, David A., and Lyle Yorks. 1983. *From Management Theory to Business Sense:
  The Myths and Realities of People at Work.* New York: American Management
  Association.

Williamson, Oliver. 1985. *The Economic Institutions of Capitalism.* New York: Free
  Press.

_____. 1975. *Markets and Hierarchies: Analysis and Antitrust Implications.* New York:
  Free Press.

Wolf, William B. 1974. *The Basic Barnard.* Ithaca, NY: Cornell University School of
  Industrial and Labor Relations.

Womack, James; Daniel Jones; and Daniel Roos. 1990. *The Machine That Changed the
  World.* New York: Rawson Associates.

Woodward, Joan. 1958. *Management and Technology.* London: HMSO.

Zuboff, Shoshana. 1984. *In the Age of the Smart Machine.* New York: Basic Books.

INDEX